I0057298

Public Health: Concerns and Strategies

Public Health: Concerns and Strategies

Edited by **Charline Ryler**

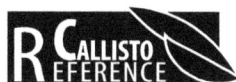

R CALLISTO REFERENCE

New York

Published by Callisto Reference,
106 Park Avenue, Suite 200,
New York, NY 10016, USA
www.callistoreference.com

Public Health: Concerns and Strategies
Edited by Charline Ryler

© 2016 Callisto Reference

International Standard Book Number: 978-1-63239-740-9 (Hardback)

This book contains information obtained from authentic and highly regarded sources. Copyright for all individual chapters remain with the respective authors as indicated. All chapters are published with permission under the Creative Commons Attribution License or equivalent. A wide variety of references are listed. Permission and sources are indicated; for detailed attributions, please refer to the permissions page and list of contributors. Reasonable efforts have been made to publish reliable data and information, but the authors, editors and publisher cannot assume any responsibility for the validity of all materials or the consequences of their use.

The publisher's policy is to use permanent paper from mills that operate a sustainable forestry policy. Furthermore, the publisher ensures that the text paper and cover boards used have met acceptable environmental accreditation standards.

Trademark Notice: Registered trademark of products or corporate names are used only for explanation and identification without intent to infringe.

Printed in the United States of America.

Contents

Preface

This book traces the progress of the field of public health and highlights some of its key concepts and applications. As a branch of science public health deals with protecting and improving the health of people by promoting better lifestyle choices, diagnosis and prevention of infectious diseases and advocating general hygiene. It has various sub-fields like community health, health economics, insurance medicine, environmental health, etc. This book elucidates the theories and innovative models around prospective developments with respect to this subject. It attempts to understand the multiple branches that fall under this discipline and how such concepts have practical applications. Most of the topics introduced in this book cover the immediate concerns and emerging strategies of public health. This text will provide comprehensive knowledge to the readers and will serve as a valuable reference guide.

This book is the end result of constructive efforts and intensive research done by experts in this field. The aim of this book is to enlighten the readers with recent information in this area of research. The information provided in this profound book would serve as a valuable reference to students and researchers in this field.

At the end, I would like to thank all the authors for devoting their precious time and providing their valuable contributions to this book. I would also like to express my gratitude to my fellow colleagues who encouraged me throughout the process.

Editor

Prevalence, Knowledge and Self-Reported Containment Practices about Bedbugs in the Resource-Limited Setting of Ethiopia: A Descriptive Cross-Sectional Survey

Kaliyaperumal Karunamoorthi[1,2*], Buzuna Beyene[1], Argaw Ambelu[1]

[1]Division of Medical Entomology and Vector Control, Department of Environmental Health Science & Technology, College of Public Health and Medical Sciences, Jimma University, Jimma, Ethiopia
[2]Unit of Tropical Diseases, Faculty of Public Health and Tropical Medicine, Jazan University, Jazan, KSA
Email: [*]karunamoorthi@gmail.com

Abstract

Over the past decade, a dramatic rise in bedbug resurgence has become one of the top potential public health hazards. This study was conducted to determine prevalence, knowledge and self-reported containment practices about bedbugs in the resource-limited setting of Ethiopia. A community based, cross-sectional survey was conducted between January and May 2014. Selected 260 respondents were interviewed by the administration of a pre-tested questionnaire on knowledge and practices about bedbug infestation in the resource-limited setting of Ethiopia. Overall, 91.6% (238/260) of the residents had ample awareness on bedbug infestation. The majority of them (97.2%) extremely bothered about infestations because of bad odors (83.8%), insomnia (79.8%), biting (66.9%), and skin rashes (56.9%). A high prevalence of infestation (72.7%) was observed. Bedrooms and main hall/salon were identified as potential high-risk areas. Chi-square exhibited a strong association between sanitary status and housing conditions (χ^2 = 40.91; df = 4; P = 0.0001). Besides, there was a strong association between respondents' monthly income (χ^2 = 42.1; df = 6; P = 0.0001) and educational status (χ^2 = 26.01; df = 5; P = 0.0001) with the presence or absence of bedbug infestation. Though the majority of respondents had adequate knowledge, they suffer with deprived practices attributable to deficient resources as well as negligence/ignorance. This study emphasizes the following key interventions: 1) community-based awareness campaigns, 2) implementation of sustainable preventive/containment strategies, 3) educational interventions to ensure translation of knowledge into practices, and 4) the implementation of appropriate poverty alleviation programs to enhance the local-residents living-standard in the future.

---

[*]Corresponding author.

Keywords

Bedbug, Bedbug Infestation, Containment and Management Practices, Ethiopia

---

1. Introduction

Bedbugs are wingless hematophagous ectoparasites. The common bedbug, *Cimex lectularius* L., the tropical bedbug, *C. hemipterus* (Fabricius), and a few closely related species of blood-feeding true bugs (Hemiptera: Cimicidae) have been the persistent pests of humans throughout recorded history [1]. While in the absence of humans, they may feed on mice, rats, chicken and other animals [2]. Usinger (1966) [3] suggested that the ancestors of bedbugs fed on cave-dwelling bats and accordingly our ancestors became an alternative host when they shared caves with bats. Subsequently, they evolved parallel to the social evolution of the human species.

In the past decade, there is a dramatic resurgence of bedbug infestation which has been observed worldwide, both in the high-income economies *viz.*, the United States, Canada, Europe, Australia, as well as among some of the low-income African and Asian countries [4]. It is fuelled by the unplanned urbanization, uncontrolled population spurt, poor personal hygiene, inadequate resources, unawareness, enhanced international travel, widespread insecticide resistance, and poor-quality housings [5] [6]. The infestation has been detected across a wide range of settings regardless of their hygienic status like single family homes, multi-unit dwellings, buses, trains, cruise ships, aircraft, hotels, schools, cinema halls, shelters, dorm rooms, and health facilities [7] [8].

Bedbugs' classic hiding niches include cracks and crevices of beds, wooden furniture, couch or sofa, floors, walls, mattress, and/or curtains [2]. During the night, they emerge and migrate up to 20 feet to feed (bite) on their preferred host, humans. They sense and seek their hosts through the perception of body heat, odor and by detection of carbon dioxide (CO_2). They recurrently feed on humans to complete their life cycle. After feeding, they defecate and leave black or brown spots, the typical signs of bedbug infestation [9]. Although bedbugs are not in as insect vector of diseases, they reduce the quality of life by causing discomfort, anxiety, insomnia, ostracism, psychological disorders or various phobias [2] [10]. The victims have often been reported to suffer from biting and a variety of cutaneous and systemic reactions [10] [11]. At the moment, elimination of the infestation is one of the Herculean tasks as emergence of resistance to pyrethroid insecticides [12]. Irrespective of their socioeconomic status, all sections of the society are at the risk of being bitten. Therefore, bedbugs have proven to be a challenging pest and so it becomes the subject of significant research and public concern.

Bedbug infestation is a quite common phenomenon in the resource-limited settings as it is inextricably linked to poverty. In Ethiopia, it is one of the most neglected, under-reported as well as under-studied health care concerns owing to the massive disease burden of the major killer diseases *viz.* Tuberculosis, HIV/AIDS and Malaria. In Ethiopia nearly 80% of the population is living in the remote rural areas with substandard housing, which imposes a severe risk to the infestation. Nevertheless, the prevalence of bedbug infestation and its public health impacts remains little-known. Besides, the information on communities' knowledge and containment practices is also quite dearth and scanty. This could lead to a serious setback to the ongoing and future effective bedbug interventions in the long term.

In this context, it is an attempt to identify potential risk indicators of bedbug infestation and control practices in an Ethiopian resource-poor setting. It could provide an opportunity to all pertinent stakeholders to recognize the bedbug infestation as a matter of public health and medical concern/nuisance. It may pave the way to detect, prevent, and control infestations by the cost-effective sustainable management/containment strategies. Besides, it could be helpful to develop the next generation tools for the bedbug resurgence surveillance, monitoring, management and control in the future.

2. Materials and Methods

2.1. Description of the Survey Setting

The survey was conducted among the Amuru town residents and it is the district [Woreda (an administrative body)] next to the village [Kebele (small administrative unit)]. It is located North West of Horo-Guduru Wollega

Zone, Oromia region, Ethiopia (**Figure 1**). It is located at nearly 320 km North West of Addis Ababa, the federal capital city of Ethiopia. It is situated at an altitude of 760 - 2505 m above the sea level and the average annual rainfall and temperature are about 800 - 1500 mm and 180C, respectively. Based on climatic conditions, the present study area classified is as one of the woienadega areas of Ethiopia. Local residents cultivate Teff (*Eragrostis tef* Zucc.), maize (*Zea mays* L.), barley (*Hordeum vulgare* L.), cereal such as sorghum (*Sorghum bicolor* L.), and wheat (*Triticum aestivum* L.). Besides, it is also well-known for the cultivation of the cash crop like khat (*Catha edulis* Forsk.) and coffee (*Coffea arabica* L.) and raising live stocks.

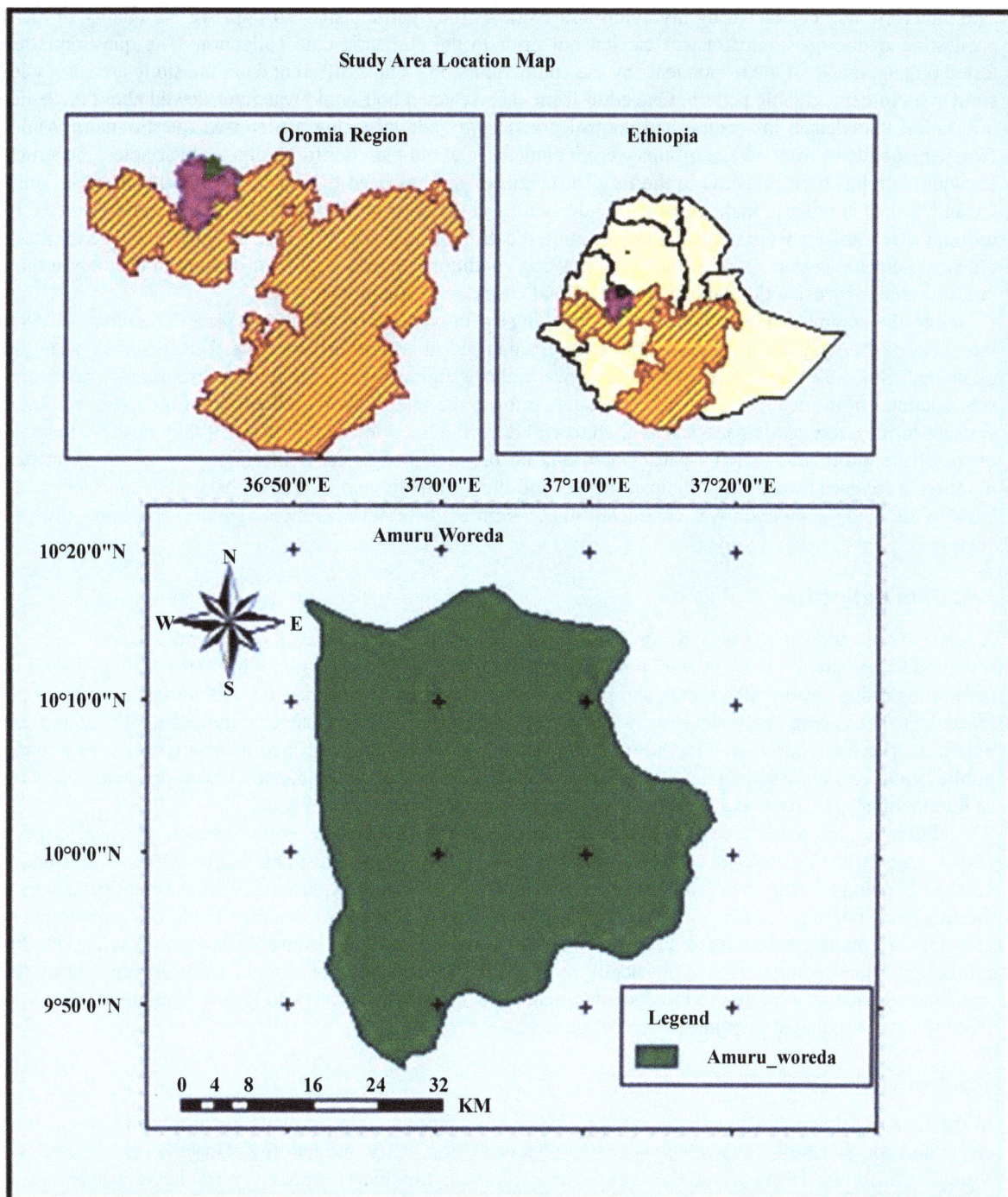

Figure 1. Location of the study area Amuru town, Wollega zone, Oromia region, Ethiopia.

2.2. Study Design and Sampling Technique

The study was a community based cross-sectional survey conducted between January and May of 2014. A stratified, systematic random sampling was used for selection of a total of 260 households from all the total existing 1164 households. The sample size was calculated by employing 95% confidence interval formula to estimate a population proportion.

2.3. Interview

The interview was conducted by involving 260 eligible study participants. To improve the quality of the data, pre-testing of the questionnaire was carried out prior to the authentic data collection. The questionnaire was tested on ten percent of the respondents by the enumerators, in an area different from the study area, but with the similar socio-demographic pattern. One adult from each selected household was interviewed about the bedbug's infestation knowledge, infestation and control practices by administering a pretested questionnaire. Male and female respondents from all age-groups were included. To avoid biased information and variables, the structured questionnaire has been prepared in the English language and has been translated into the local native language (Afan Oromo) in order to make it easy to understand and to administer by interviewers and interviewees. In addition, the researchers were trained in determining the different levels of infestation. Subsequently they made the physical personal inspection to evaluate the housing conditions and the degree of bedbug infestation in the chosen households by using the standard observational checklists [**Appendix**].

Before the commencement of the survey, meetings with community health workers, community leaders and members of the neighborhood associations were organized in which the objectives of the survey were clearly explained. Since all the selected respondents were above eighteen-years of age, the informed written consent was obtained from each of the study participants prior to the interview, with the help of an approved voluntary consent form. Every participant was assured to withdraw the interview at any phase if they wish to do so. However, all the informants actively participated and no one declined to cease the interview. Study identification numbers were used instead of participant names and the information collected has been kept confidential. Feedback to the study population was conducted in the form of dissemination meetings after the completion of the survey.

2.4. Data Collection

A team of well-trained and closely supervised local interviewers conducted the household survey using a pretested questionnaire to interview with the representative of the selected household. Interviewers collected information regarding socio-demographic and physical observation and inspection on bedbug infestation and prevalence data. The chosen respondents were invited and called upon to impart their knowledge, attitude and control practices. The main questions focused on 1) the knowledge on bedbugs, 2) bedbugs' infestation as a matter of public health concern/issue, 3) diverse health impact (psychological, allergic, and clinical presentation), 4) types of interventions practiced, and 5) name of the local plants used against bedbugs.

Additionally, the prevalence of bedbug infestation was also determined by the personal physical inspections (using suggestive key indicators like the presence of adults, nymphs, eggs, and faeces or traces of blood from crushed bedbugs) and by using the standard checklists. The surveyed households were categorized into three groups, poor, fair and good based on a classification scheme that mainly considers the housing quality (careful inspection of mattresses/fabrics and other household items like bed), and domestic and personal hygiene for the infestation. The investigators also physically removed the adults and large nymphs using forceps during the inspections. Residents were advised to decontaminate their infested materials and proper health education was offered to each respondent to minimize the infestation.

2.5. Data Management and Analysis

In the field, data were collected in a standardized questionnaire and data collection forms and was checked for errors and completeness. Data was then counterchecked before entry into DbaseV (Borland International, Scotts Valley, California, USA) using the double entry system. Summary statistics were being performed using STATA version 10 (STATA Corp., Texas, USA). The range and mean were analysed and appropriate tables, graphs and percentage details were displayed. A Chi-square analysis was performed to test the hypothesis. The level of significance was also determined by using 95% of confidence intervals and P-value.

3. Results

3.1. Socio-Demographic Characteristics of Survey Respondents

The socio-demographic characteristics of the study participants are shown in the **Table 1**. It has been estimated that nearly 91.6% (238/260) of the respondents had ample awareness of bedbug infestation and control (**Table 1**). Overall, 68.6% (179/260) and 31.4% (82/260) of the respondents had knowingly on the mode of growth/development and the rest didn't.

Table 1. Study of respondents with gender, age, ethnicity, educational status, average monthly income and knowledge of bedbug infestation and control practices in Ethiopia.

Socio-demographic variables	n	%
Gender		
Male	164	63.1
Female	96	36.9
Age in years		
18 - 20	70	26.9
21 - 30	36	13.9
31 - 40	33	12.7
41 - 50	36	13.8
51 - 60	21	08.1
>60	63	24.3
Educational status		
Illiterate	18	06.9
Can read and write	29	11.2
1 - 5th grade	39	15.1
6 - 10th grade	55	21.2
11 - 12th grade	36	13.9
Above 12th grade	83	31.9
Monthly income [Ethiopian Birr (1 USD = 18.78 Eth Birr)]		
<500	57	21.9
501 - 1000	70	26.9
1001 - 1500	55	21.2
1501 - 2000	37	14.3
2001 - 2500	31	11.9
2501 - 3000	05	02.0
>3000	05	02.0
Do you have awareness on bedbugs' infestation and control?		
Yes	23	91.6
No	22	08.4

3.2. Housing Conditions and Bedbug Infestation

Out of 260 houses 177 (68.1%) were privately owned and 83 (31.9%) were rented by the individuals/municipality. Overall, 172 (66.2%) and 81 (31.2%) of the houses were built of mud and cement, respectively. Almost, 200 (76.9%) and 50 (19.3%) houses were with bare soil floors, and the concrete, respectively. Pertaining the type of the roof, 237 (91.2%), 13 (5.1%) and 10 (3.7%) houses were constructed with the corrugated iron sheet (CIS), thatched, and a few of them with the materials like plastic sheets and tarpaulins, respectively. The investigators also made a visual personal inspection of the potential high-risk sleeping areas (rooms), cloth, and other hiding niches in order to estimate the prevalence of infestation (**Table 2**) and found that overall 72.7% (189/260) of the households were infested. The chi-square analysis exhibits a strong association between sanitary status and housing conditions ($\chi^2 = 40.91$; $df = 4$; P = 0.0001) (**Table 2**).

Both the bedrooms and main hall/salon were identified as potential risk-areas in terms of infestation (**Figure 2**). Nearly 97.2% (203/209) of the respondents were extremely concerned about the infestation due to various negative consequences, particularly bad-odour (83.8%), biting (66.9%), and social stigma (42%) (**Figure 3**).

3.3. Bedbug Management and Control Practices

The residents were noted to apply various bedbug interventions, particularly plant-based products as repellent by means of conventional intervention. Overall, 89.3% (232/260) and 83.9% (218/260) of the respondents were found to use Endod (*Phytolacca dodecantra* L'Hér.), and Tid (*Juniperus procera* L.) leaves solutions (suspensions) as repellant (**Table 3**). Besides, study participants were also applying a various environmental and chemical control interventions (**Table 3**). About, 81.2% (211/260) and 91.2% (237/260) of the respondents have

Table 2. Classification of the housing conditions based on the sanitary conditions with reference to bedbugs' infestation.

S. No.	Sanitary conditions	Good		Fair		Poor		P-value
		n	%	n	%	n	%	
1.	Personal hygiene	43	16.6	106	40.8	101	38.9	$\chi^2 = 40.91$
2.	Good-housing conditions	92	35.4	101	38.9	67	25.8	$df = 4$
3.	Environmental sanitation	97	37.4	111	42.6	52	20.1	P = 0.0001[*]

Note: [*]P < 0.05 statistically significant.

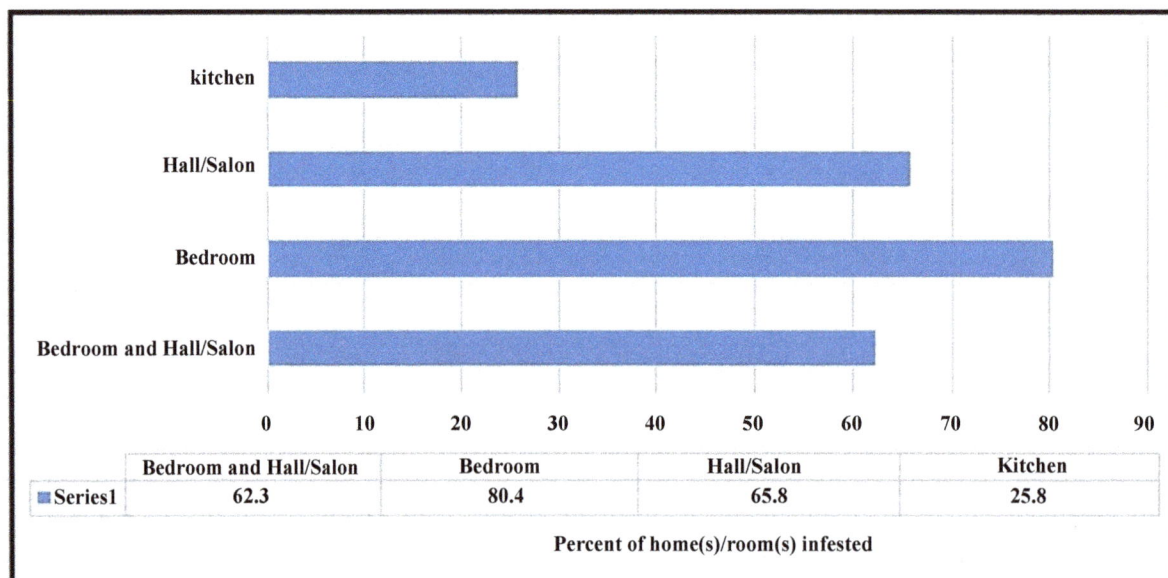

	Bedroom and Hall/Salon	Bedroom	Hall/Salon	Kitchen
■Series1	62.3	80.4	65.8	25.8

Percent of home(s)/room(s) infested

Figure 2. The prevalence of infestation in the whole houses and partition room(s). **Note:** a percent does not add up to 100, because of multiple responses.

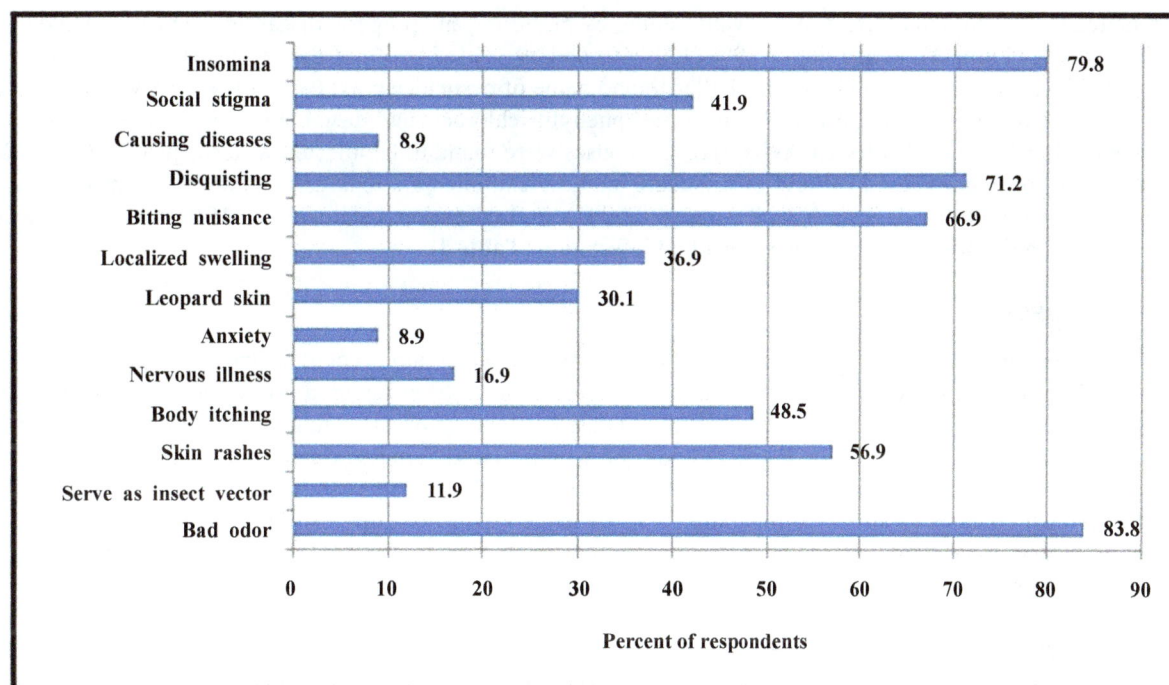

Figure 3. Respondents' perception on the physico-psycho-socio-health impacts of bedbug infestation. **Note:** a percent does not add up to 100, because of multiple responses.

Table 3. Respondents of various self-reported practices for the bedbug prevention and control.

	I. Conventional Interventions as bedbug repellent	n	Percent[a]
1.	Leaves of Eucalyptus (*Eucalyptus citriodora* Hook.) solution/dried leaves as fumigant	201	77.4
2.	Keberacho (*Echinops kebericho* Mesfin.) plants' dried roots as fumigant	198	76.2
3.	Tid (*Juniperus procera* L.) leaves suspension	218	83.9
4.	Endod (*Phytolacca dodecantra* L'Hér.) leaves solution	232	89.3
5.	Other plants' materials/products	014	05.4
	II. Environmental Interventions		
1.	Personal hygiene	141	54.3
2.	Washing the infested clothes frequently	149	57.4
3.	Proper disposal of domestic waste	237	91.2
4.	Plastering of wall cracks and crevices	211	81.2
5.	Pouring boiled water on the infested areas/materials	109	42.1
6.	Others	021	08.1
	III. Chemical Interventions		
1.	5% DDT	154	59.3
2.	Commercial insecticide products/Roach killer	174	66.9
3.	Pyrethroid-based insecticides	102	39.3
4.	Other pesticides	017	06.6

Note: a percent does not add up to 100, because of multiple responses.

repaired the cracks and crevices in the walls/ceiling by plastering and properly discarding their household waste, respectively (**Table 3**). In addition, 66.9% (174/260) and 59.3% (154/260) of the people applying several commercial insecticide products like Roach Killer [brand name of pesticide spray; (which is extensively available in the Ethiopian markets)] and 5% DDT (dichloro-diphenyl-trichloroethane) dustable powder to prevent/curb bedbugs (**Table 3**). Overall, 72.7% (189/260) of the houses were found to be infested whereas just 27.3% (71/260) of them were uninfestated (**Table 4**). Chi-square analysis exhibited a strong association between respondents' monthly income ($\chi^2 = 42.1$; $df = 6$; P-value = 0.0001), and educational status ($\chi^2 = 26.01$; $df = 5$; P-value = 0.0001) with the presence or absence of bedbug infestation (**Table 4**).

4. Discussion

Indeed, bedbugs are ecto-parasitic insects and they have been taken into account as one of the potential medical and public health hazards. Fairly large numbers of studies have been reported on various aspects of bedbug; however, to the best of our knowledge, no study to date has focused on the communities' awareness and bedbug control practices. Generally, knowledge, attitude and practice (KAP) studies are considered to be an educational diagnosis on the risk-population. They often aid to design tailored strategies suitable for the local socio-cultural and political contexts of at-risk communities [13]. In this context, this paper is aimed to identify potential key risk indicators associated with the bedbug infestation. Compounding factors like poverty, limited-resources and negligence or ignorance often cause the sustainable bedbug interventions out of reach.

The majority of informants (91.6%) had ample awareness of bedbug infestation and control (**Table 1**). The level of awareness was noted to be extremely higher than the previous study and it has been reported to be terribly lower in awareness [14] among the developed countries. This could be possibly explained that this is because the survey has been conducted in one of the resource-poor settings like Ethiopia, where poverty and unhygienic living conditions are quite widespread. Besides, many poverty interrelated issues often inflame the higher-level of infestation and the associated public health and medical risks in Ethiopia. Therefore, local residents

Table 4. The association between respondent's monthly income and educational status with presence or absence of bedbugs' infestation.

Variables	Number of Bedbugs			P-value
	Total	Presence	Absence	
Educational status				
Illiterate	18	10	08	
Read and write	29	22	07	$\chi^2 = 26.01$
1 - 5th grade	39	23	16	$df = 5$
6 - 10th grade	55	33	22	P = 0.0001*
11 - 12th grade	36	25	11	
12+	83	76	07	
Monthly income [Ethiopian Birr (1 USD = 18.78 Eth Birr)]				
<500	57	44	13	
501 - 1000	70	36	34	
1001 - 1500	55	34	21	
1501 - 2000	37	43	03	$\chi 2 = 42.1$
2001 - 2500	31	31	00	$df = 6$
2501 - 3000	05	05	00	P = 0.0001*
>3000	05	05	00	

Note: *P < 0.05 statistically significant.

might have acquired ample awareness by means of long-period of exposure/personal contact (bite). A study reported that nearly sevenfold higher number of people identified bedbugs rightly if they have had prior contact with bedbugs than those who had not [14].

The respondents have received bedbug related information from several sources via cultural knowledge transmission (*i.e.* word of mouth) from their parents/relatives (73.1%), previous experience (contact) (14.3%), health facilities (7.8%), and educational institutions/mass media (4.8%). The finding is concurrent with a very recent study conducted in Germany by Seidel and Reinhardt (2013) [14] reporting on; (a) the previous contacts with bed bugs (60%), (b) knowledge from friends or relatives (25%), and (c) school or education courses (15%). It has also been reported that the previous experience has contributed to the correct identification of bedbug. Therefore, showing the bedbugs to the people could be helpful to improve the awareness of the people [14]. It is important to note that the higher-level of awareness is one of the important social determinants of health and it can make a significant contribution to public health promotion campaigns against bedbug. Henceforth it shall often offer an ideal opportunity for us to implement sustainable community-based interventions by generating awareness in this vicinity.

In spite of the limited-resources, relatively sizable numbers of households were categorized to be good (free of infestation). However, most of the houses were poorly maintained by the residents (**Table 2**). In the developing economies, delivering quality healthcare services to all the needy peoples is a quite challenging task because of inadequate healthcare facilities, inadequate skilled personnel, and underfunding. However, the findings exhibit that leading a healthy life is relatively feasible by improving the domestic and personal hygiene of the society. These can be achieved by aggressive health education campaigns to translate their knowledge into practice to lead a healthier life. Subsequently, it can lead to attaining our ambitious Millennium Development Goals (MDGs) in the near future.

Overall, 80.4% (152/189) of the bedrooms, followed by 65.6% (124/189) of main hall/salon were observed to be infested (**Figure 2**), and they are the most potential risk-associated rooms or areas in the households. Since bedbugs hide in the cracks and crevices of walls and other materials like bed, chairs and couches, they emerge and get easy access to feed (bite) on the human at night. 15 If family size is quite bigger, all the family members cannot accommodate in the bedroom, rather some of them might prefer to sleep in the salon/main hall. These create an ideal situation for the infestation; consequently the bedrooms and salons are often infested than in any other rooms (**Figure 1**). Bedbugs are nocturnal feeders and will aggregate together in harbourages in close proximity to where their preferred host sleeps [15].

Due to the recent resurgence, it is extremely vital to understand the potential health risks associated with bedbug infestation [11]. The great majority of the respondents were worried because of a various adverse psycho-socio-economic-health consequences of infestation (**Figure 2**). A recent study reported that bedbug infestation causes serious social stigmatization and isolation too [16]. The majority of people consider that the persons with poor hygiene and low economic status might have infested [3]. Though bedbug bites are painless, it may cause severe reactions ranging from asymptomatic to itchy, swollen and blistered bites on exposed skin, sometimes resulting in secondary bacterial infections too [17].

Considerable numbers of respondents erroneously perceived that bedbug may cause several diseases and they can serve as insect vectors too (**Figure 3**). To date there are no scientific report that bedbugs can transmit the infections [17] [18], however, there are several studies indicate that they can cause severe skin irritations [19], stronger dermatological responses [20], and psychological stress [21]. Bedbugs are classified as urban pests and as a potential health hazard [4]. The infestation is quite unbearable in the hotel industry as it often tarnishes the hotel's reputations consequently cause serious negative economic consequences [14].

Since the pre-historic era the people tend to use various plants to either repel or to kill various dreadful bloodsucking insects. Even today it is one of the quite common phenomena in the resource-limited African settings like Ethiopia [22]. Respondents apply several plants as repellent to prevent/manage and control the infestation. The local-residents use the Endod, Tid, and Eucalyptus (*Eucalyptus citriodora* Hook.) leaves' solutions (suspensions) as repellant (**Table 3**). Besides, the dried leaves of Eucalyptus and the roots of Keberacho (*Echinops kebericho* Mesfin.) are also applied as fumigants. In Ethiopia, several previous studies reported that these plants can serve as potential repellents against mosquitoes and several other domestic pests [23]-[25]. In resource-limited settings, it could be one of the most viable options (strategies) to curb infestation efficiently, since these plants are easily accessible, affordable, locally known, and culturally acceptable [26]. However, further scientific analyses are also required to be warranted to isolate and to identify the responsible bio-active molecules as well as to establish their mammalian toxicity too [27].

Residents were practicing various environmental interventions like plastered the cracks and crevices of walls/ceiling to eliminate the hiding niches of bedbugs, while a few of them frequently exposed their infested materials/cloths under sunlight to inhibit infestation (**Table 3**). The great majority of the respondents has been using a variety of chemicals, particularly Roach Killer spray/fumigant and 5% of DDT powder (**Table 3**) to repel or to kill various domestic pests like cockroach, housefly, mosquitoes particularly to curb the bedbug infestation. Indeed insecticides are powerful weapons in the fight against insect vector of diseases and domestic pests. However, the haphazard and unsafe insecticide application could inflict serious negative impacts on human health, animals and the environment [28] [29]. Since insecticides are toxic in nature appropriate awareness campaigns instructing a safe use of insecticide is quite inevitable [29]. In 1950, the DDT was very effective to control the bedbugs [30], subsequently the liberal use of DDT, and changes in cultural practices had eradicated the infestations in the developed world [31]. Today, pyrethroids are one of the most commonly used insecticides to combat the bedbug infestations. However, bedbugs have developed resistance to several insecticides, including pyrethroids [30] [32] and other insecticides like malathion, diazinon, lindane, chlordane, and dichlorvos too. The recent worldwide bedbug resurgence is mainly attributable to the widespread insecticide resistance, particularly pyrethroids [30].

Chi-square analysis showed a strong association between respondents' monthly income and educational status with the presence or absence of bedbug infestation and it was statistically significant (**Table 4**) (P = 0.0001). Though the infestation cuts all the socio-economic-barriers, perhaps it is quite obvious that the economically-disadvantaged people disproportionably share a larger burden of infestation than wealthier people. The experience of a bedbug infestation of low-income people poses a significant threat to their overall health [16]. It could be possibly explained that the educated individuals are expected to have more awareness than the illiterates and it could directly reduce the degree of infestation in their homes. Therefore, it is essential for healthcare/educational institutions and national, regional and local responsible bodies to recognize the risk of infestation and the need for the development of protocols to prevent, identify, and generate awareness, and to eliminate the infestation effectively [33].

5. Conclusion

Indeed bedbugs are considered to be one of the potential medical and public health hazards in resource-constrained settings like Ethiopia. Poor quality of housing, overcrowding and other related confounding factors serve as a potential breeding ground for widespread bedbug infestation. However, it can be effectively contained with the help of the existing resources if the people are properly educated to translate their knowledge into practices. Therefore, this study calls for the following key interventions for the sustainable bedbug elimination that includes: 1) community-based awareness campaigns, 2) implementation of sustainable preventive/containment strategies, 3) educational interventions via mass media, 4) continuous monitoring and quality assurance mechanisms to be placed to ensure zero tolerance of infestation. Furthermore, implementation of suitable poverty alleviation programmes could substantially enrich the living-standard of the people in the future.

Acknowledgements

We are very much grateful to the study participants who shared their knowledge on the Bedbugs infestation. Without their contribution, this study would have been impossible. The authors would like to acknowledge Ms. L. Melita for her sincere assistance in editing the manuscript. Our last but not least heartfelt thanks go to our colleagues from the School of Environmental Health Science, Faculty of Public Health, Jimma University, Jimma, Ethiopia, for their kind support and cooperation.

References

[1] AFPMB (Armed Forces Pest Management Board) (2013) Bed Bugs-Importance, Biology, and Control Strategies. Technical Guide No. 44. http://www.afpmb.org/sites/default/files/pubs/techguides/tg44.pdf

[2] Hwang, S.W., Svoboda, T.J., De Jong, I.J., Kabasele, K.J. and Gogosis, E. (2005) Bed Bug Infestations in an Urban Environment. *Emerging Infectious Diseases*, **11**, 533-538. http://dx.doi.org/10.3201/eid1104.041126

[3] Usinger, R.L. (1996) Monograph of Cimicidae (Hemiptera-Heteroptera). Thomas Say Foundation, College Park.

[4] Harlan, H.J., Faulde, M.K. and Baumann, G.J. (2008) Bedbugs. In: Bonnefoy, X., Kampen, H. and Sweeney, K., Eds.,

Public Health Significance of Urban Pests, World Health Organization, Regional Office for Europe, Copenhagen, 131-154.

[5]   Panagiotakopulu, E. and Buckland, P.C. (1999) *Cimex lectularius* L., the Common Bedbug from Pharaonic Egypt. *Antiquity*, **73**, 908-911.

[6]   Potter, M.F. (2008) The History of Bed Bug Management. Bed Bug Supplement: Lessons from the Past. *Pest Control Technology*, **36**, 12.

[7]   Wang, C., Saltzmann, K., Chin, E., Bennett, G.W. and Gibb, T. (2010) Characteristics of *Cimex lectularius* (Hemiptera: Cimicidae), Infestation and Dispersal in a High-Rise Apartment Building. *Journal of Economic Entomology*, **103**, 172-177. http://dx.doi.org/10.1603/EC09230

[8]   Delaunay, P. (2012) Human Travel and Traveling Bedbugs. *Journal of Travel Medicine*, **19**, 373-379. http://dx.doi.org/10.1111/j.1708-8305.2012.00653.x

[9]   Wang, C. (2009) Bed Bugs. The State University of New Jersey, Rutgers, Fact Sheet FS1098.

[10] Goddard, J. and deShazo, R. (2012) Psychological Effects of Bed Bug Attacks (*Cimex lectularius* L.). *American Journal of Medicine*, **125**, 101-103. http://dx.doi.org/10.1016/j.amjmed.2011.08.010

[11] Paul, J. and Bates, J. (2000) Is Infestation with the Common Bedbug Increasing? *British Medical Journal*, **320**, 1141. http://dx.doi.org/10.1136/bmj.320.7242.1141

[12] Romero, A. (2009) Biology and Management of the Bed Bug, *Cimex lectularius* L. (Heteroptera: Cimicidae). Doctoral Dissertations, University of Kentucky, Lexington.

[13] Chinnakali, P., Gurnani, N., Upadhyay, R.P., Parmar, K., Suri, T.M. and Yadav, K. (2012) High Level of Awareness but Poor Practices regarding Dengue Fever Control: A Cross-Sectional Study from North India. *North American Journal of Medical Sciences*, **4**, 278-82. http://dx.doi.org/10.4103/1947-2714.97210

[14] Seidel, C. and Reinhardt, K. (2013) Bugging Forecast: Unknown, Disliked, Occasionally Intimate. Bed Bugs in Germany Meet Unprepared People. *PLoS ONE*, **8**, e51083. http://dx.doi.org/10.1371/journal.pone.0051083

[15] Gangloff-Kaufmann, J., Hollingsworth, C., Hahn, J., Hansen, L., Kard, B. and Waldvogel, M. (2006) Bed Bugs in America: A Pest Management Industry Survey. *American Entomologist*, **52**, 105-106. http://dx.doi.org/10.1093/ae/52.2.105

[16] Lyons, J. (2010) The Social Impacts of Bed Bugs on Inner Winnipeg. University of Manitoba, Manitoba.

[17] Goddard, J. (2009) Bed Bugs (*Cimex lectularius*) and Clinical Consequences of Their Bites. *Journal of American Medical Association*, **301**, 1358-1366. http://dx.doi.org/10.1001/jama.2009.405

[18] Doggett, S.L., Dwyer, D.E., Penas, P.F. and Russell, R.C. (2012) Bed Bugs: Clinical Relevance and Control Options. *Clinical Microbiology Review*, **25**, 164-192. http://dx.doi.org/10.1128/CMR.05015-11

[19] Reinhardt, K., Kempke, D., Naylor, R. and Siva-Jothy, M.T. (2009) Sensitivity to Bedbug Bites, *Cimex lectularius*. *Medical and Veterinary Entomology*, **23**, 163-166. http://dx.doi.org/10.1111/j.1365-2915.2008.00793.x

[20] Leverkus, M., Jochim, R.C., Schäd, S., Bröcker, E.B. and Andersen, J.F. (2006) Bullous Allergic Hypersensitivity to Bed Bug Bites Mediated by IgE against Salivary Nitrophorin. *Journal of Investigative Dermatology*, **126**, 91-96. http://dx.doi.org/10.1038/sj.jid.5700012

[21] Goddard, J. and de Shazo, R. (2012) Psychological Effects of Bedbug Attacks (*Cimex lectularius* L.). *American Journal of Medicine*, **125**, 101-103. http://dx.doi.org/10.1016/j.amjmed.2011.08.010

[22] Karunamoorthi, K., Mulelam, A. and Wassie, F. (2008) Laboratory Evaluation of Traditional Insect/Mosquito Repellent Plants against *Anopheles arabiensis*, the Predominant Malaria Vector in Ethiopia. *Parasitology Research*, **103**, 529-534. http://dx.doi.org/10.1007/s00436-008-1001-9

[23] Karunamoorthi, K., Mulelam, A. and Wassie, F. (2009) Assessment of Knowledge and Usage Custom of Traditional Insect/Mosquito Repellent Plants in Addis Zemen Town, South Gonder, North Western Ethiopia. *Journal of Ethnopharmacology*, **121**, 49-53. http://dx.doi.org/10.1016/j.jep.2008.09.027

[24] Karunamoorthi, K., Ilango, K. and Endale, A. (2009) Ethnobotanical Survey of Knowledge and Usage Custom of Traditional Insect/Mosquito Repellent Plants among the Ethiopian Oromo Ethnic Group. *Journal of Ethnopharmacology*, **125**, 224-229. http://dx.doi.org/10.1016/j.jep.2009.07.008

[25] Karunamoorthi, K. and Tsehaye, E. (2012) Ethnomedicinal Knowledge, Belief and Self-Reported Practice of Local Inhabitants on Traditional Antimalarial Plants and Phytotherapy. *Journal of Ethnopharmacology*, **141**, 143-150. http://dx.doi.org/10.1016/j.jep.2012.02.012

[26] Karunamoorthi, K., Ramanujam, S. and Rathinasamy, R. (2008) Evaluation of Leaf Extracts of *Vitex negundo* L. (Family: Verbenaceae) against Larvae of *Culex tritaeniorhynchus* and Repellent Activity on Adult Vector Mosquitoes. *Parasitology Research*, **103**, 545-550. http://dx.doi.org/10.1007/s00436-008-1005-5

[27] Karunamoorthi, K. (2012) Plant-Based Insect Repellents: Is That a Sustainable Option to Curb the Malaria Burden in Africa? *Journal of Medicinal and Aromatic Plants*, **1**, e106.

[28] Karunamoorthi, K., Mohammed, M. and Wassie, F. (2012) Knowledge and Practices of Farmers with Reference to Pesticide Management: Implications on Human Health. *Achieves of Environmental and Occupational Health*, **67**, 109-116. http://dx.doi.org/10.1080/19338244.2011.598891

[29] Karunamoorthi, K. and Yirgalem, A. (2013) Insecticide Risk Indicators and Occupational Insecticidal Poisoning in Indoor Residual Spraying. *Health Scope*, **1**, 166-173. http://dx.doi.org/10.5812/jhs.8344

[30] Potter, M.F. (2008) Bed Bug Supplement. The History of Bed Bug Management. *Pest Control Technology*, **36**, S1.

[31] Busvine, J.E. (1958) Insecticide-Resistance in Bed-Bugs. *Bulletin of World Health Organization*, **19**, 1041-1052.

[32] Douglas Reis, M. (2010) An Evaluation of Bed Bug (*Cimex lectularius* L.) Host Location and Aggregation Behavior. Master's Thesis, Virginia Polytechnic Institute and State University, Blacksburg.

[33] Adeyeye, A., Adams, A., Herring, L. and Currie, B.P. (2010) Bed Bug Infestation on a Maternity Unit in a Tertiary Care Center. *American Journal of Infection Control*, **3**, E82.

Appendix 1. Jimma University College of Public Health and Medical Science Department of Environmental Health and Technology

Questionnaire

1. PERSONAL INFORMATION OF STUDY PARTICIPANT

1.1. Age_____   Sex_____
1.2. Address region_____   Zone _____   Woreda _____   Town _____   Kebele _____
1.3. Religion:
Orthodox--------------------   Muslim-----------------   Catholic----------------------
Protestant--------------------   Others-------------------
1.4. Ethnicity:
Oromo-----------   Garage---------   Amhara----------------
Tigre---------------   Others------------
1.5. Educational Status----------------------
1.6. Occupational Status:
Farmers----------------   Merchant----------------   Daily Laborer------------
Student----------------   Government Employer-------------   Fisherman -----------
NGO worker--------------------   Others---------------
1.7. Monthly Income---------------- (Ethiopian Birr)

2. RELEVANT INFORMATION

2.1. Type of wall of the house:
Mud--------------   Concrete------------   Others (specify) ---------------
Is there any crack and crevices on the wall?
Yes---------   No--------
2.2. Type of the floor:
Mud-------   Concrete------------   Wood------------   Others (specify) ---------
Is the floor dusty?
Yes-----   No------
Are there any cracks on the floor?
Yes---   No--------
2.3. Type of roof:
Corrugated iron sheet--------   Hatched--------------   Others (specify) -------------
2.4. Type of bed and bed frames:
Wood------------   Metal---------   Others (specify) ---------
Are there any cracks and crevices on the bed and bed frames?
Yes-----   No-----
2.5. Total number of rooms or partitions of the main house-----------------
2.6. What is the total number of people live in each room? -----------------

3. ASSESSMENT OF KNOWLEDGE OF RESIDENTS TOWARDS BEDBUGS

3.1. Are there bedbugs in your house?
Yes------   No--------
3.2. If yes, $Q_{3.1}$ do you know way of transmission?
Yes------   No---------
3.3. If yes, $Q_{3.2}$ how does it be transmitted from person to person?
Yes-----   No-----
3.4. Do you know how to prevent or control bedbugs?
Yes-------   No--------
3.5. If yes, $Q_{3.4}$ how can it be prevented?
Using traditional methods----------   Using drugs---------
By washing clothes--------   Using exposing to sunlight--------

Others (specify) ---------------
3.7. Do you have any information about bedbugs?
Yes-----   No-------
3.8. If yes, $Q_{3.7}$ Where do you get treatment?
Health center's...............   Hospitals.........................
Health status.........   Community health..................
Others (specify).........
3.9. Do you know the risk of bed bugs?
Yes............   No.........
3.10. If yes $Q_{3.9}$ would you tell me what they are?
Skin rash.....................   Body itching............
Nervous illness.........   Anxiety..................
Leopard skin..................   Body swelling...............
Others (specify).............
3.11. Does the bedbugs have a role in the transmission of diseases?
Yes...........   No.........
3.12. If yes, would you mention some of diseases that the bedbugs hold for their transmission?
1. ....   2. ....
3. ....   4. ....
5. ....   6. ....
3.13. Do you know how the bedbugs multiply?
1. They lay eggs...........................   2. They directly give birth..................
3. Others (specify).........................   4. I don't know ....

4. ATTITUDES
4.1. Do you feel/worried discomfort due to presence of bedbugs in your houses?
Yes....................   No.....................
4.2. If yes, in what sense you feel discomfort due to their presences?
a.   They have a bad odor   ....
b.   Their bite is painful   ....
c.   Their presence is disgusting   ....
d.   They transmit diseases or act as vector   ....
e.   They causes diseases themselves   ....
f.   They annoy people ....
g.   They have social stigma ....
h.   Others (specify) ....
4.3. Do you feel discomfort due to control of bedbugs when using local modern methods practice?
Yes......   No.........
4.4. If yes, $Q_{4.3}$ In what cases............

5. PRACTICES
5.1. Do you know how to control the bed bugs?
Yes.........   No.........
5.2. Do you have a practice of washing your clothes regularly?
Yes.........   No.........
5.3. Did you practice any vector control around in your residential house?
Yes.........   No.........
5.4. Have you advised your family and your neighbors' to keep personal hygiene and houses clean?
Yes.........   No.........
5.5. Have you used repellant plants to avoid bedbugs?
Yes.........   No.........
5.6. If yes, Q5.5 Name the plants.........................
5.7. If it is applicable, how it is applicable?

Smoke…………..   Keeping the plant in the room………………

Spray or inside the house…………………   Others (specify)……………………..

5.8. Application time. Morning……………………

Evening……………………   Night………………………

Midday…………………   Others (specify)…………..

5.9. Which plant is more effective and its methods of application

Name of the plant ………………………   Application Method ………………………

5.10. How many times do you apply in a day?

Once times a day……………   Two times a day……………

Three times a day………………   Others (specify)……………

5.11. Modern methods to control bedbugs (Types of insecticides)

DDT………………   Roach killer…………..   Others (specify)……………

5.12. Frequency of the insecticide usage.

Six months ……………   Within six-month ……………

One year………..   Two year………………

Three year……………   Others…………………

5.13. From the local/ traditional/or modern methods, which one is your preferences? ……….

Why you prefer this method? ………………………..

5.14. What are the environmental control methods you practices so as to control bedbugs?

a.   Keeping personal hygiene…………………

b.   Washing the clothes frequently……………

c.   Manage wastes in the houses in a safe way………….

d.   Cracks and crevices in the house plugging………………

e.   Avoid sharing of clothes………………………..

f.   Pouring boiling water over beds and bed frames……………

g.   Taking all the above…………………..

h.   Others……………………

6. PREVALENCE

6.1. Are bedbugs present in your houses? (in any rooms/partitions)

Yes…….   No…….

6.2. if yes, Q6.1

a) In how many of total rooms are bedbugs prevalent?

b) Are bedbugs also prevalent in the kitchen? (have you ever noticed any on floor, on wall, on the roof,

Yes………………   No…………………..

c) Are bedbugs also prevalent in the main house?

Yes……………   No………………

d) In which room in the houses do you frequently observe? ………………………

6.3 Are there any signs of presence of bedbugs in the house?

Yes………   No……………

6.4 If yes. Q6.3 which sigs

a) live bedbugs seen…………..

b) Dead bedbugs' body seen………………

c) Egg/egg shell of the bed bugs seen……………………

6.5 If you see eggs of the bed bugs, which is the shape of it?

Circular……………………   Cylindrical………………..

Oval………………   Others (specify)……………..

Appendix 2

Observational Checklist

1. Personal hygiene of the residential households

Good ……………   Fair…………….   Poor…………………………

2. Standards of the residential houses

Good ……………   Fair……………..   Poor…………………………

3. Environmental safety around the house is acceptable?

Yes…………   No……………

4. Are there any cracks crevices, dusts and other wastes in the houses?

Yes……………………..   No…………………………

5. Checking the presences of bedbugs in the houses.

Presences of bedbugs ………………   Where it is observed? …………………..

a.   Live bedbugs

b.   Dead bedbug

c.   Egg/egg shell

6. Are there any insects which are related to the presences of bedbugs?

Yes…………………   No…………………………..

If yes, what type of insects?……………………

Thank you for your kind cooperation

2

Health, Physical Activity and the Rio de Janeiro 2016 Olympic Games: Legacy or Fallacy?

Vagner Rosa Bizarro[1], Tatiane Andreazza Lucchese[1], Amanda Maia Breis[1],
Karine Rucker[1], Minelli Salles Alves Fernandes[1], Mikele Torino Paletti[1],
Ana Luísa Conceição de Jesus[1], Raphael Calafange Marques Pereira[2],
Denise Rosso Tenório Wanderley Rocha[1], Alberto Krayyem Arbex[1,3]

[1]Division of Endocrinology, IPEMED Medical School, Rio de Janeiro, Brazil
[2]Division of Rehabilitation Sciences, UNISUAM, Rio de Janeiro, Brazil
[3]Harvard School of Public Health, Harvard University, Boston, USA
Email: vavarb@yahoo.com, albertoarbex@gmail.com

Abstract

It is generally expected that the Rio de Janeiro 2016 Olympic and Paralympic Games will bring health and social benefits to their host city and to Brazil. This assumption comes from "common sense", as a logical conclusion arising from the fact that host cities "inspire" and stimulate lifestyle changes. Benefits are also expected on tourism, self-image, architecture and the economy of the country as a whole. But are these expectations real and evidence-based? What parts of these "facts" are concrete and which ones are not? This paper suggests available ways of quantifying positive effects of hosting an Olympic Game, and puts the focus of this approach on the Rio de Janeiro 2016 Olympic Games and their true legacy, seeking scientific certainties.

Keywords

Physical Activity, Olympic Games, Paralympic Games, Olympic Legacy, Rio de Janeiro, Rio 2016

1. Introduction

Rio de Janeiro is a "sports city". This assumption arises immediately when we think of the warm weather, large beach areas and the idea of "eternal summer" that is associated with this city. Besides, it hosted many mega-events happened within a decade: the Panamerican Games (2007), the FIFA World Soccer Games (2014) and the Olympic Games (2016), the latter to be hosted in Rio de Janeiro during August and September 2016. But scientific studies do not confirm this stereotype of a "sports city". Surveys held in Brazil and specifically in Rio de Janeiro showed that more than 75% of the population of Rio "never or almost never" perform any physical activity at least 30 minutes, one day a week. Only 13% of the Brazilian population is considered "physically active" [1] [2].

Would it be possible to change this difficult scenario? May we start this change with the Olympic and Paralympic Games in 2016? These are some of the questions this article intends to answer.

2. Rio 2016: Health Legacy

The idea that such a big event as the Olympic Games could bring enormous benefits for the population's health and well-being has been used, by most of previous hosts, as one of the main arguments for receiving the Games. The huge amount of money necessary to prepare a city for the Olympics becomes more acceptable when those costs intend—at least theoretically—to improve several dimensions of a city, such as infrastructure, tourism, jobs and health promotion—the latter being possible through direct and indirect investments [3].

Since the 2012 London games [4] and continuing to 2016 Rio de Janeiro games [5] the olympic projects addressed specifically the Olympic legacy on health promotion [6]. The legacy would be the socioeconomic related determinants [6]. The health legacy was also analyzed by editors of leading scientific journals, including The Lancet and the British Medical Journal [5] [7].

A review study that has served as a reference to relate the impact of sporting events in the lives of populations was developed by UK Sport (2011). This study evaluated if the participation as spectator in three major sports events in England in the summer of 2010—"Women's Hockey Champions Trophy in Nottingham", "Triathlon World Championships Series" in Hyde Park, London, and "IRB Women's Rugby World Cup in Guildford and Twickenham", could influence stimulating physical activity. The authors concluded that mega events may inspire people, but it neither proved that this inspiration turns into real life changing and "inspires" the beginning of a physical activity, nor even encouraged people to keep up with it. A possible explanation is that behavior changes involve a multifactorial chain: they are usually not linked to one single reason [8].

The same conclusions are summarized at an exemplary systematic review of evidence based data regarding the London 2012 Olympic and Paralympic games [9]. Although there are a number of papers that discuss positive and negative legacies of mega sports events in the economic and social context, there are few studies about legacy in sports, and more specifically in physical and sports activity levels in the general population [4]-[7] [10]. The impact assessment in sports is highly difficult. Many variables may interfere with the interest of the population in these activities. Thus, it is hard to attribute a cause-effect relationship between the implementation of a particular event and the sport and physical activity levels of the population [7] [10] [11]. Another barrier for studies in the area is that as there is wide variation in research protocols that raise physical activity levels of populations, it is difficult to compare the levels pre and post events. The few published studies on this subject may be questioned due to methodological and/or ideological issues. In other words, doubts remain about the validity of some studies, not only because of the above mentioned reasons, but simply because some of them were supported by stakeholders from both government and institutions that disclose clear interests in finding positive associations [12].

A clear benefit to Brazilians would be to increase in physical activity levels, both in local, regional and national levels. This kind of legacy could be assessed using VIGITEL [11], a surveillance system of risk and protective factors for chronic non communicable diseases (NCDs). Using a simple telephone survey, this system could generate series of data measured before and after the games, but this has not been suggested so far. The Rio 2016 Olympic Games can be analyzed as a complex intervention in health, which makes the assessment of his legacy a multifaceted action [13], although some general issues are critical [7]: a) developing cost-effectiveness studies that measure outcomes of public interest and collective health; b) seeking additional effects and assigning the actions and interventions linked to the Olympic Dossier. These results should be compared to a "control" scenario model, *i.e.*, what would have happened if the Olympics had not been held at Rio. These are thrilling prospects for short term researches on the field, regarding the fact that the Olympic Games in Rio de Janeiro have still did not take place. There is time to plan and to act [14].

Health, Physical Activity and the Olympic Games

Sports and healthy living represent an investment in the long-term health of the nation. Efforts have been made to ensure a legacy which reaches beyond sport, to help to drive change in the nation's health and the way people live [15].

The concept of a health legacy of the Olympic Games was defined as: "The sustainable, positive health impacts on the host city or country, associated with the hosting of the Olympic Games", formally discussed at a symposium in Lausanne in 2002 entitled "The legacy of the Olympic Games 1984-2000" [16].

In recent years, the IOC Medical Commission has reoriented its work from a major focus on anti-doping issues, which recently have largely been taken over by the World Antidoping Agency, to focusing more on the health protection of current and future athletes and the health of the host city population [16].

The health legacy is multifaceted, with many potential long term impacts. These fall broadly into the following categories: improved capacity in traditional medical services required for hosting the Olympics; a strengthened public health system, including disease surveillance, risk management and health emergency response; an enhanced living environment for the host city citizens; and increased health awareness among athletes, visitors, and host country residents through successful health education and campaigns prior to and during the Olympic Games [16].

As previous cities hosting the Olympic Games, Beijing was also successful in providing high quality medical services. These included "athlete-friendly" health care in the polyclinics and venues, an intricate hospital network and reliable pre-hospital emergency health services, strengthened anti-doping systems in an attempt to assure a drug-free Games, and a new research project on sports injury prevention and treatment. These and many other initiatives have not only left the host city with improved health infrastructures and advanced technologies, but also an impressive resource of trained health professionals of great benefit to the host city long after the ending of the Games [16].

Another example of health impact is a research conducted on four categories of impact, largely based on a literature review and a on series of consultations and workshops with key stakeholders, especially within London: First, socio-economic health impact, which takes into account how potential socio-economic developments affect public health through their effects, for example, on levels of income and job security, on social cohesion and on access to housing and education. Second, physical health impact which traces the effects of changes in the quality of the physical environment, the amenity and the transport system. Third, mental health impact which reflects individuals' ability to balance all aspects of life arising from their social, economic, physical and emotional interactions by managing their surroundings and making choices throughout their lives. Fourth, the well-being health impact which reflects the extent to which individuals (expect to) feel contented (for examples, happy, healthy and prosperous): a negative impact can be reflected in depression, anxiety and stress [17].

3. Sports Legacy

3.1. Olympic Games

Among the welfares promoted by the Games' hosts, many of them focus on those that are sports-related. Some can be highlighted, such as increased sport participation, the creation of new sports programs and the improvement of sport infrastructure, as well as the formation of sport-related social capital intended to revitalize communities. These benefits are directed not only to the host city, but to all of the host nation [18].

The "Olympics Training Center" will emerge from the other six venues. Its goal will be to provide high-level facilities for several sports. It will also be available for those Olympic Experimental School's students as well as for other social projects [19]. As appealing as this idea of improvement may seem, however, it is not so easily achieved. So far, many were the host cities that believed in such development but were not able to prove it a reality. Studies have not revealed yet, for instance, enough evidence of improvements in health in the city of London after the Games in 2012, nor an increased participation in physical or sporting activities for host countries. The same occurs to other health benefits [7].

The Olympic Games are a major milestone in the host cities, creating an impact that has grown since the 1984 Olympics, when the Games have become larger and more expressive, involving more athletes, modalities and media [20].

The importance of sport to society can be demonstrated in several ways. In fact, the sport has a significant impact mainly in education and health of the population and may contribute to overcoming social problems experienced by the country. Moreover, it is an activity that is gaining economic importance, given the volume of funds and the growing number of companies involved. The actions for development of this activity in the country need to be comprehensive covering since the formation of athletes and construction of sports venues to create professional leagues and changes [12].

Thus, the Olympic Games, has great influence on the practice of physical activities in the countries that host the games. There is no denying the importance and value of sport among people, especially young people. With the Olympics, young people are attracted and stimulated by the practice of sport, with the spirit of competition, the cult of exuberance and physical perfection, as did the Greeks, nowadays so evident [12].

3.2. Paralympic Games

The Paralympic Games have evolved from a cultural to a true sports event, and its importance grew during the last editions. The empowerment of disabled athletes is a key goal of these games, and many studies seek to better understand how these Games arouse an increased concern from the general public, since they represent the human capability to overcome, the resiliency and the high development of rehabilitation processes. There are broad sociological questions involved with physical impairment and performance, but the Paralympic Games are clearly in a rise, and surely represent a positive movement towards a better understanding, social and sports inclusion of athletes with physical disabilities [21].

In Rio de Janeiro, there are some laboratories working specifically on paralympic performance at the Unisuam's post graduation in Rehabilitation Sciences, such as the "Lab of Human Movement Analysis" and the "Neurofunctional Performance Lab". They study the special conditions under which top para-athletes perform, in order to build scientific knowledge in this field. These research lines are highly important for Brazil, and may pose an important sports legacy for the host country, especially because Brazil traditionally performs significantly better in Paralympic Games (ranked 9th at the Beijing 2008 Paralympic Games and 7th at London Paralympics) than in Olympic Games (ranked 23th at the Beijing 2008 Olympic Games and 22th at London Olympics) [22].

The greatest legacy of the Paralympic competition is not simply to win a medal or the competition itself, but mainly the example these athletes give to hundreds of thousands of people who live stigmatized by physical and mental disabilities. Even those who do not wish to be athletes, the average citizen can find inspiration, building a parallel of their lives with those who overcome several difficulties with lots of courage, persistence and dedication towards sports. It is relevant to know that there are people who, despite difficulties of all kinds, are able the fight and win in sports. This is an attitude that shoes optimism, raises self-esteem and reorient sperspectives for many people, besides acquiring an attitude of acceptance and respect for individual differences [23].

It seems to be indeed a challenge posed by the issue of integration of disabled athletes into a high performance level sports competition. The goal to overcome difficulties through sports is clearly within the message of Olympism. Therefore, the Paralympic Games are a key part of the Rio 2016 Olympic Games, and bring along a remarkable legacy in society and culture [16].

4. Social Legacy

Last July 2015, the Rio de Janeiro city government disclosed the legacy the 2016 Olympic Games intends to leave to the city. From the start it was advertised that one of the main goals of hosting the Games was to leave a legacy for the city, with great improvements in social and economic spheres. The Games would not be their only concern, but instead, the future that would arise and become possible to build through and after the event itself [19].

The two main venue clusters will be transformed into different facilities for education, social projects, public leisure and elite-level sports. Most of the venues will remain untouched, whilst two of them, thanks to the "nomadic architecture", will become part of several new projects, such as schools and aquatics centers. Amongst those remaining untouched, some will become an Olympic Experimental School, with space for 850 full-time students. These institutions shall combine academic teaching with top-level sports training [19].

Inadequate attention to planning the post-Games period and the legacy of the Olympic Games is a risk [24]. The host cities usually focus on preparing to win the right to host the Games, planning grand and successful Olympics, but the post-Games period is neglected, because of lack of economic interest. It is important to plan what will be done with the huge infrastructure assembled for and by the Games [20].

Toronto and Vancouver, both in Canada, are also good examples of how the Olympic Games could bring positive consequences to the host cities. Their populations emphasized the idea of the need of public benefits to be brought by the games. A study held after the Vancouver Winter Games showed that hosting the game contributed to improve the image of Canada as a destination for Americans, besides increasing the feeling of pride of their own country among Canadian [25].

The legacy of investment in security infrastructure, urban revitalization, public transport, telecommunications, energy and data transmission is perhaps the greatest benefit that could happen to emerging economies like Brazil and the city of Rio de Janeiro, where huge architectural projects as the New Harbour in downtown ("Porto Maravilha") and the expansion of the subway to the western region of the city would otherwise not become viable in a short term [26].

Some authors also refer to a neoliberal influence of the organization of the games over the host country, because the dynamics of such mega-events necessarily include thorough negotiations with multinationals and the dominant economic system after all, what could be positive for the nation's growth [27].

All these achievements will also allow the city of Rio to host major international sports events, concerts and exhibitions, in a phenomenon called a "festivalisation" of the city, an inclusion of some parts of the "Global South" (Steinbrink). These are some of the heralded future benefits advertised by the Games organizers [28].

In the social sphere, the sport has pedagogical function in the individual formation process, stressing discipline, respect for hierarchy and the "rules of the game", solidarity, team spirit and other factors of human development. Can be used as social rescue tool (Italy, for example, organized a program for recovering addicts through sports) and has also been considered an antidote to violence (in New York, the Midnight leagues contributed to the decrease in crime rate). In the economic sphere, the sport involves a lot of financial resources; moves a large and diversified manufacturer specializing in the production of sports equipment, uniforms, protective equipment and footwear, among others.

The growth of the Second Time Program (STP), a program supported by the United Nations, which provides access to sports in public schools, including currently one million children. Between 2009 to 2016, the STP intends to grow to cover 3 million children [7]. In addition, the School and University Games, an initiative awarded by the International Olympic Committee (IOC), will be expanded. Of the current 2.5 million young people, the event will meet 5 million students, which will encourage the participation in Olympic sports [10].

The social importance of the Olympic Games can be assessed by parallel initiatives, such as the first World Indigenous Games, held at Palmas, Brazil, during October 2015. This innovative event counted with 21 countries, and its main goals were to empower these communities worldwide and to affirm the self-determination of indigenous people [29].

5. Olympic Games: Early and Future Examples

Hosting a mega event like the Olympics involves economic, social and environmental considerations [5]. According to Cashman [20], there are several types of impact to be expected: changes in the design of cities, changes in the physical structure and environment, representing the culture of a city and country, improvements in transportation, rising costs and taxes, potential increase in tourism and business, creation of new sites that can be used by the community after the Games, and community involvement as volunteers [20].

In this context, it becomes extremely important to study the established strategies and the possible impact before, during and after the Games because often the legacy turns into a huge public debt instead of concrete results, as the example of the 2007 Pan American Games (PAN 2007) showed [30].

About the prospects for the Olympic Games in Rio de Janeiro of 2016, a most expected legacy refers to the transport infrastructure, which aims to: improve public transport, especially high capacity, opening of new road connections in the north-south direction, increasing capacity to meet demand shifts in the east-west direction [31].

Since the nominations to previous Olympic Games and the organization of the PAN 2007, the mega sporting events has been one of local government's strategies to strengthen economic vocations of the city as the service sector, including tourism, economy linked to sport the cultural sector. Rio de Janeiro shares those similar goals with other host cities [12].

A Olympic Legacy Committee of Rio 2016—an alliance made up of government, by companies, by the Brazilian Olympic Committee and groups and community-organizations was created to oversee all projects associated with the Olympic legacy from 2009 to 2020 [9].

6. History

According to existing historic manuscripts, the first ancient Olympic Games were celebrated in 776 BC in Olympia [32].

From ancient times to the modern day and age, mankind has progressed scientifically, technologically and socially, eliminating the horrors of that time, aimed at the sport with its true value [32]. The first edition of the modern Olympic Summer Games was held in 1896 in Athens (Greece), and the first Olympic Winter Games in 1924 in Chamonix (France) [33].

It was Pierre de Coubertin who dreamt up this ambitious project. Drawing inspiration from the ancient Olympic Games, he founded the International Olympic Committee (IOC) in 1894 in Paris, with the goal of organizing the first Olympic Games of modern times [33]. Coubertin devoted his life to the reform of education and youth in France. Fascinated by the English education system, which included sport in the teaching program (a new idea at the time), he sought to convince his contemporaries in France that sport could be beneficial for young people. Coubertin brought a modern and international dimension and succeeded in re-establishing the Games. But for him, the Games were not an end in themselves. Rather they were part of a much broader project: education through sport [21].

7. Olympic Values

Olympism is a philosophy of life, exalting and combining in a balanced whole the qualities of body, will and mind. Blending sport with culture and education, Olympism seeks to create a way of life based on the joy of effort, the educational value of good example, social responsibility and respect for universal fundamental ethical principles [3].

The philosophy of Olympism is an essential element of the Olympic Movement and the celebration of the games. It is also what makes them unique. The pursuit of this ideal and the other "fundamental principles of Olympism" gives rise to a series of values, which are applicable both on the field of play and in everyday life [21].

The IOC has identified the following three Olympic values [21] [34]:

- **Excellence**. In the Olympic ideal, this value refers to giving one's best, on the field of play or in life, without measuring oneself with others, but above all aiming at reaching one's personal objectives with determination in the effort. It is not only about winning, but mainly about participating, making progress against personal goals, striving to be and to do our best in our daily lives and benefiting from the combination of a strong body, will and mind.
- **Friendship**. Men and women are at the Centre of the Olympic Movement's focus encouraging the links and mutual understanding between people. This value broadly refers to building a peaceful and better world through solidarity, team spirit, joy and optimism in sport. The Olympic Games inspire humanity to overcome political, economic, gender, racial or religious differences and forge friendships in spite of those differences. The athletes express this value by forming life-long bonds with their team-mates, as well as their opponents.
- **Respect**. In the Olympic ideal, this value represents the ethical principle that should inspire all who participate in the Olympic programs. It includes respect for oneself and one's body, respect for one another, for rules and for the environment. It thus refers to the fair play that each athlete has to display in sport, as well as avoiding doping [21] [34].

These three core values are conveyed through the Olympic symbols. The motto embodies excellence by encouraging athletes to strive to do their best. The flame symbolizes friendship between peoples with the torch relay usually travelling through different countries in the world. The rings represent respect, bringing all nations and all five continents together without discrimination. The principles shown are universality and humanism [35].

A very powerful symbol, the five rings are the visual representation of Olympism. It was Pierre de Coubertin himself who designed the symbol. The five rings represent the five continents. They are interlinked to show the universality of Olympism and how athletes from all over the world come together for the Olympic Games. On the Olympic flag, the rings appear against a white background. Combined in this way, the six colors of the flag (blue, yellow, black, green, red and white) represent all the nations. It is therefore not the case that each of the colors is associated with a particular continent. Today, the symbol is one of the most widely recognized in the world. Its use is subject to very strict rules enacted by the IOC. It is important to note that there is just one

Health, Physical Activity and the Rio de Janeiro 2016 Olympic Games: Legacy...

23

Olympic symbol. For the other identifying elements described below, other terms are needed [21] [35].

A motto is a phrase which sums up a life philosophy or a code of conduct to follow. The Olympic motto is made up of three Latin words: faster, Higher and Stronger. These three words encourage the athlete to give his or her best during competition. To better understand the motto, we can compare it with the Olympic creed: The most important thing in life is not the triumph, but the fight; the essential thing is not to have won, but to have fought well. Together, the Olympic motto and the creed represent an ideal that Coubertin believed in and promoted as an important life lesson that could be gained from participation in sport and the Olympic Games: that giving one's best and striving for personal excellence was a worthwhile goal. It is a lesson that can still be applied equally today, not just to athletes but to each one of us [21] [35].

These symbols are much more than emblems and people should immediately be able to associate them with fundamental values for sport and life in general [35].

8. Conclusions

The projects, goals and expectations for the Rio 2016 Olympic Games must be sustainable and inclusive. Otherwise, those who don't have a powerful voice in society will remain unheard and excluded from the wide improvements likely to be brought by the Games. Yet these legacies will not emerge individually simply by "the power of sport"; they need to be grounded in extensive planning and political processes meant to keep on going even after the 2016 Olympic Games are over.

One of the scopes of the Olympic ambitions of the Brazilian government, in fact, is the massification of sports in the school environment. Hosting mega sporting events may bring opportunities, and strengthen actions to encourage the population's physical activities of leisure and health promotion. These are very important in an increasing context of chronic degenerative diseases associated with a sedentary lifestyle and habits of unhealthy life, which is the case. For this purpose, governments and institutions linked to sports should use media coverage intended for mega sports events to help boost the development of the sport and the dissemination of physical activity in the country. But this is not so easily achieved-recent examples are frustrating ones.

Ribeiro stated that "the ideal legacy is what can be positive in all aspects: sport, economic, social and environmental". And that is the main challenge for a country that chooses to host a mega event such as the Olympic Games: to transform the entire investment in real growth for the host city and host country [12].

A desired legacy can only be achieved if it is based on extensive planning and if it focuses on some main points. It must be connected with existing social structures and the everyday lives of local populations.

In conclusion, a true legacy in health, as consequence of hosting the Olympic Games, should not be taken for granted. It is essential to evaluate these facts through studies with high methodological quality, based on projects developed before, during and after the event. There is a window of opportunity for many to grow and evolve, but the Games are not and should not be regarded as a solution for structural problems.

Acknowledgements

We would like to thank Prof. Dr. Jörg Königstorfer, Head of the Chair of Sports and Management at the Teschnische Universität Munich, Germany, for inspiring the idea of this paper, and for future research prospects. We also thank Raphael Calafange, from UNISUAM Brazil, for specific technical considerations regarding the Paralympic Games. Finally, we thank Professor Dr. Aline Marcadenti and Prof. Dr. Lamartine DaCosta for their lifetime examples of dedication to interdisciplinary science.

References

[1] Monteiro, C.A., Conde, W.L. and Matsudo, V.R. (2003) A Descriptive Epidemiology of Leisure-Time Physical Activity in Brasil, 1996-1997. *Revista Panamericana de Salud Pública/Pan American Journal of Public Health*, **14**, 246-254. http://dx.doi.org/10.1590/S1020-49892003000900005

[2] Dumith, S.C. (2009) Physical Activity in Brazil: A Systematic Review. *Cadernos de Saúde Pública*, Rio de Janeiro, **25**, S415-S426. http://dx.doi.org/10.1590/s0102-311x2009001500007

[3] Demarzo, M.M.P., Mahtani, K.R., Slight, S.P., Barton, C. and Blakeman, T. (2014) The Olympic Legacy for Brazil: Is It a Public Health Issue? *Cadernos de Saúde Pública*, **30**, 8-10.

[4] Mahtani, K.R., Protheroe, J., Slight, S.P., Demarzo, M.M.P., Blakeman, T., Barton, C.A., Brijnath, B., *et al.* (2013) Can the London 2012 Olympics "Inspire a Generation" to Do More Physical or Sporting Activities? An Overview of

Systematic Reviews. *BMJ Open* [Internet]. http://bmjopen.bmj.com/content/3/1/e002058.full.pdf+html

[5]   Weed, M. (2010) How Will We Know If the London 2012 Olympics and Paraolympics Benefit Health? *BMJ*, **340**, c2202. http://dx.doi.org/10.1136/bmj.c2202

[6]   Dossiê de Candidatura do Rio de Janeiro a sede dos jogos olímpicos e Paraolímpicos [Candidature Dossierfrom Rio de Janeiro to host the Olympic andParalympic games], 2016, V.1.

[7]   Welling, K., Datta, J., Wilkinson, P. and Petticrew, M. (2011) The 2012 Olympics Assensing the Public Health Effect. *Lancet*, **378**, 1193-1195. http://dx.doi.org/10.1016/S0140-6736(11)60550-3

[8]   International Olympic Committee (IOC), Implementing the Olympic Movement's Agenda 21. Sustainability through Sport. 2012.
http://www.olympic.org/Documents/Commissions_PDFfiles/SportAndEnvironment/Sustainability_Through_Sport.pdf

[9]   D Louise Mansfield, L., Wellard, I., Chatziefstathiou, D. and Dowse, S. (2009) A Systematic Review of the Evidence Base for Developing a Physical Activity and Health Legacy from the London 2012 Olympic and Paralympic Games. Department of Health, Canterbury Christ Church University, Kent.

[10] Department of Education Rio de Janeiro city. Programa de Alimentação escolar [Schoolfeedingprogram]. 2014.
www.ebc.com/noticias/2015/05/olimpiadas-vao-deixar-legado-da-alimentacao-saudavel-nas-escolas-publicas-do-rio

[11] Malta, D.C., Moura, E.C., Castro, A.M., Cruz, D.K.A., Monteiro, Neto, O.L. and Monteiro, C.A. (2009) Padrão da atividade física em adultos brasileiros: Resultado de um inquérito por entrevistas telefônicas 2006 [Pattern of Physical Activity in Brazilian Adults: Results of a Survey by Telephone Interviews in 2006]. *Epidemiologia e serviços de saúde*, **18**, 7-16.

[12] Souza, D.L. and Saks, P. (2013) Legados esportivos de megaeventos esportivos: Uma revisão da literatura (Sporting Legacy of Mega Sports Events: A Literature Review). *Motrivivência*, **41**, 42-46. http://dx.doi.org/10.1136/bmj.a1655

[13] Craig, P., Dieppe, P., Mancintyre, S., Michie, S., Nazareth, I. and Petticrew, M. (2008) Developing and Evaluating Complex Interventions: The New Medical Research Council Guidance. *BMJ*, **337**, a1655.

[14] Sampson, A., Harden, A., Tobi, P. and Renton, A. (2012) Promoting a Healthy Legacy for the Olympic Park: Findings from a Pre-Games Study. *Perspectives in Public Health*, **132**, 64-65. http://dx.doi.org/10.1177/1757913912437675

[15] Mayor of London (2013) Inspired by 2012: The Legacy from the London 2012 Olympic and Paralympic Games.
https://www.gov.uk/government/uploads/system/uploads/attachment_data/file/224148/2901179_OlympicLegacy_acc.pdf

[16] Dapeng, J., Ljungqvist, A. and Troedsson, H. (2008) The Health Legacy of the 2008 Beijing Olympic Games: Successes and Recommendations. World Health Association.
http://www.olympic.org/Documents/Commissions_PDFfiles/Medical_commission/The_Health_Legacy_of_the_2008_Beijing_Olympic_Games.pdf

[17] Department of Culture, Media and Sport of London (2005) Olympic Games Impact Study: Final Report.
http://www.gamesmonitor.org.uk/files/PWC%20OlympicGamesImpactStudy.pdf

[18] Coakley, J. and Souza, D.L. (2013) Sport Mega-Events: Can Legacies and Development Be Equitable and Sustainable? *Motriz: Revista de Educação Física*, **19**, 580-589. http://dx.doi.org/10.1590/s1980-65742013000300008

[19] Comitê Olímpico Brasileiro (2015) Rio 2016 Olympic and Paralympic Games Venues to Leave Sporting, Educational and Social Legacy to City. Comitê Olímpico Brasileiro, Brazil.
http://www.rio2016.com/en/news/rio-2016-olympic-and-paralympic-games-venues-to-leave-sporting-educational-and-social-legacy-to

[20] Cashman, R. (2002) Impact of the Games on Olympic Host Cities: University Lecture on the Olympics. Centre d'Estudis Olímpics (CEO-UAB). International Chair in Olympism (IOC-UAB), Barcelona.

[21] International Olympic Committee (IOC) (2013) The Olympic Museum, Lausanne 3rd Edition. Olympism and the Olympic Movement. http://www.olympic.org/documents/reports/en/en_report_670.pdf

[22] International Paralympic Movement (2015) www.paralympic.org

[23] Brazilian Paralympic Committee (2015) www.cpb.org.br

[24] Ribeiro, C.H.V., Soares, A.J.G. and Da Costa, L.P. (2014) Percepção sobre o legado dos megaeventos esportivos no brasil: O caso da copa do mundo FIFA 2014 e os jogos olímpicos Rio 2016. *Revista Brasileira de Ciências do Esporte*, **36**, 447-466. http://dx.doi.org/10.1590/S0101-32892014000200012

[25] Armenakyan, A. and Helsop, J.N. (2010) Does Hosting the Olympic Games Matter? Canada and Olympic Games Images before and after the 2010 Olympic Games. *International Journal of Sport Management and Marketing*, **12**, 111-140.

[26] Fonseca, M.L.M. (2011) Externalidades e Bens Públicos em Grandes Eventos Esportivos: Avaliações e Perspectivas

(Externalities and Public Goods in Major Sporting Events: Reviews and Perspectives). In: Planejamento, Patrimômino Cultural e Eventos Esportivos: Construindo Estratégias.

[27] Gaffney, C. (2010) Mega Events and Socio-Spatial Dynamics in Rio de Janeiro. *Journal of Latin American Geography*, **9**, 7-29.

[28] Steinbrink, M. (2013) FestiFAVELisation: Mega-Events, Slums and Strategic City-Staging—The Example of Rio de Janeiro. *Journal of the Geographical Society of Berlin*, **144**, 129-145.

[29] Indigenous World Games (2015). http://en.jogosmundiaisindigenas.com/

[30] Pires, S.P., Baptista, L.F.S. and Portugal, L.S. (2013) Megaeventos e o Desenvolvimento Urbano e Regional: Uma Análise das Especificidades e Impactos Provenientes dos Jogos Olímpicos e Um Panorama Para a Cidade do Rio de Janeiro (Mega-Events and the Urban and Regional Development: A Review of the Specificities and Coming Impact of the Olympic Games and an Overview for the City of Rio de Janeiro). Encontros Nacionais de ANPUR, Anais.

[31] Special Committee for Urban Legacy of Department of Urbanism of Rio de Janeiro City (2009) Plano de Legado Urbano e Ambiental: Olimpíadas Rio 2016 (Plan of Urban and Environmental Legacy: Olympics 2016). Secretaria Municipal de Urbanismo—Prefeitura da cidade do Rio de Janeiro.

[32] International Olympic Committee (IOC) (2012) The Olympic Games of Antiquity. http://www.olympic.org/documents/reference_documents_factsheets/the_olympic_games_of_game_antiquity.pdf

[33] International Olympic Committee (IOC) (2013) The Olympic Museum, Lausanne 3rd Edition. The Modern Olympic Games. http://www.olympic.org/Documents/Reports/EN/en_report_668.pdf

[34] Brazilian Olympic Committee (2014) Olimpismo. Movimento Olímpico. http://www.rio2016.com/educacao/sites/default/files/midiateca/aulas/movolimpico_aula1.pdf

[35] International Olympic Committee (IOC) (2007) The Olympic Symbols. 2nd Edition. http://www.olympic.org/documents/reports/en/en_report_1303.pdf

Perceptions on Public Health Facilities by Slum Dwellers in the Metropolitan Cities of India

Palaniappan Marimuthu[1], Grish N. Rao[2], Manoj Kumar Sharma[3], Ramasamy Dhanasekara Pandian[4]

[1]Department of Biostatistics, National Institute of Mental Health Neuro Sciences, Bangalore, India
[2]Department of Epidemiology, National Institute of Mental Health Neuro Sciences, Bangalore, India
[3]Department of Clinical Psychology, National Institute of Mental Health Neuro Sciences, Bangalore, India
[4]Department of Psychiatry Social Work, National Institute of Mental Health Neuro Sciences, Bangalore, India
Email: p_marimuthu@hotmail.com

Abstract

Rapid urbanisation and quest for better livelihood, push-pull factor of occupations education, policy changes attract large scale rural population to urban areas. It is well documented that in spite of better public health facilities including tertiary care hospitals which are available in the urban areas but the services are underutilised by the urban poor. Aim: Hence, in this paper, it is attempted to comprehend the reasons for underutilisation of available public health facilities and to compare the difference with non-slum areas of the major metropolitan cities of India. Methods: A secondary data from National Family Health Survey-III for five major metropolitan cities namely, Delhi, Hyderabad, Mumbai, Kolkata and Chennai is used for the analysis. Slum data which are classified by both the agencies, that is census of India and NFHS-III as slum households only considered for analysis. Results: In Mumbai slums about 90% of the households are having water sources from public tap or piped to yard followed by Hyderabad having better water supply and Chennai slum dwellers having minimum access to good water sources. About 11.4% of the households do not know where their toilet drainage is connected. There is a significant ($P < 0.001$) difference in the observed proportions of toilet facilities by the cities studied. Proportions of open defecation is compared among five cities and it is found that Delhi and Hyderabad have similar proportion ($P > 0.05$) 75% to 79%, Kolkata and Chennai have parallel high proportion, that is more than 95% ($P > 0.05$) and Mumbai stands as median percent age as 89.6. Apart from Delhi, about 40% to 45% of the slum population is in the opinion of "long waiting time" in the government hospitals, and the same trend of proportions is observed for "poor quality of service".

Keywords

Slums, Metropolitan Cities, Government Health Facility, Toilets, Health Schemes, Perceptions

---

1. Introduction

The United Nations predicts that the world urban population will grow nearly two billion [1] by 2030. Slums are defined by the United Nations Organizations as "a building or group of buildings and area characterized by overcrowding, deterioration in sanitary conditions, or absence of facilities and amenities, which because of these conditions or any of them endanger the health, safety or morals of its inhabitants or the community".

As per the census of India, the slums are defined as "residential areas where dwellings are in any respect unfit for human habitation by reasons of dilapidation, overcrowding, faulty arrangements and designs of such buildings, narrowness or faulty arrangement of streets, lack of ventilation, light, sanitation facilities or any combination of these factors which are detrimental to safety, health and morals [2].

In India, unprecedented slum growth in their steep magnitude and their distribution is a big challenge to the civic administration. The slum population represents a poor physical, socio-economic environment and human health of an urban city.

In a decade, cultivable areas of India shrink from 163,355 to 141,861 (000') hector [3], forcing the agriculture labour force to seek for alternate livelihood. Rural literacy rate increases to 84.98% from 68.91% in a decade [4] and this elevated literacy rate is also another push factor for large scale migration to the urban areas. Lower sex ratio in the slum area indicates that male labour forces are more migrating to urban area than their counter part. The employment opportunity in the urban areas and the migration are in direct proportions. Slum dwellers ignore their health due to low literacy level, lack of awareness and reluctant to lose wage. Effective Health service for urban poor, which is a desperate need, their unwillingness to avail the health care facility and there are some bottle necks from the supply side. This implies that cases of infections, malnourishment in women and children and deaths rates are high in slum areas.

Apart from supplying civic amenities, sometime sudden epidemic break is a big challenge to the public health authorities. Government of India implemented some programs specific to slum population welfare and their health such as Rajiv A is Yojana, which is supporting states for activities like slum surveys, GIS mapping of slums and mobile clinic etc. Recently, Government of India launches the National Urban Health Mission for addressing the health needs of urban poor. All the health policy documents are too addressed the problem of slum health and recognise the underutilisation of the available welfare programs by slum dwellers.

It is well documented that in spite of better public health facilities including tertiary care hospitals which are available in the urban areas still the services underutilised by the urban poor. Hence, in this paper, it is attempted to understand the reasons for underutilisation of available public health facilities and is attempted to compare the difference with non-slum areas of the major metropolitan cities of India, viz., Delhi, Mumbai, Kolkata, Hyderabad and Chennai.

2. Data and Method

It is a secondary data analysis; National Family Health Survey-III data for five major metropolitan cities namely, Delhi, Mumbai, Kolkata and Chennai was used for the analysis. These data were obtained from *Measuresdhs USA* [5]. The households were classified as slum and non-slum by two agencies, viz., NFHS and census of India. slum data which were classified by both the agencies, that is census of India and NFHS-III as slum households were only considered for analysis. Definition for slum household by the census of India is provided above in the introduction part [2] and the in NFHS-III slum households were identified in the eight designated cities by the interviewing team supervisor at the time of the fieldwork. Few variables which are more relevant for the public health aspects namely, source of water supply, toilet facility, health insurance, reasons for not utilising the government health facilities and possessing of BPL cards selected for this study. Sampling and sample size of slum data where explained (Health and living conditions in eight Indian cities. NFHS-3) elsewhere [6].

Chi-square test was used to test the proportions among five cities. Data were analysed using SPSS 11.0 Statistical package.

3. Results

From **Table 1**, it evident that better water supply is available for Mumbai slums about 90% of the households are having water sources from public tap or piped to yard followed by Hyderabad. From the above table it appears that Chennai slum dwellers having minimum access to good water sources. Majority of slum population is depending on the public water supply/hand pumps. Other category includes Protected well, unprotected well, Tanker truck, Cart with small tank, Bottled water. Observed difference of proportions in each city by source of water supply are significantly different ($P < 0.001$).

From **Table 2**, higher proportion of Mumbai and Kolkata slum households possess toilets with "Flush to piped sewer System" at the same time those who go for open defecation is also in higher proportion from these two cities. In general majority of the households are not having toilet facility and they mostly go for open defecation. About 11.4% of the households do not know where their toilet drainage is connected. "Other" category includes that Flush-don't know where, Pit latrine-ventilated improved pit (VIP), Pit latrine-with slab, Pit latrine-without slab/open pit and dry toilet. There is a significant ($P < 0.001$) difference in the observed proportion by each city. Proportions of the open defecation is compared [7] among the five cities it is found that Delhi and Hyderabad have similar proportions ($P > 0.05$) 75% to 79%, Kolkata and Chennai have parallel high proportion, that is more than 95% to 100% ($P > 0.05$) and Mumbai stand as medianper cent of 89.6.

In **Table 3**, it is shown that least proportion (25.8%) of Delhi slum dwellers expressed that "Facility time is not convenient" to them and highest proportion of (61.3%) form Mumbai slums also stated the same reason for not utilising the public health facility. Apart from Delhi, about 40 to 45 per cent of the slum population is in the opinion of "long waiting time" in the government hospitals. Same trend of proportions are observed for "poor quality of service" except for Delhi and Chennai. Another important reason for underutilisation of public health facility is "absence of health personnel" in the hospital and the least per cent is observed in Chennai. Others category includes Payment required, Medicine not provided reasons. Proportions of different reasons for not utilising the government health facilities by five cities are statistically significant ($P < 0.001$).

Table 1. Sources of water supply by five metropolitan cities.

	Piped into dwelling		Piped to yard/plot		Public tap/standpipe		Tube well or borehole		Other sources	
	n_1	% Slum	n_2	% Slum	n_3	% Slum	n_4	% Slum	n_5	% Slum
Delhi	8801	26.52%	605	39.01%	1830	81.09%	796	54.65%	1179	25.78%
Kolkata	2022	25.91%	2169	48.96%	3094	67.74 &	1464	32.45%	216	84.72%
Mumbai	5336	41.96%	1471	90.21%	453	90.51%	6	100.00%	3	100.00%
Hyderabad	3175	44.16%	3809	37.28%	806	62.90%	22	11.00%	144	86.81%
Chennai	552	16.85%	991	31.18%	1847	70.76%	292	44.52%	1529	40.35%
P-value	$P = 0.000$		$P = 0.000$		$P = 0.000$		$P = 0.000$		$P = 0.000$	

*Mumbai for computing χ^2-test last two categories ("tub well" and "other") merged.

Table 2. Distribution of available Toilet facility by five metropolitan cities.

	Flush-to piped sewer system		Flush-to Septic tank		Flush-to pit latrine		Flush-to somewhere else		No facility/uses bush/field		Other sources	
	n_1	% Slum	n_2	% Slum	n_3	% Slum	n_4	% Slum	n_5	% Slum	n_6	% Slum
Delhi	8987	23.93%	1399	26.80%	55	67.27%	1605	87.66%	876	74.54%	278	58.99%
Kolkata	4109	56.02%	3732	39.82%	762	37.01%	84	84.52%	80	100.00%	198	60.10%
Mumbai	6852	53.08%	177	77.40%	11	36.36%	114	100.00%	77	89.61%	30	80.00%
Hyderabad	5620	43.58%	1416	29.66%	210	59.52%	348	65.23%	94	79.79%	235	65.96%
Chennai	1939	33.47%	516	31.78%	15	46.67%	2478	56.90%	107	95.33%	156	79.49%
P-value	$P = 0.000$		$P = 0.000$		$P = 0.000$		$P = 0.000$		$P = 0.000$		$P = 0.000$	

Table 3. Opinion about Government Health Facility by five metropolitan cities.

	Facility timing not convenient		Waiting time too long		Health personnel often absent		Poor quality of care		Others	
	n_1	% Slum	n_2	% Slum	n_3	% Slum	n_4	% Slum	n_5	% Slum
Delhi	1465	25.80%	5304	34.50%	206	36.89%	3391	37..36%	204	54.41%
Kolkata	1663	47.02%	3920	46.51%	169	32.54%	3734	42.05%	385	26.75%
Mumbai	863	61.30%	2032	44.64%	119	52.94%	2251	47.80%	156	48.72%
Hyderabad	1252	40.26%	2079	46.51%	483	44.31%	2933	40.64%	196	14.29%
Chennai	930	43.01%	1125	41.60%	81	19.75%	1372	36.23%	181	34.25%
P-value	P = 0.000		P = 0.000		P = 0.000		P = 0.000		P = 0.000	

Above **Figure 1** is self-explanatory for those who are covered by some health insurance schemes, it ranges from 14% to 24%, about one-fourth of slum population in Mumbai is covered by some health insurance scheme and least proportion observed from Delhi. Further analysis it is noted that those who are covered by some health scheme majority of them are supported by ESIS scheme (data not shown). Data have three categories that is "yes" "No" and "Don't know" and the proportion from these five cities are statistically significant ($P < 0.001$).

Possessing the Below Poverty Line card is requirement for availing the government subsidised/welfare programs, by the poor people. It is noted that about 9.4% of themonly having this BPL cards in these five cities.

4. Discussion

Ample opportunities for health care, education and employment are available in the urban areas, but the newly migrated urban poor are reluctant to utilise the government facilities. The reason is that they are mainly migrated for their livelihood and they do not concentrate the available scheme or they do not know the places where to go and avail the services offered by the government. In Delhi slums, 86.50% of slum dwellers, the major source of drinking water is either tap or hand pump [8]. In another study from Delhi slums [9], it is reported that tap water is 41.2%, ground water is 56.1%, and other sources are 50.8% [9].

A study by Anita Khokhar, *et al.* [10] list the reasons for availing the government health facility which is easy available (45.3%), effective treatment (12.5%), low cost (67.3%), better service (4.4%), faith in system (6.9%), cordial behaviour (0%) and others (0%). And they also reveal that 87.3% of users in the opinion waiting time in the government health facility are more than 2 hours. In another study from Pune Slums [11], it is reported that 35.1% of the slum dwellers avail the services of government health facilities while the satisfaction level is higher with private doctors (81.6%) and the main reason for the dissatisfaction with government health facilities is long waiting time (35.8%).

Upendra Bhojani *et al.* [12] from Bangalore, have demonstrated socioeconomic gradient with people living below the poverty line at significantly greater odds of reporting chronic conditions than people living above the poverty line (OR = 3, 95%; CI = 1.5, 5.8). Private healthcare providers manage over 80% of patients. They also show that an increase in income is positively associated with the use of private facilities. They also shown that an increase in income is positively associated with the use of private health facilities. A study on access to health service comprising of four cities [13], it uncovers that majority (68%) of the respondents who are replied to the questionnaire say that there are only private health facilities in the slums. A small proportion about four percent says that there are government facilities. Most (80%) of those who consult a doctor prefer private facilities, of which about half visited private clinics, and 30% go to private hospitals and around 17% go to government hospitals. Almost no respondent choose to visit government dispensary for his or her conditions.

Archana S. Nimbalkar *et al.* [14] compare the health seeking behaviour between rural and slum samples and they report that antenatal care, hospital delivery, neonatal follow-up, health seeking, essential newborn care and exclusive breastfeeding are also lower in urban slums, as compared to villages. Health care and socioeconomic status of neonates in slums of smaller cities is poorer than in surrounding villages. BBL Sharma *et al.* [15] have demonstrated that more than 90 per cent of the population and almost all the poor are not covered by any health insurance scheme. Health care needs of these disadvantaged groups are primarily met through direct out-of

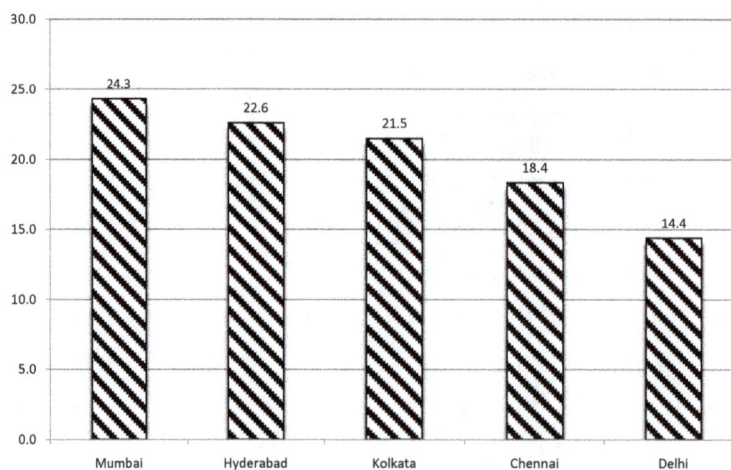

Figure 1. Members of the Households (%) covered by a health scheme or Health Insurance by Five cities.

pocket expenditure on services provided by the public and private sectors.

There are some Health supporting/insurance schemes available for the poor people by Government, they are Rashtiya Swasthiya Bima Yojana (RSBY), Employment State Insurance Scheme (ESIS), Aam Aadmi Bima Yojana (AABY), Janashree Bima Yojana (JBY), Universal Health Insurance Scheme (UHIS). But for availing benefits from these (most) schemes one should have the BPL card, it may note that, from this study we found that only 9.5% of the slum dweller are having the BPL card.

References

[1]   (2007) UN-HABITAT Report, Slum Dwellers to Double by 2030.

[2]   RGI. Census of India, Housing Stock, Amenities & Assets in Slums—Census 2011 HH-1.

[3]   Agriculture Census Division, Department of Agriculture and Cooperation (2012) All India Report on Agriculture Census 2005-06. Agriculture Census Division, Department of Agriculture and Cooperation, New Delhi.

[4]   Rao, K.H. Rural Development Statistics, 2011-12. National Institute of Rural Development, Hyderabad.

[5]   http://www.dhsprogram.com/data/available-datasets.cfm

[6]   Gupta, K., Arnold, F. and Lhungdim, H. (2009) Health and Living Conditions in Eight Indian Cities. National Family Health Survey-3, India 2005-06, Ministry of Health and Family Welfare, Government of India.

[7]   Fleiss, J.L., Levin, B. and Paik, M.C. (1980) Statistical Methods for Rates and Proportions. Wiley, USA, 138-142.

[8]   Directorate of Economics and Statistics Urban Slums in Delhi. Based on 69th Round of NSS. State Sample, Delhi-110054.

[9]   Marimuthu, P., Meitei, M.H. and Sharma, B.B.L. (2009) General Morbidity Prevalence in the Delhi Slums. *Indian Journal of Community Medicine*, **34**, 338-342. http://dx.doi.org/10.4103/0970-0218.58395

[10] Khokhar, A., Garg, S. and Singh, M.M.C. (2003) Health Care Service Utilization for Kuslsus and Diarrhoeal Diseases: A Study amongst Slum Dwellers in Delhi. *Health and Population-Perspectives and Issues*, **26**, 59-66.

[11] Banerjee, A., Bhawalkar, J.S., Jadhav, S.L., Rathod, H. and Khedkar, D.T. (2012) Access to Health Services among Slum Dwellers in an Industrial Township and Surrounding Rural Areas: A Rapid Epidemiological Assessment. *Journal of Family Medicine and Primary Care*, **1**, 20-26.

[12] Bhojani, U., Beerenahalli, T.S., Devadasan, R., Munegowda, C.M., Devadasan, N., Criel, B. and Kolsteren, P. (2013) No Longer Diseases of the Wealthy: Prevalence and Health-Seeking for Self-Reported Chronic Conditions among Urban. *BMC Health Services Research*, **13**, 306. http://dx.doi.org/10.1186/1472-6963-13-306

[13] Pradeep, I.G. (2015) Health Status and Access to Health Services in Indian Slums. *Guin Health*, **7**, 245-255.

[14] Nimbalkar, A.S., Shukla, V.V., Phatak, A.G. and Nimbalkar, S.M. (2013) Newborn Care Practices and Health Seeking Behavior in Urban Slums and Villages of Anand, Gujarat. *Indian Pediatrics*, **50**, 408-410.

[15] Sharma, B.B.L., Nair, K.S. and Bir, T. (2002) National Seminar on Development of Health Insurance in India: Current Status and Future Directions an Overview. *Health and Population-Perspectives and Issues*, **25**, 11-25.

4

Relationship of Workaholism with Stress and Job Burnout of Elementary School Teachers

Hossein Jenaabadi[1], Bahareh Azizi Nejad[2], Fatemeh Saeidi Mahmoud Abadi[3], Rezvan Haghi[4], Maryam Hojatinasab[5]

[1]Faculty of Educational Sciences and Psychology, University of Sistan and Baluchestan, Zahedan, Iran
[2]Department of Educational Science, Payame Noor University, Tehran, Iran
[3]Islamic Azad University, Tehran, Iran
[4]Allameh Tabatabai University, Tehran, Iran
[5]MA of Educational Research, University of Sistan and Baluchestan, Zahedan, Iran
Email: hjenaabadi@ped.usb.ac.ir, Bahareh19@gmail.com

Abstract

Teachers voluntarily devote a lot of time to their vocational activates. This can lead to workaholism and may result in stress and job burnout. The main objective of the current study is to examine the relationship of workaholism with stress and job burnout of elementary school teachers in Zahedan. This is a descriptive-correlational study. The sample includes 350 elementary school teachers in Zahedan whom are selected through applying stratified random sampling method and are examined using questionnaires on workaholism, occupational stress, and job burnout. To analyze the obtained data, correlation coefficient and simultaneous multiple regression analysis are applied using $SPSS_{21}$. Teachers' mean scores on workaholism, stress and job burnout are higher than the considered theoretical mean. Workaholism and its components (feeling of being driven to work, work involvement, and work enjoyment) are significantly and positively related to job burnout and occupational stress ($p < 0.01$). The results of simultaneous multiple regression analysis indicate that components of workaholism can predict teachers' occupational stress and job burnout ($p < 0.05$). Considering the results, holding training courses for teachers to become familiar with the phenomena of workaholism, stress, and job burnout, individual and organizational outcomes, methods of dealing with them and managing them effectively is highly recommended.

Keywords

Workaholism, Occupational Stress, Job Burnout, Elementary School Teachers

1. Introduction

Attendance at workplace, spending considerable amount of time doing a job, and concerns about and mental preoccupations with occupational activities lead people to voluntarily devote a lot of time to their vocational activates without having adequate rest and recreation and dedicating enough time to family and friends. These people usually experience a lot of stress and their work may cause physical and mental problems for them. These people are known as workaholics and this trait is referred to as workaholism [1]. Studies on workaholism have provided different and contradictory results. As an instance, some researchers examined workaholism with a positive attitude and concluded that workaholics were very satisfied and productive; however, others had a negative viewpoint and considered workaholism as a non-fun phenomenon which caused various difficulties for others (an individual's colleagues) [2]. As Askari and Nouri noted, Piotrowski and Vodanovich asserted that when workaholic behaviors were excessive, this phenomenon converted into workaholism which significantly endangered human health through creating stress and job burnout [3]. In this regard, the present study aims to investigate the relationship of workaholism with stress and job burnout.

The term workaholism was first used in 1968 by Wayne Oates, an American pastor and psychologist, in his book entitled "Confessions of a Workaholic". In his point of view, workaholics were those who needed to work so extreme that might cause serious threats to their health, personal happiness, interpersonal relationships and social responsibilities and roles, since they had irrational commitments to work hard and they voluntarily devoted a great amount of time to their work. Spence and Robbins (1992) offered the first academic and practical definition of the term "workaholism". From their perspective, workaholism originated from a series of people's attitudes and perceptions. They considered a person workaholic when he/she was highly involved with his/her work. He/she had extraordinary inner compulsion to work hard and scantly enjoyed his/her work [4].

According to the typology, Spence and Robbins (1992) characterized workaholism by the amount and degree of the following components: 1. Work involvement; 2. Feeling of being driven to work; and 3. Work enjoyment. In workaholics, the degree of work involvement was really high and they were really eager to work; however, they barely enjoyed their work [4]. In contrast, people who were eager to work were involved with the work and enjoyed it; however, they did not have any excessive tension towards it. Scott, Moore, and Miceli (1997) identified three workaholism patterns including compulsive-dependent, perfectionist, and achievement-oriented [5]. Compulsive-dependent workaholics experienced a lot of anxiety and stress. Their work caused various physical and psychological problems. These people had low levels of satisfaction with their life and job and had low job performance. Perfectionist workaholics experienced a high level of stress, mental and physical problems, established hostile and ineffective interpersonal relations, had many absents and turnovers voluntarily and had low job satisfaction and job performance. Finally, achievement-oriented workaholics had high levels of job satisfaction, life satisfaction, mental and physical health, job performance and organizational citizenship behaviors and they had low stress and low voluntarily turnovers.

Occupational stress was initially considered by Hans Selye, emphasizing its importance in the educational environments. Occupational stress is the interaction between working conditions and an employee in a way that the person cannot cope with related pressures which endanger the mental health of the employee and result in physical burnout and job dissatisfaction [6]. In general, stress has greatly been taken into the consideration in recent years such that this century is known as the age of stress. Teaching profession is one of the most stressful professions and in this regard, over the past thirty years in various countries, a large number of researchers have expressed the concern that teachers experience severe stress and conducted different studies on this matter. In terms of responsibility for students' welfare and well-being, teachers have a unique profession. This is why teachers experience a different form of stress which needs to be defined. Teachers' occupational stress can be defined as negative and unpleasant emotions including anger, hopelessness, anxiety, depression, and nervousness which are created as the result of their occupation. Stress is a common phenomenon in the teaching profession. All teachers have been reported some degrees of occupational stress from mild to severe in different time periods. Based on previously conducted studies, teaching is regarded as one of the world's top ten most stressful careers and one-third of teachers believe that teaching is highly stressful [7]. Moreover, these studies reported high levels of job dissatisfaction and depression among teachers, mentioning that stress is a part of teaching. While some degrees of stress can increase and improve people's performance, high levels of stress can lead to numerous consequences such as physical illnesses and mental fatigue. If stress persists, in long term, it can endanger personnel's health and alter them to impotent and incapable people, the negative impacts of which are reflected in their performance [8]. Accordingly, stress management aids teachers to improve their physical, psychological, social and occupational performance.

Burnout contains fatigue and exhaustion in jobs helping people, especially social work professions. As stated in Amiri, Asadi, and Delbari Ragheb (2011), Jackson and Maslesh mentioned that burnout includes a feeling of losing energy, powerlessness, incapability, despair, failure and disability [9]. It is a state of physical, emotional and mental exhaustion in repose to stressors in an organization. Emotional exhaustion refers to an individual's reduction of emotional ability when the person does not have enough energy to perform his/her tasks. In depersonalization, people feel indifferent towards their job, performance, and colleagues. In the lack of personal accomplishment, people's perception of their abilities decrease and in this case, they cannot fulfill their responsibilities like before [10]. Burnout has various stages. In the first stage, a person loses his/her feelings. In the second stage, he/she experiences the deterioration of character or depersonalization. In the final stage, he/she considers himself/herself useless and inefficient, despises his/her work and thinks that no one appreciates his/her efforts, considering himself/herself unsuccessful. These feelings may cause negative attitudes towards the person, his/her job and life. These attitudes may decrease his/her occupational performance, interaction with others, level of commitment, and job satisfaction and increase his/her absences and turnovers [11].

Considering what was mentioned earlier, it can be accepted that one of the most significant indicators of organizations' success, in addition to financial resources, is employing healthy, capable, and committed labor force. Particularly in a profession like teaching in which one provides some human services, this issue is of great importance. In addition to external rewards, teachers, due to intrinsic motivations, somehow become workaholics [12]. Moreover, due to the nature of their job, teachers are encountered with various stressors, such as insufficient salaries and students' lack of interest in education; however, the main problem occurs when teachers' capabilities are not sufficient for fulfilling their workplace demands [13], such that these stressors may eventually lead to job burnout. Therefore, the main issues of this research were to indicate how is the status of elementary school teachers in Zahedan, considering workaholism, stress and job burnout? And what is the relationship of workaholism with stress and job burnout of elementary school teachers in Zahedan?

2. Methods

The present study had two main aspects: objectives and methods of collecting data. This was an applicable study. Moreover, considering the main issue of the current study, *i.e.* examining the relationship of workaholism with teachers' stress and job burnout, this study was a descriptive-correlational study (using regression) with regard to the relationship between the variables. The statistical population included all elementary school teachers in Zahedan in the academic year 2014-2015 (N = 3756). Using cluster and stratified random sampling methods proportional to the size, based on the Cochran's formula, 350 elementary school teachers (80 males and 270 females) were selected. In this study, three questionnaires were used to collect data.

A. Spence and Robbins' Workaholism Inventory (1992): This inventory includes 20 questions and 3 components including work involvement (6 questions), feeling of being driven to work (7 questions), and work enjoyment (7 questions). This inventory is designed based on a 5-point Likert type scale and is scored from 1 (totally disagree) to 5 (totally agree). Closer scores to 100 indicate symptoms of workaholism and vice versa.

B. Dua's Occupational Stress Survey (1994): This survey contains 21 items which examine employees' job stress. This scale is designed based on a 5-point Likert type scale and is scored from 1 (completely agree) to 5 (completely disagree). Closer scores to 105 show symptoms of having more occupational stress and *vice versa.*

C. Job Burnout Inventory of Alexander-Stamatios *et al.* (2003): This Inventory includes 20 questions that investigate job burnout. This scale is designed based on a 5-point Likert type scale and is scored from 0 to 4 (0 = never, 1 = sometimes, 2 = half of the time, 3 = usually, and 4 = always). Closer scores to 80 show symptoms of having more job burnout and *vice versa.*

To examine the validity of these questionnaires, content validity was applied. In this regard, the validity of these questionnaires was confirmed by professors of psychology at University of Sistan and Baluchestan, ensuring that these questionnaires evaluate the attributes considered by the researcher and are valid. To determine their reliability, Cronbach's alpha coefficient was used, the results of which are presented as follows: work involvement (0.641), feeling of being driven to work (0.619), work enjoyment (0.644), workaholism (0.671), occupational stress (0.814), and job burnout (0.76). These coefficients indicated that these questionnaires have the required reliability. The obtained data was analyzed in both descriptive and inferential levels. In the descriptive level, frequency, percentage,

3. Results

In the current study, 350 elementary school teachers participated, among which 77.1% were females, 84.86% were married, 56.9% had a BA degree and 70.41% had more than 10 years of service. To realize the descriptive status of variables under study, mean and standard deviation were used, the results of which are presented in **Table 1**. This finding indicates that teachers' mean scores on all the variables under study are higher than the considered theoretical mean, *i.e.* 3, which is worrying.

To answer the first research question, *i.e.* what is the relationship between workaholism and teachers' occupational stress? Pearson correlation coefficient and simultaneous multiple regression analysis were used, the results of which are presented in **Table 2** and **Table 3**.

Based on the results demonstrated in **Table 2**, all correlation coefficients of workaholism and its three components with occupational stress are significant and positive ($p < 0.01$). Therefore, it is confirmed that workaholism and its components are significantly and positively related to teachers' occupational stress. It can be concluded that with an increase in teachers' workaholism, their occupational stress increases. To predict teachers' occupational stress based on the components of workaholism, simultaneous multiple regression analysis was used, the results of which are presented in **Table 3**.

Based on **Table 3**, the amount of F is significant at the level of 0.000. Therefore, the null hypothesis, *i.e.* the regression is not significant, is rejected at the 0.99 confidence level and it is confirmed that the linear regression model fits. According to the regression model, the coefficient of determination of R^2 is equal to 0.559, indicating that workaholism can explain 55.9% of the variance of occupational stress. Moreover, beta coefficient demonstrates that with one unit increase in work involvement, occupational stress increases 1.126, with one unit increase in feeling of being driven to work, occupational stress increases 0.503, and with a unit increase in work enjoyment, occupational stress increases 0.886.

To answer the second research question, *i.e.* what is the relationship between workaholism and teachers' job burnout? Pearson correlation coefficient and simultaneous regression analysis were applied, the results of which are presented in **Table 4** and **Table 5**.

Based on the results demonstrated in **Table 4**, all correlation coefficients of workaholism and its three components with job burnout are significant and positive ($p < 0.01$). Therefore, it is confirmed that workaholism and

Table 1. Descriptive status of the variables under study.

Variable	M (from 5)	SD
Work involvement	3.87	0.71
Feeling of being driven to work	4.01	0.62
Work enjoyment	4.03	0.6
Workaholism	3.97	0.64
Occupational stress	3.33	0.74
Job burnout	3.48	0.79

Table 2. Correlation coefficients of workaholism (and its components) with teachers' occupational stress.

Variable	Occupational stress	
	R	Sig
Work involvement	0.739	0.000
Feeling of being driven to work	0.743	0.000
Work enjoyment	0.73	0.000
Workaholism (the overall index)	0.74	0.000

Table 3. Results of regression analysis conducted to predict occupational stress based on components of workaholism.

	Non-standard coefficients		Standard coefficients	T	Sig
	B	Std. error	Beta		
Work involvement	1.17	0.505	1.126	2.322	0.021
Feeling of being driven to work	0.614	0.257	0.503	2.388	0.017
Work enjoyment	1.08	0.532	0.886	2.032	0.043

$R = 0.748$; $R^2 = 0.559$; F = 146.07; Sig = 0.000.

Table 4. Correlation coefficients of workaholism (and its components) with teachers' job burnout.

Variable	Job burnout	
	R	Sig
Work involvement	0.737	0.000
Feeling of being driven to work	0.739	0.000
Work enjoyment	0.728	0.000
Workaholism (the overall index)	0.738	0.000

Table 5. Results of regression analysis conducted to predict job burnout based on components of workaholism.

	Non-standard coefficients		Standard coefficients	T	Sig
	B	Std. error	Beta		
Work involvement	1.313	0.54	1.185	2.429	0.016
Feeling of being driven to work	0.566	0.275	0.436	2.057	0.040
Work enjoyment	1.144	0.57	0.88	2.008	0.045

$R = 0.744$; $R^2 = 0.554$; F = 142.92; Sig = 0.000.

its components are significantly and positively related to teachers' job burnout. It can be concluded that with an increase in teachers' workaholism, their job burnout increases. To predict teachers' job burnout based on the components of workaholism, simultaneous multiple regression analysis was used, the results of which are presented in **Table 5**.

Based on **Table 5**, the amount of F is significant at the level of 0.000. Therefore, the null hypothesis, *i.e.* the regression is not significant, is rejected at the 0.99 confidence level and it is confirmed that the linear regression model fits. According to the regression model, the coefficient of determination of R^2 is equal to 0.554, indicating that workaholism can explain 55.4% of the variance of job burnout. Moreover, beta coefficient demonstrates that with one unit increase in work involvement, job burnout increases 1.185, with one unit increase in feeling of being driven to work, job burnout increases 0.436, and with a unit increase in work enjoyment, job burnout increases 0.88.

4. Discussion and Conclusion

The present study aimed to examine the relationship of workaholism with stress and job burnout in elementary school teachers in Zahedan. The results of the current study indicated that workaholism and its components were significantly and positively related to teachers' occupational stress. The results of simultaneous multiple regressions demonstrated that workaholism could predict teachers' occupational stress. These findings were in line with the results of Shariat, Taboli, and Shokou Saljooghi (2012) [14], Schaufeli, Bekker, Vander Heijden, and Prins (2009) [15], Srivastava (2012) [16], Aziz and Cunningham (2008) [17], Morgan (2006) [18], Saiedi and Asadi (2012) [19], and Gholipur *et al.* (2008) [12]. To explain these findings, it could be noted that workaholism imposed a great pressure on a person, the consequence of which was occupational stress and as the result of occupational stress, the person's physical and mental energy gnawed. Due to threats caused for the resources including time, facilities, social opportunities and supports, the individual became exhausted. Other words, workaholism imposed a great burden on the individual and this burden increased tension, fatigue, and burnout and decreased job satisfaction. Teachers had numerous tasks and as a result of high workload and a wide variety of duties they had, they bear a high level of working pressure. On the other hand, lack of promotion opportunities for this group imposed them to occupational stress. Workaholic teachers spent most of their time and energy at work and devoted little time to their life and other matters. In fact, these people neglected their need to rest and ignored other issues related to their daily life which might lead to incidence of some negative emotions impacting one's behavior and progress. Additionally, with increasing school responsibilities and altering its environment to a more complex one, teachers were expected to perform their tasks in a whole different level and this expectation put an increasing pressure on teachers endangering their health and personal comfort. Therefore, it was likely that teachers, in addition to external rewards, due to internal motivations became workaholics. These people usually devoted most of their time to their educational and professional work. This was why they became workaholics and as a result they experienced higher levels of stress and involvement with their work [12].

Morgan (2006) considered workaholism as the main reason causing anxiety and mental pressures in organizations and indicated that workaholism could lead to high blood pressure, stress, anxiety and occupational stress [18]. Robbinson (2007) stated that workaholism increased mental and physical illnesses and endangered an individual's health [20]. Anderson concluded that a person who experienced lower levels of workaholism (due to lower occupational stress) had better mental and physical health and had a better opportunity to improve himself/herself [21]. Mudrak stated that although workaholics mighty enjoy their work, work enjoyment was not regarded as a core component of workaholism. People who worked under pressure might not do their job based on their interests and willingness; however, due to high levels of pressure, they experienced a sense of tension, coercion and compulsion to work [22]. Workaholics experienced a lot of stress and anxiety, and were encountered with various physical and mental problems, had low levels of life and job satisfaction, and had low job performance (Scott et al., 1997). In addition, Karask demonstrated that if employees were allowed to control their work and the variable of control on the job was considered, employees would experience less stress and felt more committed to their job and organization [23].

Other findings of the current study indicated that workaholism and it components were significantly and positively correlated with teachers' job burnout. The results of simultaneous multiple regression analysis indicated that workaholism could predict teachers' job burnout. These findings are consistent with the results of Schaufeli et al. (2009) [15], Aziz and Cunningham (2008) [17], ShabaniBahar, and Mahmudiyan (2012) [21], Burke and Kraut (2009) [24], Taris [25], and Robbinson (2007) [20]. To explain these results, it can be noted that workaholics resist on working to improve themselves and to become satisfied and they search for happiness and joy in their work. These people have strong intrinsic motivation to work, against which they cannot resist. This independent motivation may cause due to environmental conditions including financial situations, atmosphere of the organization, pressure caused by one's administrator, job promotion and/or escaping from the family. Since workaholics have destructive behaviors, their behaviors may cause various physical and psychological consequences and impact their relations. These people spend a little time to rest and over time, they become exhausted cognitively and emotionally. Since they always work, even when they are not at work, they experience sympathetic arousal and become emotionally disturbed and as a result, they mostly report various mental disorders and physical complaints. When a person suffers from burnout, he/she is permanently tired, aggressive, cynical, and angry. He/she has negative thoughts and is irritable and bored. He/she becomes angry with the slightest discomfort, and is frustrated and feels hopelessness. Teachers who are eager to spend a lot of time at work enter their work lives into their personal lives unintendedly and usually loss the balance between their work lives and personal lives. Due to this severe exhaustion which is caused to the nature of teaching, teachers are faced with burnout symptoms including reduced effectiveness, fatigue, and spending a lot of time at work. As a result, workaholic teachers become exhausted faster and this in turn may affect the quality of their service and may lead to dissatisfaction of school administrators, students, and parents.

Workaholism is a kind of addiction which can be pleasant and at the same time tedious and problematic such that some researchers considered this state as a disease. These people do not necessarily love their jobs; however, they cannot live without it. They think that they are the only people who can handle that job and that they do the job in a pretty particular way. Due to this extreme indulge in work, they become workaholics. Since workaholics experience high workload including high occupational demands, little by little, they loss their mental energy [15], especially when employees increasingly involve themselves in the process of doing things and weaken themselves in this way. Meanwhile, since workaholics are not willing to delegate their power and duties, they are in conflict with their colleagues and as a result, their work becomes much more complicated. When workaholics spend a lot of time on doing their work, their energy is weakened and they suffer from occupational burnout [26]. In a study, Gholipur *et al.* (2008) indicated that people who are involved in their work are more prone to mental and physical traumas compared to others, since they devote a lot of mental energy and time to their work [12]. This means that they neglect their personal affairs and spend most of their time at work. Therefore, the more the intensity of the work and the more the job's demands, the more the employees' burnout. The results of this study are consistent with these results and showed that since workaholics are more involved with their work, they feel that they are more driven to work; hence, they are more prone to occupational burnout.

Overall, results showed that with increasing teachers' workaholism, they experience more stress and occupational burnout. Compulsive-dependent workaholics experience a lot of anxiety and stress. Their work causes various physical and psychological problems. These people have low levels of satisfaction with their life and job and have low job performance. Perfectionist workaholics experience a high level of stress, mental and physical problems, establish hostile and ineffective interpersonal relations, have many voluntary absents and turnovers and have low job satisfaction and job performance. Therefore, not only they experience stress, but also they experience occupational burnout. When workaholics spend a lot of time on doing their work, their energy is weakened and they suffer from occupational burnout [26]. Therefore, not only these people harm themselves, but also they harm their organization. In this regard, attempting to find a solution to decrease this phenomenon and it consequences seems essential. Considering the results of the current study, holding training courses for teachers to become familiar with the phenomena of workaholism, stress, job burnout, individual and organizational outcomes, methods of dealing with them and managing time effectively (aiding at devoting time to work, family and oneself) is of great importance. It is recommended that other researchers conduct studies to investigate other educational levels and other organizations and also examine the relationship of workaholism with other occupational consequences based on demographic characteristics (gender, age, marital status, level of education, etc.). These studies can be conducted using a qualitative method or both qualitative and quantitative methods. Moreover, since the questionnaires used in this study were developed in other countries, developing such questionnaires in accordance with the condition of our country is highly recommended. Since this study was carried out on elementary school in Zahedan, hence, generalizing its results has its own limitations. Therefore, when generalizing these results to other teachers and employees, great caution should be taken.

References

[1]   Ahmadi, P., Tahmabi, R., Babashahi, J. and Fatahi, M. (2010) The Role of Personality Factors in Workholism Formation. *Transformation Management Journal*, **2**, 46-67.

[2]   Burke, R.J., Oberklaid, F. and Burgess, Z. (2006) Workaholism among Australian Women Psychologists: Antecedents and Consequences. *International Journal of Management*, **21**, 263-277.

[3]   Askari, A. and Nouri, A. (2011) Investigating the Relationship between Workaholic and Dimensions of General Health in the Employees of an Organization in Isfahan. *Iran Occupational Health*, **8**, 237-245.

[4]   Spence, J.T. and Robbins, A.S. (1992) Workaholism: Definition, Measurement, and Preliminary Results. *Journal of Personality Assessment*, **58**, 160-178. http://dx.doi.org/10.1207/s15327752jpa5801_15

[5]   Scott, K.S., Moore, K.S. and Miceli, M.P. (1997) An Exploration of the Meaning and Consequences of Workaholism. *Human Relations*, **50**, 287-314. http://dx.doi.org/10.1177/001872679705000304

[6]   Keramati, M.R. (2012) The Relation between Teachers' Perception of School Atmosphere and Their Occupational Stress. *Quarterly Journal of Business Management*, **8**, 103-140.

[7]   Allison, M.G. (2007) Identifying the Types of Student and Teacher Behaviors Associated with Teacher Stress. *Teaching and Teacher Education*, **23**, 624-640. http://dx.doi.org/10.1016/j.tate.2007.02.006

[8]   Pourghane, P., Sharifazar, E., Zaersabet, F. and Khorsandi, M. (2010) Survey the Effect of Religious Beliefs in Stress Reduction in Students of Langroud Faculty of Medical Sciences. *Journal Holistic Nursing and Midwifery*, **20**, 10-15.

[9]   Amiri, M., Asadi, M.R. and Delbari Ragheb, F. (2011) Identification and Ranking Effective Factors on the Internet Shopping use of Fuzzy ANP. *Quarterly Journal of Business Management*, **3**, 37-56.

[10] Rostami, A., Noruzi, A., Zarei, A., Amiri, M. and Soleimani, M. (2008) Exploring the Relationships between the Bur-

nout and Psychological Wellbeing, among Teachers While Controlling for Resiliency and Gender. *Iran Occupational Health*, **5**, 68-75.

[11] Amiri, H., Mirhashemi, M. and Parsamoein, K. (2011) Relationship between Perceived Job Characteristics, Job Roles and Burnout. *Journal of Modern Industrial/Organization Psychology*, **2**, 53-69. (In Persian)

[12] Gholipur, A., Nargeseyan, A. and Tahmasbi, R. (2008) Workaholism: The New Challenge of Human Resource Management. *Danesh e Modiriyat*, **21**, 91-110. (In Persian)

[13] Talaei, A., Mokhber, N., Mohammad Nejad, M. and Samari, A.A. (2008) Burnout and Its Related Factors in Staffs of University Hospitals in Mashhad. *Koomesh*, **9**, 237-245. (In Persian)

[14] Shariat, H., Taboli, H. and Shokuh Saljooghi, Z. (2012) The Relation between Workaholism & Occupational Stress: A Case Study about Welfare Organization Personnel of Kerman, Iran. *Interdisciplinary Journal of Contemporary Research in Business*, **4**, 151-168.

[15] Schaufeli, W.B., Bakker, A.B., Vander Heijden, F.M. and Prins, J.T. (2009) Workaholism, Burnout and Well-Being among Junior Doctors: The Mediating Role of Role Conflict. *Work and Stress*, **23**, 155-172. http://dx.doi.org/10.1080/02678370902834021

[16] Srivastava, M. (2012) Stress, Workaholism and Job Demands: A Study of Executives in Mumbai. *NMIMS Management Review*, **XXII**, 94-116.

[17] Aziz, S. and Cunningham, J. (2008) Workaholism, Work Stress, Work-Life Imbalance: Exploring Gender's Role. *Gender in Management: An International Journal*, **23**, 553-566. http://dx.doi.org/10.1108/17542410810912681

[18] Morgan, G. (2006) Images of Organization. Sage Publications, London.

[19] Saiedi, L. and Asadi, A. (2012) Workaholism, Work Stress. *Journal of Management*, **23**, 32-37. (In Persian)

[20] Robbinson, B.E. (2007) Chained to the Desk: A Guidebook for Workaholics, Their Partners and Children, and the Clinicians Who Treat Them. New York University Press, New York.

[21] ShabaniBahar, G. and Mahmudiyan, Z. (2012) The Relationship between Workaholism and Job Burnout of Sport Teachers in Kermanshah. *Journal of Sport Management and Motor Behavior*, **8**, 129-147. (In Persian)

[22] Hasani, M. and Shohudi, M. (2013) The Relationship between the Components of the Circuit's Security Leadership and Mental Security with Dimensions of Workaholism: Urmia University Personnel. *Journal of Executive Management*, **5**, 85-106. (In Persian)

[23] Khaef Elahi, A.A., Nargesian, A. and Babashahi, J. (2012) Investigating the Relationship between Workaholism and Organizational Citizenship Behavior (Case of: Nurses in Tehran City). *Transformation Management Journal*, **4**, 21-37. (In Persian)

[24] Burke, M. and Kraut, R. (2008) Mopping up: Modeling Wikipedia Promotion Processes. *Proceedings of the 2008 ACM Conference on Computer Supported Cooperative Work*, San Diego, 8-12 November 2008, 27-36. http://dx.doi.org/10.1145/1460563.1460571

[25] Taris, T.W., Schaufeli, W.B. and Verhoeven, L.C. (2005) Workaholism in the Netherlands: Measurement and Implications for Job Strain and Work-Nonwork Conflict. *Applied Psychology: An International Review*, **54**, 37-60. http://dx.doi.org/10.1111/j.1464-0597.2005.00195.x

[26] Sonnentag, S. and Zijlstra, F.R. (2006) Job Characteristics and Off-Job Activities as Predictors of Need for Recovery, Well-Being, and Fatigue. *Journal of Applied Psychology*, **91**, 330-350. http://dx.doi.org/10.1037/0021-9010.91.2.330

Health-Related Physical Fitness in Female Models

Salime Donida Chedid Lisboa[1], Rodrigo Sudatti Delevatti[1,2], Ana Carolina Kanitz[1,3], Thais Reichert[1], Cláudia Gomes Bracht[1], Alexandra Ferreira Vieira[1], Luiz Fernando Martins Kruel[1]

[1]Universidade Federal do Rio Grande do Sul, Porto Alegre, Brazil
[2]Faculdade Sogipa de Educação Física, Porto Alegre, Brazil
[3]Universidade Federal de Uberlândia, Uberlândia, Brazil
Email: sa.lisboa@hotmail.com

Abstract

The model profession uses the appearance for the representation of products and brands via events. For some individuals that are included in this medium, plus a laboral activity, modeling becomes a lifestyle, the search for the status and work opportunities turn a dream for a thousands of children and teenagers because the profession has particulars experiences. To win this, many girls change physical and eating behaviors which are harmful to health. The objective of this study was to analyze the health-related physical fitness in female models comparing them with non-models. The study was conducted at the Caxias do Sul, Rio Grande do Sul, Brazil. Participated of the study female runway and commercial models bokered in Cast One Models, with age between 15 - 25 years old. The non-models were students from public and private schools or university students. The health-related physical fitness, the physical activity levels and dietary intake were assessed of all participants. The data were described as mean and standard deviation. For comparison between models and non-models was used t independent test for variables normally distributed and U Mann-Whitney test for not normally distributed variables, adopting a level of significance (α) of 0.05. It was found difference in total energy between model group and non-model (GM: 1509.78 kcal, NM: 2292.51 Kcal; p = 0.014). There were no differences between groups in the others variables analyzed (p > 0.05). In conclusion, the profession model seems not interfere in variables that make up the health-related physical fitness.

Keywords

Models, Health, Exercise

1. Introduction

Adolescence is comprised between the age group from 10 and 19 years old [1], phase of life which is characterized by several changes in social, cultural and economic fields [2]. In this way, a proper nutrients ingestion and regular performance of physical activities become crucial, in order to obtain appropriate health levels. In this period, physical size and body shape become issues of concern for adolescents, because leanness has a big tendency for acceptance before society. Besides that, there are some professions with particular physical requirements, like athletes, ballet dancers and models, which are daily charged about the maintenance and/or weight reduction, which may become risk professions [3] [4].

The professional model term, in theory and practice, is a beauty model, a person who uses his/her appearance to represent products and brands, through publicity and events, what can many times become a lifestyle and/or professional career [5]. To be able to reach the status of being a model as a work career is a dream of thousands of children and adolescents, being these age groups in which the intensification of this dream increases, because this profession provides a glamour life to the ones who are successful and private experiences in each work done [6].

The required body measurements for models depend on the classification in which they are included. The classic categories are: photographic (commercial) and runaway model (fashion). Commercial models are characterized by performing mostly advertising works, like magazines, outdoors and television commercials. The attributions for this group, for both sexes, are to be photogenic along with well cared hair and skin. In relation to the body, measurements must be proportional, meeting the requirements of the contractor, depending on the required appeal for sealing of a particular product [7]. In regards to runaway models, they perform fashion parades and present season collections made by stylists, besides performing commercial works, like the photographic ones. The prerequisites to this kind of work are more rigorous, because the girls must begin with ages between 13 and 18, minimum height of 1.74 m, hip measure 90 cm and waist about 60 cm. Body weight must be reduced, approximately 20 kg less than the considered optimal for the age group. The other measures (bust and foot) vary according to body shape [8].

Discussions about models daily life conditions become increasingly delicate and explored by study fields like nutrition, psychology and physical education, since that besides being a profession with big turnovers due to contracts; it generates long working days, what can cause reductions in quality of life. Many sacrifices are adopted to reach the goals, because the girls start to give less importance to studies and the vast majority adopts eating and physical behaviors which are harmful to health. To the favoring of the leanness, adolescents from all over the world follow their own concepts of care, making them more susceptible to diseases and impairing their health in all the fields included in it [9].

The aforementioned state of health is not only characterized by a state of absence of diseases but as a general state of balance in different aspects as psychological, biological, emotional, social, mental and intellectual, thus enabling a well-being sensation that will be along with improvements in physical fitness of the individual and his/her relation to health, because physical activities practice is determined by physical fitness and health levels [10]. Guedes [11] defines physical fitness as a "the dynamic state of energy and vitality that permits to each person not only the performance of daily tasks, the active occupations of leisure time and to deal with unexpected emergencies without excessive fatigue, but also to avoid the appearance of hypokinetic functions, while operating at the peak of the intellectual capacity and feeling the enjoyment of living". To obtain this, it is necessary to maintain the continuous practice of physical exercises and the search for the maintenance of physical fitness levels and its components when related to health (cardiorespiratory capacity, muscle strength/resistance and flexibility) [12].

Physical inactivity for lack of time and lack of stimulus along with bad eating habits, for care with appearance, are crucial points for the accomplishment of this work, because isolated evaluation of body composition, nutritional state and quality of life of adolescent models have already been found in the literature. However, we could not find studies that relate these variables in a same study, in adolescent and young adult models, because even with the advancement of exercise sciences, the importance of health-related physical fitness and the relation between exercise practice to quality of life in models are still little explored outcomes.

Therefore, the objective of the present study was to evaluate the health-related physical fitness, the physical activity levels and dietary intake in female models in comparison with non-models.

2. Methods

2.1. Subjects

The sample of the study was composed by runaway and/or commercial female models between the ages of 15 and 25 from Cast One Models agency from the city of Caxias do Sul, Rio Grande do Sul, Brazil and also by adolescent and young adult students from public/private schools and universities from Caxias do Sul, Rio Grande do Sul, Brazil. The sample of the study was selected by convenience, being made contact with 16 models from Cast One Models agency, in which 10 accepted to participate in the study. After the selection of the models, a total of 8 non model girls were invited to participate in the study, of which 8 accepted it and were part of the study. These girls were also selected by convenience, in compliance with the same age groups and home city of the models, only avoiding the inclusion of obese girls, by believing that this would generate a huge comparative bias, once obesity is associated with physical activity level and physical fitness.

2.2. Procedures

The test protocols were performed at Estação Saúde gym in Caxias do Sul, Rio Grande do Sul, Brazil. 3 days were used for data collection, being the first day designated to the signature of a free and informed consent form, completing of an anamnetic record, body composition evaluation, filling of questionnaires about physical activity level, delivery and explanation of dietary records and familiarization with physical fitness tests (mensuration of peak oxygen consumption (VO_{2peak})), flexibility, maximum dynamic muscle strength (1RM) of knee extensors and elbow flexors, resistant strength (muscular endurance) of knee extensors and elbow flexors). On the second day, a second familiarization with 1 RM and muscular endurance tests was made and the cardiorrespiratory and flexibility tests were performed. On the third day, the 1RM and muscular endurance tests were performed, finalizing the experimental procedures. The reading and the signature of the consent form were made individually (for girls over the age of 18 years) and with the company of those responsible for them (for girls under the age of 18). An assent form was also filled to secure agreement between the study and the locals of the subjects' recruitment. In all the procedures, there were between two and three physical education professionals performing the aforementioned procedures.

Individuals attended to evaluation location according to the schedule, with two-piece suits. Firstly, height (HEI) and body weight (BW) measurements were made. With these values, their body mass index (BMI) was calculated, using the formula body weight (Kg)/height^2 (m). After this, the measurements of the seven skinfolds were made: triceps, subscapularis, supra-iliac, abdominal, leg, middle axillary line and thigh. Based on the obtained values, body density was estimated utilizing the equation of the seven skinfolds proposed by Jackson *et al.* [13] for women.

For the evaluation of cardiorrespiratory fitness, a treadmill of Olympikus brand was utilized, with resolution of speed and inclination of 0.1 Km·h^{-1} e 1%, respectively, portable gas analyzer of mixing box type VO2000, INBRAMED brand, pneumotachograph, ranging from 2 to 225 L·min^{-1} for low, medium and high flows, neoprene mask and a heart rate monitor FT1 model, POLAR brand. Study subjects performed a familiarization session with the treadmill, the neoprene mask and the heart rate monitor that would be further used in the test. The maximum test on the treadmill was performed for the determination of the peak oxygen consumption (VO_{2peak}) of the samples. For the accomplishment, individuals were instructed to stand with feet apart on the treadmill, where the neoprene mask would be put. To start the test, the respiratory exchange ratio (RER) should be under 0.85. We utilized a protocol that consisted of an initial speed of 4 km/h during two minutes, with increments of 1 km/h at each two minutes, with fixed inclination (1%). This protocol test was created for the conducting of the present study, aiming that the models reached the maximum effort without big increments in the inclination of the treadmill. Heart rate was recorded at each 10 seconds and the exertion perception was also registered at the end of each stage of the test. The test was conducted until voluntary exhaustion (signalized by manual gests). The evaluation was considered valid when one of the following criteria was reached at the end of the test [14]: 1) obtaining of the estimated HR_{max} (220-age); 2) occurrence of a plateau in the VO_2 with the increased velocity of the treadmill; 3) obtaining of a RER higher than 1.1; 4) perceived exertion higher than 17 (very intense—Borg's Scale of RPE).

The measurement of the maximal dynamic strength was obtained after a familiarization period of two sessions, with 1 RM tests for knee extension and elbow flexion. In these tests, individuals executed one repetition in each proposed exercise supporting the maximal possible load. The execution rhythm was controlled by a metronome (QUARTZ brand), being 1.5 seconds for the concentric phase and 1.5 seconds for the eccentric phase. Previously to the test, the girls performed a warm-up period (5 minutes) in cycle ergometer during five minutes, and after this an initial load was selected, in which the participants wouldn't be able to perform more than 10 maximum repetitions. After this series, the load was being adjusted with the corresponding of the 1RM through the values proposed by Lombardi [15] until the girls reached the maximal load. Up to 5 attempts were made, with an interval of 5 minutes between each one.

For the conduction of the dynamic muscular resistance test a load corresponding to 60% of 1 RM of the knee extension and elbow flexor was utilized. For these tests, the individual should perform the maximal number of repetitions possible. The execution rhythm was controlled by a metronome, being 1.5 seconds designated for the concentric phase and 1.5 seconds for the eccentric phase.

The determination of the flexibility was made through a test utilizing the Wells Bench, which is in box format with the dimensions $30.5 \times 30.5 \times 30.5$ cm, containing in its upper flat a wooden board. The fixed scale is graded 1 by 1 cm. The test was intended to measure the degree of flexibility of the hip, back and posterior muscles of the lower members. The evaluated individual was barefoot and assumed a sitting position, facing the equipment with the soles of the feet flat on the Wells Bench, with the knees fully extended. The arms were extended on the box surface with the hands overlapped one on another. The individual extended her body forward along the fixed scale, trying to reach the greatest possible distance. Three attempts were made and that for each one of them, the distance reached in the scale was maintained for at least 1 second long. The greatest value reached after all the attempts was considered [16].

The International Physical Activity Questionnaire (IPAQ) short version was utilized as indicator of the physical activity level of the study subjects, which investigates the physical activity level of the responders on the last seven days. This questionnaire consists of questions regarding the frequency of rigorous or moderate physical activity and walking activities performed in the last week by the responder. The present questionnaire can be classified categorically and/or in a continuous way, being estimated the metabolic units (METS) spent weekly (Met.min) in walking, moderate and vigorous physical activity, and the sum of these three conditions [17].

The feeding control was performed through the application of a feeding record of three days. The recording procedure was made through the following manner: each model registered three days of the week, non-consecutive, being two business days (typical days) and one weekend day (atypical day). The feeding records were filled during the collection period. The meals were described with the schedules, the quantities in household measures, and, when possible, the brand of the feeding products. After the filling of the records made by the girls, all of the notes were checked by a trained researcher, so that no doubt would happen in regarding to the described records. The feeding records were thereafter calculated with the aid of the Nutrition Software DietWin Professional (Brubins, CAS, Brazil) in order to quantify the content of the consumed food by the models and non models.

2.3. Statistical Analysis

As descriptive statistics the mean and standard deviation values were used for normally distributed continuous variables and the median and interquartile range values were used for continuous variables that were not normally distributed. Categorical variables were presented by the sample n. The normality and homogeneity of the data were evaluated by the Shapiro-Wilk and Levene tests, respectively. For the comparison between the variables of the models and the non models it was used the independent t-test for normally distributed variables and the Mann-Whitney U test for variables that were not normally distributed. When comparing categorical variables, we used Fisher's exact test. It was adopted a 5% significance level. All analyzes were performed using SPSS program, version 20.0.

3. Results

3.1. Flow of Participants

24 girls were contacted, 16 of them were models and eight were non models. A total of six subjects left the study (six of MG, three because of contact impossibility, one because of family problems, one refused to participate and one because of address change). The adherence of the tests for the MG was impaired during the collection

sessions due to the big turnover and long working days that are required by the profession, which caused absence of some models in some of the proposed protocols. In this way, the final population of the study consisted of 18 subjects performing the tests protocols (MG; n = 10) and (NM; n = 8). In **Figure 1**, the flowchart of the individuals over the study can be visualized.

3.2. Participants

All the girls who proposed to participate in the study were born and created in the same region, frequenting similar places. In MG, all the models were contracted by the same agency, with patterned solicitations and charges for all of them. It is noteworthy to mention the great importance that the MG components gave to the collection of the data (a large number of the models performed the collection procedures in order to obtain more information about their own body and thus try to reach the measures imposed by the agency in a healthy manner). In the same way, the non models participated in the study in order to obtain information that would favor their daily performance.

3.3. Sample Characterization

The characterization of the final sample (analyzed subjects) is presented on **Table 1**.

3.4. Health-Related Physical Fitness

All of the components of health-related physical fitness did not show any difference between the groups (p > 0.05). These analyses are demonstrated on **Table 2**.

3.5. Physical Activity Level

The results found for scores of physical activity levels are presented on **Table 3**. The variables also did not show any difference between the groups (p > 0.05).

3.6. Dietary Intake

The results related to food consumption are presented on **Table 4**. A significant difference was found only for the total energetic value.

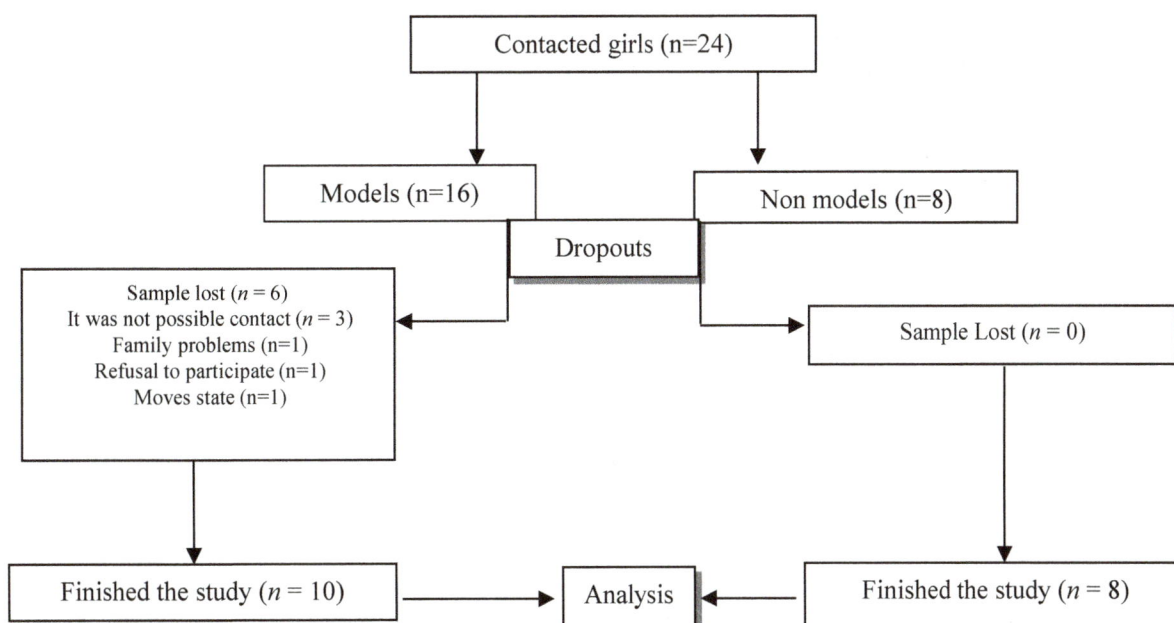

Figure 1. The flow of the participants.

Table 1. Sample characterization.

	MG ($n = 10$)	NM ($n = 8$)
Age (years)	20.5 (16.2 - 21.7)	21.5 (20.2 - 23.0)
Career Duration (months)	49.8 ± 30.7	——
Nutritional monitoring	2	2
Psychic monitoring	3	4
Education		
Fundamental Incomplete	0	0
Fundamental Complete	0	0
Medium Incomplete	3	0
Medium Complete	2	1
Superior Incomplete	5	6
Superior Complete	0	1

Age data are presented as median and interquartile range; Career duration is presented as mean ± SD; The others variables are presented by n of each group.

Table 2. Variables related to physical fitness and health in models (MG) and non models (NM).

	MG ($n = 10$)	NM ($n = 8$)	p value
VO$_{2pico}$	33.20 (32.90 - 34.10)	31.60 (26.95 - 32.60)	$p = 0.073$
1RM knee extension (Kg)	70.00 (65.00 - 72.50)	65.00 (55.00 - 72.50)	$p = 0.383$
1RM bending elbows (Kg)	16.00 (16.00 - 19.00)	18.00 (16.00 - 18.00)	$p = 0.902$
Resistant strength of knee extension (rep)	9.00 (8.00 - 11.00)	12.00 (10.00 - 12.50)	$p = 0.128$
Resistant strength of bending elbows (rep)	10.00 (8.50 - 13.50)	10.00 (8.50 - 12.00)	$p = 0.902$
Flexibility (cm)	26.90 ± 8.95	26.25 ± 4.77	$p = 0.856$
Weight (kg)	54.87 ± 3.50	53.38 ± 5.02	$p = 0.484$
Height (m)	1.74 (1.73 - 1.76)	1.65 (1.63 - 1.70)	$p = 0.002$
BMI (kg/m^2)	18.33 ± 1.44	19.19 ± 1.57	$p = 0.239$
Waist circumference (cm)	67.50 (66.00 - 68.70)	67.25 (65.12 - 70.62)	$p = 0.758$
Waist/height ratio	0.38 (0.38 - 0.40)	0.40 (0.39 - 0.42)	$p = 0.252$
Fat percentage	16.37 ± 3.04	19.71 ± 3.61	$p = 0.066$
Percentage of lean mass	83.63 ± 3.04	80.29 ± 3.61	$p = 0.066$
Fat mass (kg)	9.03 ± 2.01	10.5 ± 2.70	$p = 0.234$
Lean mass (kg)	45.83 ± 2.49	42.35 ± 3.27	$p = 0.030$
Σ7DC	86.40 (78.15 - 94.40)	98.50 (87.42 - 114.60)	$p = 0.114$

1RM: one repetition maximum; rep: repetitions. VO$_{2peak}$ data, 1RM knee extension, elbow flexion 1RM, resistant strength of knee extension, resistant strength of bending elbows, height, waist circumference and Σ7DC are presented as median and interquartile range (Mann-Whitney); The other variables are presented as mean ± SD (independent t test). α: 0.05.

Table 3. The level of physical activity rating by IPAQ questionnaire for Group models (MG) and non models (NM).

	MG ($n = 10$)	NM ($n = 8$)	p value
Mets.min.walking	297.00 (148.50 - 569.25)	264.00 (185.63 - 305.25)	$p = 0.965$
Metsmin.PAmoderate	360.00 (0.00 - 1080.00)	300.00 (225.00 - 560.00)	$p = 0.573$
Mets.min.PAvigorous	360.00 (0.00 - 1260.00)	480.00 (450.00 - 480.00)	$p = 0.897$
Mets.min.PAsum	1306.50 (572.25 - 2219.25)	1079.25 (957.00 - 1349.38)	$p = 0.897$

PA: physical activity; Mets: metabolic unities. Data are presented as medians and interquartile ranges (Mann-Whitney). α: 0.05.

Table 4. Variable feed control through food records of three days to the model group (MG) and the group non models (NM) in percentage (%) daily and grams (g) daily.

	MG (*n* = 10)	NM (*n* = 8)	p value
Mean energetic value (kcal)	1509.78 ± 531.83	2292.51 ± 552.12	p = 0.014
Carbohydrates (g)	202.20 ± 80.61	295.02 ± 85.17	p = 0.046
Protein (g)	63.17 ± 20.98	91.78 ± 26.81	p = 0.032
Lipids (g)	47.00 ± 18.41	79.00 ± 20.34	p = 0.006
Carbohydrates (%)	64.15 ± 6.30	62.97 ± 6.59	p = 0.727
Protein (%)	20.72 ± 4.96	19.86 ± 3.76	p = 0.721
Lipids (%)	15.12 ± 3.10	17.16 ± 3.97	p = 0.270

Data are presented as mean ± DE. α: 0.05. (Independent t test).

4. Discussion

The main findings of the present study were that besides the supposed similarity found between models and non models, the girls who act like models showed some anthropometric differences (height and lean mass) and also a lower total energetic consumption. Rodrigues *et al.* [18] compared a group of models (n = 33) with non models (n = 33), aged between 15 and 18, pairing them by age and BMI, analyzing body composition variables utilizing the plethysmography technique, resting metabolic rate (RMT) through indirect calorimetry and food consumption through three alternating days, and observed that many adolescents were showing their BMI under the recommended values for their age group, which corroborates the data found in our study, in which although any difference was found between the groups, in the MG the value was classified as low weight (18.3), while in NM the values correspond to the appropriate weight (19.2), according with the patterns of the Ministério da Saúde [19]. In this way, these body particularities of the MG also reflect on the fat percentages, because although only a statistical tendency exists (p = 0.06), the mean values of MG are 4% lower than those found in MG, showing tendency of the models to pursuit normative fat percentages values, to the point of being similar to the mean levels of fat (%) of the non models.

Discussions regarding body dimensions are being increasingly made. By analyzing the models population, this discussion is related to the body that would be the one which contemplates the ideals of a body considered pattern. This is clearly exposed by Norton [20] who shows in this study the influence that a famous toy can cause in the construction of the body ideal of children and adolescents. By pointing some body measures of the Barbie doll, the researcher compared it to academic women (18 to 35 years old), to photographic and runaway models (seen as carriers of the ideal body) and also to anorexic girls. The results show that runaway models are leaner than academic women, and the anorexic girls, as was expected by disease questions, are leaner than all the other evaluated ones, and when the values of the doll are observed, a big difference is presented of body measures in comparison to the other groups of the study. The doll, which became an unconsciously imposed example for children, is criticized for being too lean, even when compared to the reference samples of the study, with similar measures found in less than 1 at each 100,000 adult women. The measures which showed more extreme values were neck circumference, wrist, waist, hip and waist hip ratio. This big restriction of body measures that used to be carried over from the doll to fashion runaways, and this way of thinking seem to be modified after the decade of 90, and mainly, in the actual years due to rigid laws and rules that are being imposed to the models and their contractors, like the law against excessive leanness created by the National Assembly of France or agreements like the one made by the founder of the São Paulo Fashion Week, which vetoes the participation of people under 16 in the event. We believe in the efficacy of the laws and agreements through the results found in our variables, because there were no many differences found between models and non models, which can be indicating a new phase in the fashion world, in which the health is not necessarily detached from the model profession.

By analyzing the results obtained in the cardiorespiratory variables, there were no significant differences found in regards to the peak oxygen consumption (VO_{2peak}) just as in the muscle strength and resistance and in flexibility. Possibly, no differences were found because of the similar number of exercise practitioners between the groups (MG: 6; NM: 5), which demonstrates that far beyond the chosen profession, the fact of carrying out a determined exercise modality seems to be fundamental for the fitness levels found, either cardiorrespiratory or neuromuscular ones. It demonstrates that much more than the profession, the adoption of a structured and supervises physical training can have a stronger implication in physical fitness than the labor activities of the individuals. Particularly in women, this is of fundamental importance, helping in the prevention of highly prevalent diseases in the female sex, as osteoporosis, that must be thought about since adolescence, a phase in which occurs the deposition of a big part (around 90%) of the mineral bone content found in adult age [21].

In relation to physical activity levels, no significant differences were found between MG and NM, being both groups in scores corresponding to the sufficiently active classification (between 600 and 1499 mets.min.week), demonstrating that despite different labor occupations, the women of the present study had good physical activity levels, which is fundamental for health, because high levels of this outcome can reduce the incidence of many diseases, as well as mortality rates [22]. Our findings were satisfactory when compared to the findings of Hallal *et al.* [23] who studied the determinants of physical activities in the regional adolescence between the ages of 10 and 12, and obtained 58.2% of sedentary lifestyle scores, besides of, in the comparison between boys vs. girls, obtained scores of 40% and 67% respectively, pointing a likely higher prevalence of sedentary lifestyle for the female sex.

Moreover, the study of [18], aimed to evaluate the energetic expenditure of Brazilian models (33 models and non models aged between 15 and 18 years), found reports of up to 63.6% of the models and 60.6% of the non models performing regular physical activities, verifying that the models used to accomplish more activities when compared to control group (non models) (5.0 hours/week (IC 95% = 3.9 - 4.9 hours/week) *versus.* 2.0 hours/week (IC 95% = 2.0 - 3.8 hours/week; p < 0.01). Even that this is a different unit for evaluation, our results corroborate to the aforementioned, because even without significant statistical differences, the values found in the models are shown to be more expressive tan the ones found for the non models (1306.50; 572.25; 2219.25 mets.min *versus.* 1079.25; 957.00; 1349.38 mets.min; p = 0.897).

Regarding to food consumption, the mean energetic value (kcal) ingested by the models is found next to 782.73 less daily kcal when compared to the non models, this lower caloric ingestion can be explained by the need and exigency of maintenance and many times of the loss of body mass daily requested by the models agency. The lower energetic consumption value of MG (MG: 1509.78 ± 531.83; NM: 2292.51 ± 552.12) can even explain the big tendency of difference (p = 0.066) between the groups in the %F. It demonstrates that the food rigidity imposed in the model profession ends to be really adopted and has an impact not only in area measurements, as in perimeters and BMI, but also in the accumulation of body fat. The difference between models and non models in the food consumption corroborates to the findings of Rodrigues *et al.* [24], that found significant differences in the caloric ingestion of models and non models (1480.93 kcal/day ± 582.95 *versus* 1973.00 kcal/day ± 557.63 respectively, (p = 0.001), showing that this difference does not seem to be an isolated fact, but a real difference of the profession in question when compared to general population.

Analyzing the daily percentages indicated by the recommendations of nutrition for adolescents [25], both MG and NM are ingesting above the recommended quantities of carbohydrates suggested for adolescents, that is between 55% to 60% (MG: 64.15% ± 6.30%; NM: 62.97% ± 6.59%). The same case happens for proteins, which has as suggested intake of 12% to 15% (MG: 20.72% ± 4.96%; NM: 19.86% ± 3.76%) and for lipids, with recommendations of 30% (MG: 15.12% ± 3.10%; NM: 17.16% ± 3.97%).

It must be also noted that many girls who act as models are young and unprepared in questions of life, which causes the incorrect ingestion of foods (instant foods), being this action performed in order to gain time, contributing to a feeding considered not to be healthy, a worrying fact due to the evaluated age group and still, questions of altered ingestions, such as less fat than the recommended quantity, can implicate in injuries to women health in the future, because female hormones like estrogen and progesterone are synthesized based on fat [26].

As limitations of the present study, we highlight the reduced sample size, which is only representative of a profile of models and non models. Due to that, one should exercise caution in the interpretation of the results, being necessary to enlarge the observation of the health-related physical fitness, of the physical activity levels and of the nutritional profile in models of different levels, regions and ages.

5. Conclusions

Based on the results found in our study, we observed that the model profession can result in some anthropometric differences like greater height and lean mass, in addition to a lower energetic consumption. The comparison between models and non models showed a big similarity between the groups in aspects related to health-related physical fitness and physical activity levels. The findings of the study point that the model profession does not interfere in questions of health and its relation to physical fitness.

However, even reaching satisfactory results, we believe that this population has the need to be closely accompanied in all the ambits of life, due to the age group (adolescence and beginning of adult life) be a period of formation and consolidation of many questions of life and also because of the physical and psychological particularities that these adolescents are daily affected by, in order to avoid future problems in the health of these girls.

References

[1] The WHOQOL Group (1995) The World Health Organization Quality of Life Assessment (WHOQOL): Position Paper from the World Health Organization. *Social Science & Medicine*, **41**, 1403-1410. http://dx.doi.org/10.1016/0277-9536(95)00112-K

[2] Pires, L., Rodrigues, A.M., Fisberg, M., Costa, R.F. and Schoen, T.H. (2012) Quality of Life of Adolescent Professional Models. *Psicologia: Teoria e Pesquisa*, **28**, 71-76. http://dx.doi.org/10.1590/S0102-37722012000100009

[3] Braggion, G.L., Matsudo, S.M.M. and Matsudo, V.K.R. (2000) Food Consumption, Physical Activity and Perception of the Body Appearance in Adolescents. *Rev. Bras. Ciê. e Mov. Brasília*, **8**, 15-21.

[4] Rodrigues, A.M., Costa, R.F. and Fisberg, M. (2008) Anthropometric Characteristics of Candidates of a Selective Competition of a Big Agency from São Paulo. Centro de Estudos e Pesquisa Sanny.

[5] Pascolato, C. and Lacombe, M. (2003) How to Become a Successful Model—What It Is and How You See.

[6] Rodrigues, A.M., Cavalieri, M.C., Branco, L.M., Passos, M.A.Z., Cintra, I.P. and Fisberg, M. (2004) Anthropometric and Body Composition Profile of Adolecent Models. *J. Brazilian Soc. Food Nutr.*, **27**, 31-41.

[7] Libardi, M. (2004) Model Profession: In Search of Fame. SENAC SP, São Paulo.

[8] Castro, A.L. (2004) Body Worship: Identity of Life.

[9] Saikali, C.J., Soubhia, C.S., Scalfaro, B.M. and Cordás, T.A. (2004) Body Image in Eating Disorders. *Revista de Psiquiatria Clinica*, **31**, 164-166. http://dx.doi.org/10.1590/S0101-60832004000400006

[10] Araújo, D.S.M.S. and Araújo, C.G.S. (2000) Physical Fitness, Health and Quality of Life Related to Health in Adults. *Revista Brasileira de Medicina do Esporte*, **6**. Bouchard, C., Shephard, R.J., Stephens, T., Sutton, J.R. and Mcpherson, B.D. (1990) Exercise, Fitness, and Health: The Consensus Statement. In: Bouchard, C., Shephard, R.J., Stephens, T., Sutton, J.R., McPherson, B.D., Eds., *Exercise, Fitness, and Health: A Consensus of Current Knowledge*, Champaign, Human Kinetics, 3-28.

[11] Guedes, D.P. (1996) Physical Activity, Physical Fitness and Health. In: Carvalho, T., Guedes, D.P. and Silva, J.G., Orgs., *Orientações Básicas sobre Atividade Física e Saúde para Profissionais das Áreas de Educação e Saúde*, Ministério da Saúde e Ministério da Educação e do Desporto, Brasília.

[12] Malina, R. (2007) Pediatric Fitness, Secular Trends and Geographic Variability. Tomkinson, G.R., Olds, T.S., Eds., Tarleton State University, Stephenville.

[13] Jackson, A.S., Pollock, M.L. and Ward, A. (1980) Generalized Equations for Predicting Body Density of Women. *Medicine & Science in Sports & Exercise*, **12**, 175-182. http://dx.doi.org/10.1249/00005768-198023000-00009

[14] Howley, E.T., Basset Jr., D.R. and Welch, H.G. (1995) Criteria for Maximal Oxygen Uptake: Review and Commentary. *Medicine & Science in Sports & Exercise*, **27**, 1292-1301. http://dx.doi.org/10.1249/00005768-199509000-00009

[15] Lombardi, V.P. (1989) Beginning Weight Training: The Safe and Effective Way. Brown & Benchmark Pub, Dubuque.

[16] Charro, M.A., Bacurau, R.F.P., Navarro, F. and Pontes Jr., F.L. (2010) Physical Evaluation Manual. Phorte, São Paulo.

[17] Matsudo, S., Araújo, T., Matsudo, V., Andrade, D., Andrade, E., Oliveira, L. and Braggion, G. (2001) International Questionnaire of Physical Activity (IQPA): Study of Validity and Reproducibility in Brazil. *Revista Atividade Física & Saúde*, **6**, 5-18.

[18] Rodrigues, A.M., Cintra, I.P., Santos, L.C., Mello, M.T., Tufik, S. and Fisberg, M. (2009) Body Composition, Energy Expenditure and Food Consumption in Brazilian Models. *Revista Brasileira de Cineantropometria e Desempenho Humano*, **11**, 1-7.

[19] Ministério da Saúde (2004) Food and Nutritional Surveillance, Série A. Standards and Manual Techniques.

[20] Norton, K.I., Olds, T.S., Olive, S. and Dank, S. (1996) Ken and Barbie at Life Size. *Sex Roles*, **34**, 287-294. http://dx.doi.org/10.1007/bf01544300

[21] Bouchard, C., Shephard, R.J. and Stephens, T. (Eds.) (1994) Physical Activity, Fitness, and Health. In: Bouchard, C.,

Shephard, R.J. and Stephens, T., Eds., *International Proceedings and Consensus Statement*, Human Kinetics Publishers, Champaign, 931-942. http://dx.doi.org/10.1249/00005768-199401000-00024

[22] Vina, J., Sanchis-Gomar, F., Martinez-Bello, V. and Gomez-Cabrera, M.C. (2012) Exercise Acts as a Drug; the Pharmacological Benefits of Exercise. *British Journal of Pharmacology*, **167**, 1-12.

[23] Hallal, P.C., Bertoldi, A.D., Gonçalves, H. and Victora, C.G. (2006) Sedentary Lifestyle Prevalence and Associated Factors in Adolescents Aged between 10-12 Years. *Cadernos de Saúde Pública*, **22**, 1277-1287. http://dx.doi.org/10.1590/S0102-311X2006000600017

[24] Rodrigues, A.M., Cintra, I.P., Santos, L.C., Martini, L.A., Mello, M.T. and Fisberg, M. (2010) Adolescent Runaway Models: How Is the Food Consumption of This Group? *Revista Paulista de Pediatria*, **28**, 326-332. http://dx.doi.org/10.1590/S0103-05822010000400007

[25] Gianinni, D.T. (2007) Nutritional Recommendations of the Adolescent: Adolescence and Health. Vol. 4.

[26] Mottini, D.U., Cadore, E.L. and Kruel, L.F.M. (2008) Exercise Effects on the Bone Mineral Density. *Motriz: Revista de Educação Física*, **14**, 85-95.

6

The Effect of Circuit Training on Resting Heart Rate Variability, Cardiovascular Disease Risk Factors and Physical Fitness in Healthy Untrained Adults

Adamos Vrachimis[1,2], Marios Hadjicharalambous[2]*, Chris Tyler[1]

[1]School of Human & Life Sciences, Roehampton University, London, UK
[2]Department of Life & Health Sciences, University of Nicosia, Nicosia, Cyprus
Email: *hadjicharalambous.m@unic.ac.cy

Abstract

The purpose of the present study was to examine the effect of circuit training (CT) on resting heart rate variability (HRV) and other cardiovascular disease (CVD) risk factors such as blood lipids and blood glucose and on fitness components. Twenty-four healthy untrained adults (age 26.5 ± 5.1 years; height 1.67 ± 8.4 m; weight 66.8 ± 15.1 kg; 26.3% ± 5.2%; maximum oxygen uptake (VO_{2max}) 48.5 ± 10.0 ml·kg^{-1}·min^{-1}) were assigned to either CT (n = 12) involving bodyweight exercises, or control (CON, n = 12) groups. Prior to the start and following the end of the six-week training period, time-, frequency-domain and nonlinear measures of resting HRV, arterial blood pressure, body composition, fasting blood lipids, lipoproteins and glucose, VO_{2max}, upper body muscular endurance (UBME) and abdominal and hip flexor (AHFME), back strength (BS) and handgrip were assessed. None of the resting HRV measures (P > 0.05) were affected by the CT intervention. However, diastolic blood pressure decreased (P = 0.03), lean body weight (P = 0.03) increased, VO_{2max} (P = 0.03), UBME (P < 0.001), AHFME (P = 0.04), and BS (P = 0.03) were significantly higher following CT, whereas the other variables were not influenced by the CT. Six-week of CT involving bodyweight exercises has no significant impact on resting HRV. However, this type of training might decrease the risk for development of CVD by reducing arterial blood pressure and by improving body composition, aerobic capacity, muscular endurance and strength.

Keywords

Heart Rate Variability, Circuit Training, Healthy Untrained Adults

*Corresponding author.

1. Introduction

According to the World Health Organization (WHO), more people die annually from cardiovascular diseases (CVD) than from any other cause [1]. In particular, an estimated 17.3 million people died from CVD in 2008, representing 30% of all global deaths. Of these 17.3 million deaths, an estimated 7.3 million were due to coronary heart disease and 6.2 million were due to stroke. Almost 23.6 million people are expected to die from cardiovascular diseases in 2030, mainly due to heart disease and stroke [1]. One non-invasive clinical predictor of CVD morbidity and mortality is heart rate variability (HRV) [2]-[4]. HRV is the variation in time between beats [5] and, in particular, the variation in time of the R-R intervals, which is the distance between two R peaks on the QRS complex of an electrocardiography (ECG) wave. Originally, HRV was analyzed by the use of linear methods (time- and frequency-domain) but these means resulted in loss of information on the dynamic patterns used by cardiovascular regulation systems to adjust heart rate (HR) and blood pressure [6]. Nonlinear methods, which were developed recently, may provide additional information on cardiovascular autonomic regulation [6]. Loss of HRV has been associated with increased risk of new cardiac events (angina pectoris, myocardial infarction, or congestive heart failure) [7], coronary heart disease [8] and mortality of all causes [9]. Concomitantly, increased HRV is linked to improved prognosis and lower CVD mortality [7]. This suggests that HRV could be a valuable tool in predicting future cardiac events, and that any type of exercise intervention that is proven to improve HRV might reduce the risk of such events.

Several studies have reported the positive effect of aerobic exercise training on resting HRV measures. De Meersman [10] found that high-intensity aerobic training increases parasympathetic tone at rest in young athletes. Levy et al. [11] reported the same finding after intensive aerobic training in both healthy older and young men. Whereas, Melanson and Freedson [12] found that moderate-to-vigorous-intensity endurance training induces increases in most time- and frequency-domain measures of HRV in adult males.

Concerning strength training and HRV, studies have produced conflicting results. Carter et al. [13] reported that whole body resistance training does not cause a significant change in sympathetic tone in young subjects. In addition, Van Hoof et al. [14] and Cooke and Carter [15] found that strength training does not affect neural control of neither HR nor blood pressure, and vagal-cardiac control or cardiovagal baroreflex sensitivity, respectively. However, Heffernan et al. [16] reported a positive effect in nonlinear dynamics of HR complexity apart from a non-significant effect in spectral measures of HRV after six weeks of resistance training. Tatro et al. [17] found that lower body resistance training can cause a chronic increase in sensitivity and resetting of carotid-cardiac baroreflex in healthy males. Taylor et al. [18] also, reported a hypotensive response and a simultaneous increase in vagal modulation in older adults with hypertension as a result of isometric handgrip training at moderate intensity. To the best of our knowledge, studies investigating the effect of circuit (CT) on all three measures of resting HRV (time-, frequency-domain and nonlinear) do not exist.

CT appears to have multiple benefits on health and fitness, as various studies have shown that it may elicit significant increases in aerobic capacity muscular strength, muscular endurance, lean body weight, and significant decreases in resting diastolic blood pressure and body fat [19]-[26]. The effect of CT on some other CVD risk factors such as fasting blood glucose, and blood lipids and lipoproteins remain under-investigated.

Since CT has been associated with increases in aerobic capacity and as aerobic training has been shown to increase resting HRV measures, we hypothesized that CT may increase resting HRV measures in healthy untrained adults aged 18 - 35 years old. In addition, given that CT has been shown to improve various CVD risk factors and fitness components, we tested another hypothesis, that CT improves some other CVD risk factors and fitness components, not yet investigated. The purpose therefore of the present study was to examine the effect of six weeks of CT on a) resting HRV measures, b) blood metabolites and c) fitness components.

2. Materials and Methods

2.1. Subjects

Based on Cohen's standard effect size for a "large effect" of 0.8 [27], we estimated a sample size of 24 subjects required to test our hypothesis $(1 - \beta = 0.95, a = 0.05)$. Subjects were recruited following the distribution of a relevant advertisement leaflets at the University of Nicosia and randomly at two big private health clubs in the city of Nicosia, Cyprus. The subjects voluntarily accepted to participate in the present study. All participants gave their written informed consent to take part in the study, which was approved by the Roehampton University ethics committee. The CT group [n = 12 (10 female, 2 male); age 23.3 ± 3.2 years; height 1.67 ± 8.4 m; weight 67.6 ± 16.7 kg; body fat 27.6% ± 5.1%; maximum oxygen uptake ($\dot{V}O_{2max}$) 45.1 ± 7.71 ml·kg^{-1}·min^{-1}] and the control (CON) group [n = 12 (6 female, 6 male); age 29.8 ± 4.5 years; height 1.68 ± 8.7 m; weight 66.1 ± 14.1 kg; body fat 25.0% ± 5.3%; $\dot{V}O_{2max}$ 51.7 ± 11.1 ml·kg^{-1}·min^{-1}] comprised male and female untrained healthy subjects. They were classified as untrained if they had no background in regular endurance or resistance training or competitive sports for the last six months. Thirty-seven (n = 37) subjects initially participated in the study. However, twelve of them withdrew. Ten withdrew from the CT group; two withdrew right after the pre-training measurements and the other eight withdrew during the training phase. Subjects within the CT group had to attend at least 16 out of 18 sessions in total (90%) in order to include their data in the analysis. One of the thirteen subjects did not complete the minimum number of sessions so that set of data was excluded from the analysis. The remaining two subjects withdrew from the CON group after the first set of measurements. All subjects completed a health history questionnaire in order to confirm their healthy status and the fact that they were normotensive and were not taking any medication, which would alter cardiovascular control [22].

2.2. Circuit Training

An induction session took place just before the start of the six-week intervention training, in order to familiarize subjects with the testing equipment and the correct technique of all the exercises. Both the induction and the training sessions were undertaken by a qualified instructor. The subjects were able to train on their own, whenever they could not attend the scheduled supervised sessions by the instructor. Based on previous studies [19]-[26], CT involved a six-week training program, according to which subjects had to train three times per week. In weeks 1 and 2, 3 and 4, and 5 and 6 they had to complete 1, 2, and 3 circuits per session respectively [20] [22]. In weeks 1, 3 and 5 and weeks 2, 4 and 6 the objective was to complete 15 and 20 repetitions respectively for each exercise [20] [22]. The subjects performed both the concentric and eccentric contraction phase of each exercise in 1 second [21]. Rest between exercises (stations) was the minimum time required for subjects to move from one station to another (<15 seconds), and rest between circuits for weeks 3 - 6 was three minutes of active recovery [21]-[24].

The subjects were using only their body weight to perform the exercises [26]. The training protocol consisted of the following exercises:

1. Squats;
2. Static lunges;
3. Shoulder bridge;
4. Standing single leg calf raises;
5. Push-ups;
6. Incline bench push-ups;
7. Tricep dips;
8. Crunches;
9. Side crunches;
10. Back raises;
11. Step-ups;
12. Side-to-side jumps over skipping rope.

Female subjects performed push-ups and bench push-ups on their knees, whereas male subjects had to perform these exercises on their toes [28] [29]. If subjects could not complete 15 or 20 repetitions continuously they could rest for a few seconds and then complete the remaining repetitions [28] [29]. During the six-weeks training period, subjects were instructed to refrain from any other type of exercise; all participants included into the statistical analysis comply with this particular instruction.

2.3. Data Collection and Processing

The whole study period lasted for 16 months. During the data collection process, body composition and fitness assessment always followed HRV and blood pressure measurements. Blood samples were collected on a separate day of the same week. The first set of data was collected during the week right before the training commenced and the second set of data was collected during the week right after the end of the training period. All measurements were taken by one investigator to ensure consistency of measurement. A Hosand HR Monitor

MC030 (Hosand Technologies S.r.l., Verbania, Italy), was used to record resting HRV data with the subject sitting quietly for 5 minutes. The HR was detected by using two single-use adhesive electrodes, which were applied directly on skin, just below the pectoral muscles and fastened to the HR monitor with snaps. Prior to data collection, subjects rested comfortably in a seated position for 10 minutes.

All measurements were taken in the morning, between the hours of 7 a.m. and 10 a.m., in order to minimize diurnal effects. Subjects were overnight fasted and refrained from any excessive activity and from any caffeine consumption in the morning, prior to reporting to the laboratory. Recordings were analysed using a Hosand MC Software version 1.1.0.25 (Hosand Technologies, Verbania, Italy). Time-, frequency-domain and nonlinear analyses were used to assess HRV in this study. The time-domain measures recorded were: mean HR, standard deviation of R-R intervals (SDRR), number of adjacent R-R intervals more than 50 milliseconds (ms) different (NN50) and proportion of adjacent R-R intervals more than 50ms different (pNN50). The frequency-domain measures, which were determined by spectral analysis using fast Fourier transform, were: low frequency power (LF, 0.04 - 0.15 Hz), high frequency power (HF, 0.15 - 0.4 Hz) and low frequency power to high frequency power ratio (LF/HF). Finally, nonlinear measures were analyzed by using the Poincare plot. The measures recorded were: standard deviation calculated on the vertical axis of the Poincare plot (SD1), standard deviation calculated on the horizontal axis of the Poincare plot (SD2) and the ratio of SD1 to SD2 (SD1/SD2).

An Omron M6 Digital Automatic Blood Pressure Monitor (Omron Healthcare, Kyoto, Japan) was used to measure systolic and diastolic blood pressure. The Omron M6 device has been deemed to be in accordance with the International Protocol criteria and has been recommended for use by adults [30]. Measurements were always taken from the left upper arm in a seated position.

Body weight was measured using a digital weighing scale accurate to the nearest 0.1 kg and height was measured using a measuring pole to the nearest 0.1 cm. Percent body fat was assessed by measuring skinfolds to the nearest 0.5 mm, at four sites of the body using a Harpenden Skinfold Caliper (Baty International, West Sussex, U.K.). The method of skinfolds is considered to be a reasonably accurate tool for measuring subcutaneous fat [31] [32]. A minimum of two measurements was taken at each site (biceps, triceps, subscapular, suprailiac). However, if the difference between the two values was greater than 1 mm, the test was repeated and the two values closer to each other were recorded. The final value recorded was the average of the two values. The body fat percentage was calculated using the following equations:

$$\text{Body density}\,(\text{BD}) = C - \left[M\left(\log 10 \text{ sum of all four skinfolds}\right)\right] \quad [31] \tag{1}$$

The result of the above formula (BD) was used in the Siri equation to calculate body fat percentage.

$$\text{Body fat}\,(\%) = \left[\left(4.95/\text{BD}\right) - 4.5\right] \times 100 \;\;(\text{Siri equation}) \quad [31] \tag{2}$$

Lean body weight was calculated by subtracting fat weight from total body weight.

An estimated value of $\dot{V}O_{2\max}$ was determined after conducting the Queens College step test. Subjects had to step up and down on a step 16.25-inch high for 3 minutes at a steady pace of 24 steps per minute for male subjects and 22 steps per minute for female subjects. A Wittner 812 K Metronome (Wittner GmbH, Isny, Germany) was used to indicate the appropriate pace and a Polar RS400 HR Monitor (Polar Electro Oy, HQ, Kempele, Finland) was used to record the HR at the end of the 3-minute test. The Queen's College step test correlation between recovery HR and $\dot{V}O_{2\max}$ is r = −0.75, and test retest reliability for recovery HR is r = 0.92 [33].

A Takei TKK 5402 Digital Back Dynamometer (Takei Scientific Instruments, Tokyo, Japan) was used to measure back strength to the nearest 0.1 kg. Each subject had two attempts and the maximum value was recorded [34]. Handgrip strength was measured to the nearest 0.1 kg by using a Takei TKK 5401 Digital Handgrip Dynamometer (Takei Scientific Instruments, Tokyo, Japan). Measurements were performed twice each with the left and right hands alternately and the mean value of the highest values of the forces of both hands was recorded [34].

The YMCA Push-up Test was conducted to assess upper body (e.g. arm, shoulder muscular endurance. Male subjects performed the test on their toes, female subjects performed the test on their knees but both kept their hips and back straight [28] [29].

Abdominal and hip flexor muscular endurance was assessed by using the National Coaching Foundation (NCF) Abdominal Curl Conditioning Test (Coachwise Ltd., Leeds, UK), which is a progressive sit up test. It has been reported that sit-up tests in general have high reliability when measuring abdominal and hip flexor muscular endurance [29]. Subjects were required to perform as many sit ups as possible, keeping in time to the beeps emitted from a NCF Abdominal Curl Conditioning Test audio CD. The total number of sit ups completed correctly and the time from the start of the test until the subject could no longer keep in time with the beeps or when the sit ups were not performed correctly was recorded. Subjects were encouraged during the fitness tests for maximum effort.

Venous blood samples (4 ml) were collected in the morning between 7.00 am and 8.30 am after a 14-hour overnight fast. Following centrifugation, blood samples were analyzed for total cholesterol, HDL, LDL, triglycerides and glucose using an Olympus AU2700 Chemistry Analyzer (Beckman Coulter, Brea, CA, USA) [35].

2.4. Statistical Analysis

A separate repeated measures ANOVA was used to assess the effect of CT on each of the resting HRV measures and the rest of the variables. The statistical significance was accepted at 5% ($P < 0.05$). Data were expressed as means ± SD. All data were analyzed using the SPSS Statistical Software Package version 17.0 (SPSS, Inc., Chicago, IL, USA).

3. Results

Several HRV parameters were assessed and their P values are reported separately below and/or in **Table 1**.

HR ($F_{1,21} = 2.0$, $P = 0.17$), SDRR ($F_{1,21} = 2.1$, $P = 0.17$), NN50 ($F_{1,21} = 0.8$, $P = 0.38$), PNN50 ($F_{1,21} = 0.3$, $P = 0.59$), VLF ($F_{1,2} = 2.8$, $P = 0.11$), LF ($F_{1,21} = 0.03$, $P = 0.87$), HF ($F_{1,21} = 0.7$, $P = 0.40$), LFnu (normalized units) ($F_{1,21} = 0.8$, $P = 0.39$), HFnu ($F_{1,21} = 0.8$, $P = 0.39$), LF/HF ($F_{1,21} = 1.7$, $P = 0.20$), SD1 ($F_{1,21} = 0.7$, $P = 0.40$), SD2 ($F_{1,21} = 2.2$, $P = 0.16$) and the ratio SD1/SD2 ($F_{1,21} = 0.002$, $P = 0.97$) were not affected by training (**Table 1**). There was a significant group effect in SDRR ($F_{1,21} = 7.0$, $P = 0.02$), LF ($F_{1,21} = 8.4$, $P = 0.01$), SD2 ($F_{1,21} = 7.6$, $P = 0.01$), while there was no significant time effect in any of the measures ($P \geq 0.05$; **Table 1**).

Table 1. Means (±SD) for HRV measures.

Variable	CT (n = 12)		CON (n = 12)		P value		
	Pre	Post	Pre	Post	Time effect	Group effect	Interaction time·group
HR (bpm)	74.4 (7.9)	75.5 (5.9)	73.6 (6.7)	79.1 (7.7)	0.05	0.59	0.17
SDRR (ms)	62.9 (18.5)	67.0 (16.3)	53.0 (15.3)	46.7 (14.9)	0.77	0.02*	0.17
NN50	53.9 (54.6)	56.0 (36.5)	32.3 (35.4)	22.8 (34.2)	0.57	0.10	0.38
PNN50 (%)	18.1 (20.6)	17.5 (13.1)	9.9 (10.3)	6.9 (10.6)	0.40	0.10	0.59
VLF (ms²/Hz)	610 (297)	936 (448)	639 (597)	501 (393)	0.50	0.13	0.11
LF (ms²/Hz)	661 (457)	572 (393)	322 (274)	213 (79)	0.14	0.01*	0.87
HF (ms²/Hz)	370 (502)	258 (280)	151 (116)	115 (120)	0.11	0.13	0.40
LFnu	72.8 (15.9)	69.4 (12.2)	66.2 (16.5)	70.6 (15.5)	0.91	0.55	0.39
HFnu	27.2 (15.9)	30.6 (12.2)	33.8 (16.5)	29.4 (15.5)	0.91	0.55	0.39
LF/HF	4.2 (3.4)	2.8 (1.9)	2.7 (2.1)	3.5 (2.3)	0.69	0.54	0.20
SD1 (ms)	28.8 (19.0)	27.9 (11.6)	21.5 (6.3)	17.7 (7.8)	0.20	0.08	0.40
SD2 (ms)	83.5 (21.1)	90.4 (20.8)	71.6 (21.6)	63.3 (20.7)	0.90	0.01*	0.16
SD1/SD2	0.32 (0.13)	0.31 (0.06)	0.31 (0.09)	0.29 (0.10)	0.44	0.71	0.97

*Significantly different ($P < 0.05$). Pre, pre-training; Post, post-training; HR, heart rate; SDRR, standard deviation of R-R intervals; NN50, number of adjacent R-R intervals more than 50 ms different; PNN50 (%), proportion of adjacent R-R intervals more than 50 ms different; VLF, very low frequency power; LF, low frequency power; HF, high frequency power; nu, normalized units; SD1, standard deviation calculated on the vertical axis of the Poincare plot; SD2, standard deviation calculated on the horizontal axis of the Poincare plot.

Diastolic blood pressure ($F_{1,22} = 5.5$, P = 0.03) and lean body weight ($F_{1,22} = 5.2$, P = 0.03) were significantly improved in the CT group compared to the CON group, whereas the rest of the variables did not change after training (**Table 2**). In addition, there was a significant time effect in body fat ($F_{1,22} = 4.7$, P = 0.04) but there was no significant group effect in any of the variables (P $\geq$ 0.05).

None of the fasting blood variables changed significantly in the CT group after training, compared to the CON group (P $\geq$ 0.05; **Table 3**). However, triglycerides ($F_{1,22} = 8.3$, P = 0.01), and LDL ($F_{1,19} = 5.4$, P = 0.03) were significantly different between groups, while the variables between pre- and post-training measurements did not change (**Table 3**).

There was a main interaction (time × group) effect in $\dot{V}O_{2max}$ ($F_{1,22} = 5.2$, P = 0.03), UBME ($F_{1,22} = 101.3$, P < 0.001), AHFME ($F_{1,21} = 5.0$, P = 0.04), BS ($F_{1,22} = 5.5$, P = 0.03) which all increased significantly with training. However, HS ($F_{1,22} = 0.2$, P = 0.65) was not different following the training period (**Table 4**). UBME significantly also increased over-time comparing between pre- and post-training period in the CT group, ($F_{1,22} = 80.5$, P < 0.001). There was no significant group effect in any of the components.

4. Discussion

The primary finding of the present study was that CT, involving bodyweight exercises, significantly reduced diastolic blood pressure, increased lean body weight, aerobic capacity, and upper body, abdominal and hip flexor muscular endurance and back strength. However, CT did not influence resting HRV.

4.1. HRV

To our knowledge, this is the first study to investigate the effect of CT on all resting HRV measures: time-, frequency-domain and nonlinear measures. The non-significant effect on resting HRV is consistent with the find-

Table 2. Means (±SD) for body weight (BW), body fat % (BF%), lean body weight (LBW), systolic blood pressure (SBP) and diastolic BP (DBP).

Variable	CT (n = 12)		CON (n = 12)		P value		
	Pre	Post	Pre	Post	Time effect	Group effect	Interaction time·group
BW (kg)	67.6 (17)	67.9 (17)	66.1 (14)	65.6 (13)	0.77	0.77	0.29
BF%	27.6 (5)	26.6 (4)	25.0 (5)	24.7 (5)	0.04*	0.27	0.24
LBW (kg)	48.9 (12)	49.7 (12)	49.6 (11)	49.4 (10)	0.13	0.98	0.03*
SBP (mmHg)	115.8 (11)	110.6 (8)	110.2 (9)	110.3 (7)	0.14	0.39	0.13
DBP (mmHg)	71.9 (5)	67.8 (5)	67.5 (7)	68.8 (4)	0.24	0.43	0.03*

*Significantly different (P < 0.05). Pre, pre-training; Post, post-training.

Table 3. Means (±SD) for fasting blood triglycerides (TGL), cholesterol (CHL), high density lipoprotein (HDL), low density lipoprotein (LDL) and glucose.

Variable	CT (n = 12)		CON (n = 12)		P value		
	Pre	Post	Pre	Post	Time effect	Group effect	Interaction time·group
TGL (mg/dL)	60.8 (22)	66.7 (32)	108 (55)	111.7 (49)	0.44	0.01*	0.81
Total CHL (mg/dL)	164.8 (30)	166.6 (28)	197 (39)	184 (30)	0.22	0.06	0.11
HDL (mg/dL)	48.1 (12)	49.7 (13)	52.3 (19)	49.3 (17)	0.64	0.78	0.13
LDL (mg/dL)	95 (29)	96.0 (29)	123 (31)	112.3 (19)	0.34	0.03*	0.25
Glucose (mg/dL)	83.8 (8)	86.8 (6)	88.2 (9)	89.2 (9)	0.30	0.26	0.61

*Significantly different (P < 0.05). Pre, pre-training; Post, post-training.

Table 4. Means (±SD) for maximum oxygen uptake ($\dot{V}O_{2max}$, $ml \cdot kg^{-1} \cdot min^{-1}$), upper body (UBME) and abdominal and hip flexor muscular endurance (AHFME), back strength (BS) and handgrip strength (HS).

Variable	CT (n = 12)		CON (n = 12)		P value		
	Pre	Post	Pre	Post	Time effect	Group effect	Interaction time·group
$\dot{V}O_{2max}$	45.1 (7)	46.5 (7)	51.7 (11)	50.3 (10)	0.99	0.18	0.03*
UBME (rep.)	11.3 (9)	21.4 (9)	9.7 (9)	9.1 (9)	0.001*	0.08	0.001*
AHFME (rep.)	27.7 (17)	35.4 (29)	26.9 (12)	24.6 (13)	0.25	0.45	0.04*
BS (kg)	98.8 (54)	108.7 (53)	100.8 (35)	99.8 (34)	0.07	0.85	0.03*
HS (kg)	33.4 (14)	33.8 (13)	31.8 (9)	31.7 (10	0.74	0.71	0.65

*Significantly different (P < 0.05). Pre, pre-training; Post, post-training. UBME increased over-time comparing between pre- and post-training period in the CT group.

ings reported by previous studies [13]-[16], with reference to the effect of strength training on the spectral measures of HRV. However, Heffernan *et al.* [16] also found that the intervention increased HR complexity—a nonlinear method of assessing HR, not used in the present study—and the researchers postulated that this could be because of increased parasympathetic and/or reduced sympathetic cardiac autonomic control. Previous studies have reported that greater reductions in overall HRV and greater elevations in HR after a single bout of acute resistance exercise versus acute endurance exercise may be attributed to greater reductions in cardiac parasympathetic tone [36]. In addition, a reduction in HF spectral power of HRV after an acute resistance exercise bout was found to be related to reduce HR complexity [37]. Despite these findings, Heffernan *et al.* [16] postulated that these potentially negative acute responses do not appear to transpose to a state of permanence and could lead to positive adaptations after repeated exposure. In addition, Tatro *et al.* [17] reported a chronic increase in sensitivity and resetting of carotid-cardiac baroreflex in healthy males (32 ± 3 years old) as a result of lower body resistance training. Specifically, the researchers observed an increase in resting HRV that paralleled the increased responsiveness of the vagally mediated carotid-cardiac baroreflex. However, Tatro *et al.* [17] could not provide a clear interpretation for the increase in parasympathetic cardiac control since they found no significant change in baseline R-R interval (resting HR).

4.2. Arterial Blood Pressure

The most important finding of this study was the decrease in resting diastolic blood pressure following CT training period. These results are in agreement with several previous studies [19] [23] [38] which reported a significant decline in resting diastolic blood pressure but no change in resting systolic blood pressure, as a result of CT intervention. In Hurley *et al.* [38] study, the resistive training program used was classified as high intensity, however it could be considered as a CT program due to the short rest intervals (<15 seconds) between each exercise. Our findings are strongly supported by the meta-analysis study by Fagard [39]. In his review, Fagard [39] mentions that aerobic power increased by 10.5% in six resistance training study groups in which it was measured, which suggests that the types of resistance exercise used in most protocols comprised an aerobic component to some extent. The circuit format of resistance training used in our study with minimal rest between stations (<15 seconds) could be considered as an aerobic component, which is further supported by the training-induced significant increase in $\dot{V}O_{2max}$ (P = 0.03). It is important to note that Carter *et al.* [13] and Ray and Carrasco [40] reported that the reduction in both systolic and diastolic was not coupled to resistance and isometric handgrip respectively, exercise-induced decreases of sympathetic neural activity. This finding is consistent with the current results, given that there was not a significant change in low frequency power.

Contrary to the above results, the study by Reid *et al.* [41] showed no effect of resistance training on resting arterial blood pressure. In this study the rest period between stations in all groups was approximately 10 seconds, which was almost similar to the rest period used in our intervention. Moreover, the researchers observed a significant increase in $\dot{V}O_{2max}$ in two of the groups (endurance and strength 2), something also found in the CT group of out study. Although, there was no significant change in resting arterial blood pressure after the training, there was a trend towards an increase in diastolic blood pressure in all four groups. Reid *et al.* [41] speculated that this was due to the continual use of the Valsavamanoeuvre (expiring against a closed glottis results in an increase in intrathoracic pressure which causes an increase in both systolic and diastolic pressure) which was often observed in subjects of all groups despite admonition. In the current study, subjects were instructed in advance to breathe properly and it was made certain throughout the sessions that they were not using the Valsavamanoeuvre.

Aerobic endurance training decreases arterial blood pressure through a reduction of systemic vascular resistance, in which the sympathetic nervous system and the renin-angiotensin system appear to be involved [39]. According to the review by Fagard [39] some studies have addressed the underlying mechanisms responsible for the decrease in blood pressure in response to resistance training, but failed to bring these mechanisms to light. In our study there was no significant change in high and low frequency power, thus no change in cardiac autonomic activity. More research is needed to address the blood pressure-lowering mechanism of resistance training.

4.3. Body Composition

The significant increase in lean body weight and the no change in body fat observed in the current study are in agreement with several previous reports [19] [20] [23] [24] [37] [41] respectively. However, Wilmore *et al.* [19] and Gettman *et al.* [20] [22] reported significant reductions in body fat as a result of circuit weight training. Pollock [42] has suggested that exercise programs of duration less than 8 to 10 weeks cause insignificant changes in body composition. The training period in the studies by Wilmore *et al.* [19] and Gettman*et al.* [20] [22] was 10, 12 and 20 weeks respectively. However, in the case of Harris & Holly [23], Harber *et al.* [24], Hurley *et al.* [38], Reid *et al.* [41] and the current study the corresponding duration of the training period was 9, 10, 16, 8 and 6 weeks respectively. In the studies by Harber *et al.* [24] and Hurley *et al.* [38], there would be a significant decrease in body fat since the training period was 10 and 16 weeks respectively. However, the subjects in the study by Harber *et al.* [24] performed on average two sets for each exercise over the 10 weeks of the program and the subjects in the study by Hurley *et al.* [38] performed only one set per exercise over the 16-week training period. In contrast, the subjects in the studies by Wilmore *et al.* [19] and Gettman *et al.* [20] performed 3 circuits and in the study by Gettman *et al.* [22] even though the subjects performed 2 circuits, the duration of this study was the longest of all (20 weeks). Consequently, the lower training volume of the studies by Harber *et al.* [24] and Hurley *et al.* [38] compared to the studies by Wilmore *et al.* [19] and Gettman *et al.* [20] [22] may explain why body fat did not change significantly in those studies.

The non-significant decrease in body fat observed in the current study may be partially explained by the relatively small amounts of total energy expended in exercise over these shorter training periods (<8 - 10 weeks). Wilmore *et al.* [43] estimated a caloric expenditure of 9.0 kcal·min^{-1} during a 10-station circuit weight program. Based on these estimates, our subjects expended approximately 90 kcal·session^{-1} in the first week (total 270 kcal); 110 kcal·session^{-1} in the second week (total 330 kcal); 205 kcal·session^{-1} in the third week (total 615 kcal); 225 kcal·session^{-1} in the fourth week (total 675 kcal); 325 kcal·session^{-1} in the fifth week (total 975 kcal); 385 kcal·session^{-1} in the sixth week (total 1155 kcal); or 4000 kcal for the whole 6-week training period. This amount of kcal represents the equivalent loss of approximately 0.520 kg of fat, which is very close to the actual loss of 0.600 kg in body fat mass observed in our study.

4.4. Maximum Oxygen Uptake

The significant increase in $\dot{V}O_{2max}$ is concordant with the findings of several studies [19]-[21] [23]. Harris & Holly [23] noted that short rest intervals and adequate training stimulus appear to be keys to eliciting changes in aerobic capacity. Rest intervals between sets in our study were less than 15 seconds. Considering the training stimulus, we did not record the HR at any point during the sessions, so we do not have any information about this parameter. Nevertheless, it appears that the volume of training (number of repetitions, sets, and workload) provided adequate training stimulus to eliciting a significant improvement in aerobic capacity of the untrained subjects.

4.5. UBME, AHFME, BS and HS

The current results indicate that CT may increase UBME and AHFME confirming the particular tested hypotheses. The present findings are consistent with the positive effect of CT on muscular endurance observed by Wilmore et al. [19] and Kaikkonen et al. [21]. In addition, the present results are confirmed by several previous studies (e.g. [20]-[24] [26]), which were found that a circuit regime is an ideal methods for muscular endurance training. According to Rose and Rothstein [44] muscular endurance training (either aerobic endurance or low resistance weight training with several repetitions) was found to improve the oxidative capacity of the muscle.

The back strength improvements are consistent with whole body strength improvements found in other circuit weight programs [19] [20] [22]-[24]. Consequently, the hypothesis that CT would have a positive effect on back strength was confirmed. The circuit training-induced improvement in back strength could be explained by an increase in myofibrillar proteins, resulting in enlarged or hypertrophic muscle fibers [44]. The training-induced muscle hypertrophy can be supported by the fact that there was a significant increase in lean body weight.

Contrary to our findings regarding HS, two studies by Taniguchi [47] and Saito et al. [48] found increases in maximal handgrip force after resistance training. It should be noted, however, that the training interventions in these studies consisted of isometric handgrip training. In our study there was no handgrip exercise training involved so most probably that was the reason why this variable did not change.

4.6. Fasting Blood Variables

A review study by Hurley [45] reported that most longitudinal studies investigating the effect of resistive training on lipid profiles have showed that lipid profiles, especially HDL and LDL, are improved as a result of this intervention. Regarding fasting blood glucose, there is very little data examining this dose-response relationship between resistance exercise and this variable in healthy subjects. Williams et al. [46] found that community based resistance training significantly decreased fasting blood glucose levels in healthy older individuals. Our results on fasting blood variables are in disagreement with these findings; hence the hypotheses about these variables were not confirmed. Nevertheless, due to methodological limitations and design flaws from many of the studies involving resistive training there is not enough information to determine whether this type of exercise is effective for risk factor intervention [45].

5. Conclusion

In conclusion, the present study suggests that CT involving bodyweight exercises, as opposed to aerobic endurance training has no significant impact on resting HRV time-, frequency-domain and nonlinear measures. However, the fact that this type of training caused a significant reduction in arterial blood pressure, suggested that it might prevent the development of CVD through other mechanisms. This means that aerobic endurance and CT, or resistance training in general, should complement each other, as they seem to prevent the development of CVD through different mechanisms. Increases in aerobic capacity, lean body weight, muscular endurance and strength indicate additional benefits.

6. Study Limitations

Some limitations should be taken into consideration when interpreting the results of the current study. A) The present findings may not be applicable to older adults or clinical populations, due to the fact that age and cardiovascular diseases appear to be interrelated to resting HRV [7] [8] [49]; B) In most of the studies investigating the effect of resistance training on resting HRV measures, data was collected with the subjects resting in supine position. However in the current study, data was collected in seated position. This could partially influence the results. A study by Ribeiro et al. [50] however, showed no significant differences in HRV indexes in the supine or seated position in both young and postmenopausal women. C) In the present study, breathing patterns were not controlled during the HRV measurements since we aimed at obtaining data from a condition as close to real life as possible. However, a study by Bloomfield et al. [51] showed that when collecting HRV data in both healthy subjects and/or patients with heart disease, there is no need to control breathing.

Acknowledgements

We would like to thank Dr Jackie Dabinett for her valuable contribution, Mr. Claudio De Marco for his assistance in the HRV analysis and Ms. Maria Lazarou for her assistance in the blood sampling analysis. We also thank the participants for their excellent cooperation and commitment.

References

[1] WHO (2012) Cardiovascular Diseases. World Health Organization, Geneva. http://www.who.int/

[2] Molgaard, H., Sorensen, K.E. and Bjerregaard, P. (1991) Attenuated 24-h Heart Rate Variability in Apparently Healthy Subsequently Suffering Sudden Cardiac Death. *Clinical Autonomic Research*, **1**, 233-237. http://dx.doi.org/10.1007/BF01824992

[3] Tsuji, H., Venditti Jr., F.J., Manders, E.S., Evans, J.C., Larson, M.G. and Feldman, C.L., *et al.* (1994) Reduced Heart Rate Variability and Mortality Risk in an Elderly Cohort. The Framingham Heart Study. *Circulation*, **90**, 878-883. http://dx.doi.org/10.1161/01.CIR.90.2.878

[4] Liao, D., Sloan, R.P., Cascio, W.E., Folsom, A.R., Liese, A.D., Evans, G.W., *et al.* (1998) Multiple Metabolic Syndrome Is Associated with Lower Heart Rate Variability. *Diabetes Care*, **21**, 2116-2122. http://dx.doi.org/10.2337/diacare.21.12.2116

[5] Achten, J. and Jeukendrup, A.E. (2003) Heart Rate Monitoring Applications and Limitations. *Sports Medicine*, **33**, 517-538. http://dx.doi.org/10.2165/00007256-200333070-00004

[6] Kuusela, T.A., Jartti, T.T., Tahvanainen, K.U. and Kaila, T.J. (2002) Nonlinear Methods of Biosignal Analysis in Assessing Terbutaline-Induced Heart Rate and Blood Pressure Changes. *American Journal of Physiology-Heart and Circulatory Physiology*, **282**, H773-H783. http://dx.doi.org/10.1152/ajpheart.00559.2001

[7] Tsuji, H., Larson, M.G., Venditti Jr., F.J., Manders, E.S., Evans, J.C., Feldman, C.L., *et al.* (1996) Impact of Reduced Heart Rate Variability on Risk for Cardiac Events. The Framingham Heart Study. *Circulation*, **94**, 2850-2855. http://dx.doi.org/10.1161/01.CIR.94.11.2850

[8] Liao, D., Cai, J., Rosamond, W.D., Barnes, R.F., Hutchinson, R.G., Whitsel, E.A., *et al.* (1997) Cardiac Autonomic Function and Incident Coronary Heart Disease: A Population-Based Case-Cohort Study. *American Journal of Epidemiology*, **145**, 696-706. http://dx.doi.org/10.1093/aje/145.8.696

[9] Dekker, J.M., Schouten, E.G., Klootwijk, P., Pool, J., Swenne, C.A. and Kromhout, D. (1997) Heart Rate Variability from Short Electrocardiographic Recording Predicts Mortality from All Causes in Middle-Aged and Elderly Men. The Zutphen Study. *American Journal of Epidemiology*, **145**, 899-908. http://dx.doi.org/10.1093/oxfordjournals.aje.a009049

[10] De Meersman, R.E. (1992) Respiratory Sinus Arrhythmia Alteration Following Training in Endurance Athletes. *European Journal of Applied Physiology*, **64**, 434-436. http://dx.doi.org/10.1007/BF00625063

[11] Levy, W.C., Cerqueira, M.D., Harp, G.D., Johannessen, K.A., Abrass, I.B., Schwartz, R.S., *et al.* (1998) Effect of Endurance Exercise Training on Heart Rate Variability at Rest in Healthy Young and Older Men. *American Journal of Cardiology*, **82**, 1236-1241. http://dx.doi.org/10.1016/S0002-9149(98)00611-0

[12] Melanson, E.L. and Freedson, P.S. (2001) The Effect of Endurance Training on Resting Heart Rate Variability in Sedentary Adult Males. *European Journal of Applied Physiology*, **85**, 442-449. http://dx.doi.org/10.1007/s004210100479

[13] Carter, J.R., Ray, C.A., Downs, E.M. and Cooke, W.H. (2003) Strength Training Reduces Arterial Blood Pressure but Not Sympathetic Neural Activity in Young Normotensive Subjects. *Journal of Applied Physiology*, **94**, 2212-2216. http://dx.doi.org/10.1152/japplphysiol.01109.2002

[14] Van Hoof, R., Macor, F., Lijnen, P., Staessen, J., Thijs, L., Vanhees, L., *et al.* (1996) Effect of Strength Training on Blood Pressure Measured in Various Conditions in Sedentary Men. *International Journal of Sports Medicine*, **17**, 415-422. http://dx.doi.org/10.1055/s-2007-972871

[15] Cooke, W.H. and Carter, J.R. (2005) Strength Training Does Not Affect Vagal-Cardiac Control or Cardio-Vagal Baroreflex Sensitivity in Young Healthy Subjects. *European Journal of Applied Physiology*, **93**, 719-725. http://dx.doi.org/10.1007/s00421-004-1243-x

[16] Heffernan, K.S., Fahs, C.A., Shinsako, K.K., Jae, S.Y. and Fernball, B. (2007) Heart Rate Recovery and Heart Rate Complexity Following Resistance Exercise Training and Detraining in Young Men. *American Journal of Physiology-Heart and Circulatory Physiology*, **293**, H3180-H3186. http://dx.doi.org/10.1152/ajpheart.00648.2007

[17] Tatro, D.L., Dudley, G.A. and Convertino, V.A. (1992) Carotid-Cardiac Baroreflex Response and LBNP Tolerance Following Resistance Training. *Medicine and Science in Sports Exercise*, **24**, 789-796. http://dx.doi.org/10.1249/00005768-199207000-00009

[18] Taylor, A.C., McCartney, N., Kamath, M.V. and Wiley, R.L. (2003) Isometric Training Lowers Resting Blood Pressure and Modulates Autonomic Control. *Medicine and Science in Sports Exercise*, **35**, 251-256. http://dx.doi.org/10.1249/01.MSS.0000048725.15026.B5

[19] Wilmore, J.H., Parr, R.B., Vodak, P.A., Barstow, T.J., Pipes, T.V., Ward, P., *et al.* (1976) Strength, Endurance, BMR,

and Body Composition Changes with Circuit Weight Training. *Medicine and Science in Sports Exercise*, **8**, 59-60. http://dx.doi.org/10.1249/00005768-197621000-00073

[20] Gettman, L.R., Ward, P. and Hagan, R.D. (1982) A Comparison of Combined Running and Weight Training with Circuit Weight Training. *Medicine and Science in Sports Exercise*, **14**, 229-234. http://dx.doi.org/10.1249/00005768-198203000-00014

[21] Kaikkonen, H., Yrjama, M., Siljander, E., Byman, P. and Laukkanen, R. (2000) The Effect of Heart Rate Controlled Low Resistance Circuit Weight Training and Endurance Training on Maximal Aerobic Power in Sedentary Adults. *Scandinavia Journal of Medicine and Science in Sports*, **10**, 211-215. http://dx.doi.org/10.1034/j.1600-0838.2000.010004211.x

[22] Gettman, L.R., Ayres, J.J., Pollock, M.L. and Jackson, A. (1978) The Effect of Circuit Weight Training on Strength, Cardiorespiratory Function, and Body Composition of Adult Men. *Medicine and Science in Sports Exercise*, **10**, 171-176.

[23] Harris, K.A. and Holly, R.G. (1987) Physiological Response to Circuit Weight Training in Borderline Hypertensive Subjects. *Medicine and Science in Sports Exercise*, **19**, 246-252. http://dx.doi.org/10.1249/00005768-198706000-00011

[24] Harber, M.P., Fry, A.C., Rubin, M.R., Smith, J.C. and Weiss, L.W. (2004) Skeletal Muscle and Hormonal Adaptations to Circuit Weight Training in Untrained Men. *Scandinavia Journal of Medicine and Science in Sports*, **14**, 176-185. http://dx.doi.org/10.1111/j.1600-0838.2003.371.x

[25] Willardson, J.M. (2006) A Brief Review: Factors Affecting the Length of the Rest Interval between Resistance Exercise Sets. *Journal of Strength Conditioning Research*, **20**, 978-984. http://dx.doi.org/10.1519/00124278-200611000-00040

[26] Klika, B. and Jordan, C. (2013) High-Intensity Circuit Training Using Body Weight: Maximum Results with Minimal Investment. *ACSM's Health and Fitness Journal*, **17**, 8-14. http://dx.doi.org/10.1249/FIT.0b013e31828cb1e8

[27] Thalheimer, W. and Cook, S. (2002) How to Calculate Effect Sizes from Published Research Articles: A Simplified Methodology. Work-Learning Research. http://www.work-learning.com/

[28] American College of Sports Medicine (2005) ACSM's Guidelines for Exercise Testing and Prescription. 7th Edition, Lippincott Williams & Wilkins, Philadelphia.

[29] Augustsson, S.R., Bersas, E., Thomas, E.M., Sahlberg, M., Augustsson, J. and Svantesson, U. (2009) Gender Differences and Reliability of Selected Physical Performance Tests in Young Women and Men. *Advances in Physiotherapy*, **11**, 64-70. http://dx.doi.org/10.1080/14038190801999679

[30] Altunkan, S. (2007) Validation of the Omron M6 (HEM-7001-E) Upper-Arm Blood Pressure Measuring Device According to the International Protocol in adults and Obese Adults. *Blood Pressure Monitoring*, **12**, 219-225. http://dx.doi.org/10.1097/MBP.0b013e3280f813d0

[31] Durnin, J. and Womersley, J. (1974) Body Fat Assessed from Total Body Density and Its Estimation from Skinfold Thickness: Measurements on 481 Men and Women Aged 16 to 72 Years. *British Journal of Nutrition*, **32**, 77-97. http://dx.doi.org/10.1079/BJN19740060

[32] Duz, S., Kocak, M. and Korkusuz, F. (2009) Evaluation of Body Composition Using Three Difference Methods Compared to Dual-Energy X-Ray Absorptiometry. *European Journal of Sport Science*, **9**, 181-190. http://dx.doi.org/10.1080/17461390902763425

[33] McArdle, W.D., Katch, F.I., Pechar, G.S., Jacobson, L. and Ruck, S. (1972) Reliability and Interrelationships between Maximal Oxygen Intake, Physical Work Capacity and Step-Test Scores in College Women. *Medicine and Science in Sports*, **4**, 182-186. http://dx.doi.org/10.1249/00005768-197200440-00019

[34] Coldwells, A., Atkinson, G. and Reilly, T. (1994) Sources of Variation in Back and Leg Dynamometry. *Ergonomics*, **37**, 79-86. http://dx.doi.org/10.1080/00140139408963625

[35] Juricek, J., Derek, L., Unic, A., Serdar, T., Marijancevic, D., Zivkovic, M., *et al.* (2010) Analytical Evaluation of the Clinical Chemistry Analyzer Olympus AU2700 Plus. *Biochemia Medica*, **20**, 334-340. http://dx.doi.org/10.11613/bm.2010.043

[36] Heffernan, K.S., Kelly, E.E., Collier, S.R. and Fernhall, B. (2006) Cardiac Autonomic Modulation during Recovery from Acute Endurance versus Resistance Exercise. *European Journal of Cardiovascular Prevention and Rehabilitation*, **13**, 80-86. http://dx.doi.org/10.1097/00149831-200602000-00012

[37] Heffernan, K.S., Sosnoff, J.J., Jae, S.Y., Gates, G.J. and Fernhall, B. (2008) Acute Resistance Exercise Reduces Heart Rate Complexity and Increases QTc Interval. *International Journal of Sports Medicine*, **29**, 289-293. http://dx.doi.org/10.1055/s-2007-965363

[38] Hurley, B.F., Hagberg, J.M., Goldberg, A.P., Seals, D.R., Ehsani, A.A., Brennan, R.E., *et al.* (1988) Resistive Training Can Reduce Coronary Risk Factors without Altering VO_{2max} or Percent Body Fat. *Medicine and Science in Sports and*

Exercise, **20**, 150-154. http://dx.doi.org/10.1249/00005768-198820020-00008

[39] Fagard, R.H. (2006) Exercise Is Good for Your Blood Pressure: Effects of Endurance Training and Resistance Training. *Clinical and Experimental Pharmacology and Physiology*, **33**, 853-856. http://dx.doi.org/10.1111/j.1440-1681.2006.04453.x

[40] Ray, C.A. and Carrasco, D.I. (2000) Isometric Handgrip Training Reduces Arterial Pressure at Rest without Changes in Sympathetic Nerve Activity. *American Journal of Physiology-Heart and Circulatory Physiology*, **279**, H245-H249.

[41] Reid, C.M., Yeater, R.A. and Ullrich, I.H. (1987) Weight Training and Strength, Cardiorespiratory Functioning and Body Composition of Men. *British Journal of Sports Medicine*, **21**, 40-44. http://dx.doi.org/10.1136/bjsm.21.1.40

[42] Pollock, M.L. (1973) The Quantification of Endurance Training Programs. In: Wilmore, J.H., Ed., *Exercise and Sports Science Reviews*, Academic Press, New York, 155-188. http://dx.doi.org/10.1249/00003677-197300010-00010

[43] Wilmore, J.H., Parr, R.B., Ward, T.J., Vodak, P.A., Barstow, T.J., Pipes, T.V., *et al.* (1978) Energy Cost of Circuit Weight Training. *Medicine and Science in Sports and Exercise*, **10**, 75-78.

[44] Rose, S.J. and Rothstein, J.M. (1982) General Concepts and Adaptations to Altered Patterns of Use. *Physical Therapy*, **62**, 1773-1787.

[45] Hurley, B. (1982) Effects of Resistive Training on Lipoprotein-Lipid Profiles: A Comparison to Aerobic Exercise Training. *Medicine and Science in Sports Exercise*, **21**, 689-693. http://dx.doi.org/10.1249/00005768-198912000-00012

[46] Williams, A.D., Almond, J., Ahuja, K.D.K., Beard, D.C., Robertson, I.K. and Ball, M.J. (2011) Cardiovascular and Metabolic Effects of Community Based Resistance Training in an Older Population. *Journal of Science and Medicine in Sport*, **14**, 331-337. http://dx.doi.org/10.1016/j.jsams.2011.02.011

[47] Taniguchi, Y. (1997) Lateral Specificity in Resistance Training: The Effect of Bilateral and Unilateral Training. *European Journal of Applied Physiology*, **75**, 144-150. http://dx.doi.org/10.1007/s004210050139

[48] Saito, M., Iwase, S. and Hachiya, T. (2009) Resistance Exercise Training Enhances Sympathetic Nerve Activity during Fatigue-Inducing Isometric Handgrip Trials. *European Journal of Applied Physiology*, **105**, 225-234. http://dx.doi.org/10.1007/s00421-008-0893-5

[49] Aubert, A.E., Seps, B. and Beckers, F. (2003) Heart Rate Variability in Athletes. *Sports Medicine*, **33**, 889-919. http://dx.doi.org/10.2165/00007256-200333120-00003

[50] Ribeiro, T.F., Azevedo, G.D., Crescencio, J.C., Maraes, V.R.F.S., Papa, V., Catai, A.M., *et al.* (2001) Heart Rate Variability under Resting Conditions in Postmenopausal and Young Women. *Brazilian Journal of Medical Biology Research*, **34**, 871-877. http://dx.doi.org/10.1590/S0100-879X2001000700006

[51] Bloomfield, D.M., Magnano, A., Bigger, J.R., Rivadeneira, H., Parides, M. and Steinman, R.C. (2001) Comparison of Spontaneous vs. Metronome-Guided Breathing on Assessment of Vagal Modulation Using RR Variability. *American Journal of Physiology*, **280**, H1145-H1150.

7

Salt Preference and the Incidence of Cardiovascular Disease in a Japanese General Population: The Jichi Medical School Cohort Study

Saki Tadenuma[1,2], Hideyuki Kanda[1*], Shizukiyo Ishikawa[3], Kazunori Kayaba[4],
Tadao Gotoh[5], Yosikazu Nakamura[6], Eiji Kajii[3]

[1]Department of Environmental Health and Public Health, Faculty of Medicine, Shimane University, Shimane, Japan
[2]Department of Anesthesiology, Faculty of Medicine, Shimane University, Shimane, Japan
[3]Division of Community and Family Medicine, Center for Community Medicine, Jichi Medical University, Tochigi, Japan
[4]Graduate School of Saitama Prefectural University, Saitama, Japan
[5]Wara National Health Insurance Clinic, Gifu, Japan
[6]Department of Public Health, Jichi Medical University, Tochigi, Japan
Email: *h-kanda@med.shimane-u.ac.jp

Abstract

Dietary salt intake has been reported to be associated with cardiovascular disease (CVD). However, there were few studies that assessed the relationship of salt preference with CVD. We examined the association between salt preference and the incidence of CVD and its subtypes in a Japanese general population. Based on the prospective Jichi Medical School Cohort Study, data were analyzed from 11,394 eligible participants. A baseline survey of the preference for salt was obtained by questionnaire and health examinations from April 1992 through July 1995 in 12 communities in Japan. The participants were followed up until December 2005 (mean follow-up period, 10.7 ± 2.4 years). Subjects were divided into three categories according to their preference for salt: favor, so-so, and disfavor. A Cox proportional hazards model was used to calculate hazard ratios (HRs) of the incidence of CVD according to the preference categories. We observed 485 cardiovascular events (258 in men and 227 in women). Among the men, the multivariable adjusted HRs for incidence of myocardial infarction and subarachnoid hemorrhage for favor versus so-so salt preference were 0.34 (95% confidence interval, 0.17 - 0.71) and 7.10 (0.88 - 56.84), respectively.

*Corresponding author.

Among the women, age-adjusted HRs for the incidence of CVD, total stroke, cerebral hemorrhage, and cerebral infarction for the favor preference were 1.41 (1.02 - 1.95), 1.36 (0.97 - 1.91), 1.79 (0.87 - 3.71), and 1.40 (0.89 - 2.19), respectively. The data indicated that preference for salt may be associated with an increase in the incidence of CVD in women.

Keywords

Salt Preference, Cardiovascular Disease, Cohort Study, Japanese

1. Introduction

Cardiovascular diseases (CVD), such as coronary heart disease (CHD) and stroke, are common causes of death and disabilities for elders in developed countries, including Japan, after hypertension and atherosclerosis. An estimated 17.5 million people died from CVD in 2012 (31% of all global deaths). Tobacco use, unhealthy diet and obesity, physical inactivity and harmful use of alcohol, diabetes and hyperlipidemia, hypertension and atherosclerosis are established risk factors for CVD. One of main causes on hypertension is much more salt intakes. Salt intakes influence individual salt preferences strongly [1].

Excessive salt intake affects the incidence and prevalence of hypertension, and subsequently influences the prevalence of cardiovascular disease (CVD) [2]. High salt intake has also been associated with increased CVD mortality and incidence [3]-[6]. The Japanese are known to have higher salt intake than many other populations [7]. In Japan, the mean salt intake among adults was 10.2 g per day (men, 11.3 g per day; women, 9.4 g per day) according to a national nutrition survey in 2013 [8]. Now, a new goal has been set to improve the level of salt intake among Japanese to within 8 g per day [9]. Therefore, dietary sodium restriction must be recommended to a considerable number of people. It is important to estimate salt intake and advice participants who consume excessive amounts of salt to reduce their salt intake. In general, daily salt intake may be estimated by a food frequency questionnaire or by measurement of 24 hour urinary sodium excretion [10]. However, both methods seem inconvenient for general use in mass screening. For these reasons, at health check-up centers or outpatient clinics, salt intake is usually estimated by a questionnaire on salt preference [11] [12].

Salt preference is thought to be associated with salt intake [13]. In a prospective study that examined the relationship between salt preference and CVD, salt preference was significantly positively associated with dietary sodium intake. Compared to the low salt preference group, the high salt preference group showed a relation to higher mortality from stroke [11]. However, few researches have attempted to assess the effects of salt preference on CVD. We could find no studies that clarified the relationships between salt preference and mortality from subtypes of CVD. As far as we know, no previous studies have reported an association of salt preference with the incidence of CVD and its subtypes.

Therefore, the aim of this study was to clarify the relationships between salt preference and the incidence of CVD and CVD subtypes using about 10 years of follow-up data from a large-scale prospective population-based cohort study conducted in Japan.

2. Subjects and Methods

2.1. Subjects

The Jichi Medical School (JMS) Cohort Study is a population-based prospective study that was started in 1992 to investigate the risk factors for CVD in 12 rural areas in Japan. A total of 12,490 people (4911 men and 7579 women) were enrolled in this study. Mass screening examinations for CVD have been conducted in Japan since 1982 under the direction of the Health and Medical Service Law for the Aged, and we used this system to collect the data. The baseline data were obtained from April 1992 through July 1995. Baseline examinations consisted of physical and blood examinations and a self-administered questionnaire. A detailed description of the standardized collection of baseline examinations was published previously [14].

Among the 12,490 participants, 95 (0.8%) declined follow-up and 7 (0.06%) could not be contacted after baseline examination, after which 12,388 subjects (4869 men and 7519 women) remained. We excluded participants with a history of CVD (96 men and 74 women) and those with missing data on salt preference (356 men and 468 women). Ultimately, 11,394 subjects (4417 men and 6977 women) were analyzed in the present study. Written informed consent to participate in the study was obtained individually from all of the participants in the mass screening. This study was approved by the Institutional Review Board of Jichi Medical School.

2.2. Baseline Examination

The health checkup was carried out in all 12 communities using same protocols. The body height of all participants was measured without shoes. Body weight while fully clothed was recorded; 0.5 kg in summer or 1 kg in other seasons was subtracted from the recorded weight. Body mass index (BMI) was calculated as weight (kg)/ height (m)^2. Systolic blood pressure (SBP) and diastolic blood pressure (DBP) at baseline were measured with a fully automated sphygmomanometer (BP203RV-II; Nippon Colin, Komaki, Japan), which was placed on the right arm of the participant after resting for at least 5 minutes in a sitting position. Serum cholesterol concentration was measured by taking a blood sample from the antecubital vein of the seated participants. Total cholesterol was measured using an enzymatic method, and high density lipoprotein cholesterol (HDL-C) was measured using the phosphotungstate precipitation method (Wako, Osaka, Japan; inter-assay coefficient of variation, 1.5%).

Information on age, lifestyle, and medical history was obtained from responses to the baseline questionnaire. Salt preference was ascertained with the following question: "Do you like salty foods?" Participants answered with 1 of 5 multiple choice options: "highly favor", "favor", "so-so", "moderately disfavor", or "disfavor". Subjects were divided into three categories of salt preference according to their response: favor: "highly favor" or "moderately favor"; so-so: "so-so"; and disfavor: "moderately disfavor" or "disfavor".

Smoking habit and alcohol drinking habit were determined from the baseline questions on current smoking and current drinking. Histories of hypertension, diabetes, and hyperlipidemia were determined from questions on the medical history of each illness. Response to the number of years of education was in terms of consecutive years; the response was then categorized as ≥9 years or <9 years.

2.3. Follow-Up

The national mass screening system used to obtain the baseline data for the JMS Cohort Study was also used to follow the subjects each year. Subjects were asked whether they had a history of CVD after enrolling. Follow-up was conducted from 1995 to 2005. The mean follow-up period ± standard deviation (SD) was 10.7 ± 2.4 years. Subjects who did not attend a follow-up examination were contacted by mail or telephone. If an incident case of stroke or myocardial infarction (MI) was suspected, those subjects with such histories were asked when and which hospital they visited. Medical records pertaining to stroke and MI were checked if the subjects were hospitalized for any reason, and incident cases were recorded. If both MI and stroke had occurred during the follow-up period, each of the endpoints of stroke and MI was counted as the first for each disease. The CVD endpoint was defined as stroke or MI, whichever occurred first. Death from CVD was also included in the CVD incidence data. Information on death was obtained from death certificates, which were collected at public health centers with the official permission from the Japanese Ministry of General Affairs and the Ministry of Health, Labour and Welfare until the end of 2005. Data on subjects who moved out of the study area during the follow-up period were obtained annually from the municipal government.

2.4. Diagnostic Criteria

If a CVD event was suspected, we requested duplicate images from computed tomography or magnetic resonance imaging (in cases of stroke) or electrocardiograms (in cases of MI). The diagnoses were determined independently by a diagnosis committee in the JMS Cohort Study Group composed of a radiologist, a neurologist, and two cardiologists. Criteria for stroke were a focal and nonconvulsive neurological deficit of sudden onset persisting longer than 24 hours. Stroke subtypes were categorized as cerebral hemorrhage, cerebral infarction, or subarachnoid hemorrhage (SAH) according to the criteria of the National Institute of Neurological Disorder and Stroke [15]. MI was diagnosed according to the criteria of the World Health Organization Multinational Monitoring of Trends and Determinants in Cardiovascular Disease (MONICA) Project [16].

2.5. Statistical Analysis

All analyses were conducted according to subject gender. Descriptive parameters are shown as the mean, standard deviation, or proportion (%). We compared characteristics between salt preference groups by the chi-square test or one-way analysis of variance. Finally, Cox proportional hazards models were used to calculate hazard ratios (HRs) with 95% confidence intervals (CIs) for the incidence of CVD according to salt preference, after adjusting for age, smoking habit, alcohol drinking habit, history of hyperlipidemia, and years of education (HR-all*) for men, and after adjusting for age, smoking habit, and alcohol drinking habit, BMI, HDL-C, and years of education (HR-all†) for women, which were considered to be potential confounding factors. HRs of each incidence of stroke, stroke subtypes, and MI were calculated by same statistical models. All p values were two-tailed, and a probability value < 0.05 was considered statistically significant. All analyses were performed using the Statistical Package for Social Science (SPSS) for Windows, version 16.0 (SPSS Inc., Japan).

3. Results

During a mean follow-up period of 10.7 years, we documented 485 CVD events (258 in men, 227 in women): 415 strokes (210 in men, 205 in women), including 264 cerebral infarctions (150 in men, 114 in women), 94 hemorrhagic strokes (47 in men, 47 in women), and 56 SAHs (13 in men, 43 in women), and 76 MIs (52 in men, 24 in women).

The baseline characteristics of the subjects by salt preference group are shown in **Table 1**. In both men and women, favor salt preference was positively associated with smoking ($p < 0.01$ for men; $p = 0.01$ for women) and alcohol drinking ($p < 0.01$ for men; $p = 0.02$ for women). Among the men, those in the favor salt preference group tended to be younger, more highly educated (both, $p < 0.01$), and less likely to have hyperlipidemia ($p = 0.04$). Among the women, those in the favor salt preference group tended to be older, less well educated (both, $p < 0.01$) and more likely to have both a higher incidence of CVD ($p = 0.046$) and higher BMI ($p < 0.01$) and a lower serum concentration of HDL-C ($p < 0.01$).

The incidence and HRs for CVD by salt preference category are shown in **Table 2**. After adjustment for age, there were no significant associations between salt preference and CVD or total stroke among the men. Our data showed 11 MIs, and the HR for MI was significantly lower in the favor salt subjects compared with so-so subjects (HR, 0.34; 95% CI, 0.17 - 0.68). After further multiple adjustment for smoking status, alcohol drinking status, history of hyperlipidemia, and years of education, the HR for MI was 0.35 (0.17 - 0.71). Among women, the HR for CVD was significantly higher in the favor salt subjects compared with the so-so subjects (HR, 1.41; 95% CI, 1.02 - 1.95) after adjustment for age. After further adjustment for smoking status, alcohol drinking status, BMI, HDL-C, and years of education, the HR was 1.15 (0.81 - 1.63). The HR for total stroke was also high (1.36; 95% CI, 0.97 - 1.91) in the favor salt subjects among women. After multivariate adjustment (HR-all†), HR was 1.08 (0.74 - 1.57). No significant association was found between salt preference and MI in the women, although a significant association was found in the men.

We also analyzed the respective association between salt preference and the incidences of stroke subtypes (**Table 3**). Among the men, there were 9 SAHs, and the HR was 8.09 (1.02 - 63.84) in the favor salt subjects after adjustment for age. After multivariate adjustment (HR-all*), the HR of SAHs was 7.10 (0.88 - 56.84). Among the women, age-adjusted HRs for cerebral hemorrhage and cerebral infarction were 1.79 (0.87 - 3.71) and 1.40 (0.89 - 2.19), respectively, in the favor salt subjects. After multivariate adjustment (HR-all†), HRs were 1.59 (0.74 - 3.44) and 1.07 (0.65 - 1.78), respectively.

4. Discussion

We investigated the association between salt preference and the incidence of CVD in a Japanese general population. We found that salt preference was positively associated with an increased risk of SAH and a decreased risk of MI in men. For women, salt preference was positively associated with an incidence of CVD after age-adjustment. HRs for incidences of cerebral hemorrhage and cerebral infarction were also higher, although not with significance. To our knowledge, this study is the first prospective study to provide evidence of the relationship of salt preference with the incidence of stroke.

We found that salt preference was associated with an increased incidence of CVD in the women. We examined CVD incidence data rather than mortality data as endpoints. Because the incidence of CVD occurs earlier

Table 1. Baseline characteristics of study participants by salt preference categories.

	Favor	So-so	Disfavor	
(Men) number (n)	1813	1585	1019	p-value[a]
Number of CVD incidence	91 (5.0)	102 (6.4)	65 (6.4)	0.15
Number of Stroke incidence	81 (4.5)	76 (4.8)	53 (5.2)	0.68
Number of MI incidence	11 (0.6)	29 (1.8)	12 (1.2)	<0.01**
				p-value[b]
Age (year)	54.5 (11.5)	54.6 (12.1)	56.7 (12.4)	<0.01**
Systolic blood pressure (mmHg)	131.6 (20.6)	131.1 (21.0)	131.0 (21.0)	0.66
Diastolic blood pressure (mmHg)	79.3 (12.3)	79.0 (12.1)	79.0 (12.6)	0.71
Total-cholesterol (mg/dl)	183.8 (34.4)	186.3 (33.7)	185.3 (34.7)	0.10
HDL-cholesterol (mg/dl)	49.3 (13.6)	49.0 (13.6)	48.1 (13.0)	0.08
Body mass index (kg/m^2)	23.0 (2.9)	23.0 (2.9)	22.9 (2.9)	0.51
Current Smokers	55.8	49.2	43.4	<0.01**
Current Drinkers	78.2	75.5	70.4	<0.01**
History of hypertension	8.8	9.8	10.7	0.27
History of diabetes mellitus	1.9	2.7	3.0	0.12
History of hyperlipidemia	0.7	1.4	1.8	0.04*
Education years (over 9 years)	88.5	88.7	83.4	<0.01**
(Women) number (n)	1618	2885	2474	p-value[a]
Number of CVD incidence	67 (4.1)	80 (2.8)	80 (3.2)	0.046*
Number of stroke incidence	60 (3.7)	74 (2.6)	71 (2.9)	0.09
Number of MI incidence	7 (0.4)	8 (0.2)	9 (0.4)	0.68
				p-value[b]
Age (year)	55.8 (11.0)	54.8 (11.0)	55.5 (11.5)	<0.01*
Systolic blood pressure (mmHg)	128.9 (21.5)	127.9 (20.9)	127.6 (21.0)	0.15
Diastolic blood pressure (mmHg)	76.8 (12.3)	76.2 (12.0)	76.0 (12.1)	0.08
Total-cholesterol (mg/dl)	196.5 (34.1)	197.2 (35.5)	197.1 (34.5)	0.81
HDL-cholesterol (mg/dl)	51.5 (12.0)	52.5 (12.5)	53.8 (12.7)	<0.01**
Body Mass Index (kg/m^2)	23.5 (3.3)	23.1 (3.1)	23.0 (3.2)	<0.01**
Current smokers	6.9	5.1	5.0	0.01*
Current drinkers	26.9	25.6	23	0.02*
History of hypertension	12.9	11.6	12.4	0.39
History of diabetes mellitus	1.2	1.6	2.0	0.14
History of hyperlipidemia	1.5	2.3	2.1	0.16
Education years (over 9 years)	75.9	81.2	80.0	<0.01**

Data are expressed as a mean (standard deviation) for variables or as a percentage of the population. [a]Chi-square test; [b]Analysis of variance (ANOVA); *p values were < 0.05; **p values were < 0.01.

Table 2. Hazard ratios and 95% CIs of incidence from cardiovascular disease and myocardial infarction with gender difference by salt preference categories.

	Salt preference category		
	Favor	So-so	Disfavor
Men			
Cardiovascular disease[§]			
N	91	102	65
HR-age	0.80 (0.60 - 1.06)	1.00	0.83 (0.61 - 1.13)
HR-all[*]	0.75 (0.57 - 1.01)	1.00	0.84 (0.61 - 1.17)
Total-stroke			
N	81	76	53
HR-age	0.97 (0.71 - 1.33)	1.00	0.9 (0.63 - 1.28)
HR-all[*]	0.90 (0.64 - 1.25)	1.00	0.89 (0.62 - 1.28)
Myocardial infarction			
N	11	29	12
HR-age	0.34 (0.17 - 0.68)	1.00	0.55 (0.28 - 1.09)
HR-all[*]	0.35 (0.17 - 0.71)	1.00	0.64 (0.33 - 1.24)
Women			
Cardiovascular disease[§]			
N	67	80	80
HR-age	1.41 (1.02 - 1.95)	1.00	1.11 (0.81 - 1.51)
HR-all[†]	1.15 (0.81 - 1.63)	1.00	1.14 (0.83 - 1.57)
Total-stroke			
N	60	74	71
HR-age	1.36 (0.97 - 1.91)	1.00	1.06 (0.78 - 1.47)
HR-all[†]	1.08 (0.74 - 1.57)	1.00	1.09 (0.78 - 1.52)
Myocardial infarction			
N	7	8	9
HR-age	1.44 (0.52 - 3.98)	1.00	1.38 (0.54 - 3.50)
HR-all[†]	1.37 (0.49 - 3.82)	1.00	1.29 (0.50 - 3.36)

HR-age: hazard ratios adjusted for age. HR-all[*]: hazard ratios adjusted for age, smoking status and drinking status, history of hyperlipidemia, and education years. HR-all[†]: hazard ratios adjusted for age, smoking status and drinking status, BMI, HDL-choesterol, and education years. [§]: The case which occurred both stroke and myocardial infarction is included.

than that of mortality, our study was significant in that we captured the risk of CVD at an earlier stage. With respect to Japanese studies, the Japan Collaborative Cohort Study for Evaluation of Cancer Risk (JACC Study) reported an association between salt preference and mortality from stroke among Japanese men and women [11]. In that study, subjects were divided into three categories according to their preference answer. Compared to the low salt preference group, the salt preference group was associated with higher mortality from stroke after 16.4 years of follow-up: The multivariable HRs for CVD were 1.05 (0.92 - 1.20) for men and 1.05 (0.92 - 1.19) for

Table 3. Hazard ratios and 95%CIs of incidence of subtypes of stroke with gender differrence by salt preference categories.

	Salt preference category		
	Favor	So-so	Disfavor
Men			
Cerebral hemorrhage			
N	18	17	12
HR-age	0.96 (0.49 - 1.87)	1.00	0.92 (0.44 - 1.91)
HR-all[*]	0.84 (0.41 - 1.70)	1.00	0.86 (0.40 - 1.88)
Cerebral infarction			
N	54	58	38
HR-age	0.85 (0.59 - 1.24)	1.00	0.84 (0.56 - 1.26)
HR-all[*]	0.80 (0.54 - 1.17)	1.00	0.86 (0.56 - 1.32)
Subarachnoid hemorrhage			
N	9	1	3
HR-age	8.09 (1.02 - 63.84)	1.00	4.12 (0.42 - 39.78)
HR-all[*]	7.10 (0.88 - 56.84)	1.00	2.62 (0.24 - 29.10)
Women			
Cerebral hemorrhage			
N	15	14	18
HR-age	1.79 (0.87 - 3.71)	1.00	1.42 (0.70 - 2.85)
HR-all[†]	1.59 (0.74 - 3.44)	1.00	1.59 (0.78 - 3.27)
Cerebral infarction			
N	36	42	36
HR-age	1.40 (0.89 - 2.19)	1.00	0.93 (0.59 - 1.45)
HR-all[†]	1.07 (0.65 - 1.78)	1.00	0.94 (0.59 - 1.49)
Subarachnoid hemorrhage			
N	8	18	17
HR-age	0.78 (0.34 - 1.81)	1.00	1.10 (0.56 - 2.14)
HR-all[†]	0.65 (0.27 - 1.56)	1.00	1.05 (0.54 - 2.07)

HR-age: hazard ratios adjusted for age. HR-all[*]: hazard ratios adjusted for age, smoking status and drinking status, history of hyperlipidemia, and education years. HR-all[†]: hazard ratios adjusted for age, smoking status and drinking status, MI, and HDL-cholesterol, and education years.

women. HRs for stroke were 1.21 (0.99 - 1.49) for men and 1.22 (1.00 - 1.49) for women. It is possible that the discrepancies in the results between the JACC Study and our study were due to differences in the number of participants, follow-up period, and examination end points. Our study suggested the possibility that salt preference was associated with the stage of CVD incidence rather than mortality, with gender differences.

High salt preference may result in a long-term, high-sodium intake, then leading to high blood pressure and an increased risk of CVD. Several previous studies reported positive associations between salt preference and salt intake [12] [17] [18] and between salt intake and the incidence of CVD or mortality [3]-[6]. Several explanations for the associations between sodium intake and CVD have been put forward. High salt intakes influence

CVD by altering left ventricular mass [19] or increasing blood flow and vascular reactivity [20] [21]. In our study, the incidence of CVD was high for women. Our targets among women were almost local residents. So, the incidence of CVD may be slightly higher than the previous study. For women, high salt preference tended to be less well educated. Therefore, subjects with high salt preference may have behavioral risk factors, leading to higher risk of CVD in the women. Accordingly, women with a high salt preference may intake much more salt than those with a low salt preference. Further investigations are necessary to clarify sex difference in cardiovascular risk factors.

In our study, favor salt preference was positively associated with smoking and alcohol drinking in both men and women. The men in the favor salt preference group tended to be younger and more highly educated, whereas the women in the salt preference group tended to be older, less well educated, and more likely to have a higher BMI and lower serum concentration of HDL-C. Despite these results, salt preference was not associated with CVD risk factors such as SBP, DBP, and a history of hypertension. Our results suggest that salt preference may be one of the risk factors of premature CVD. It is also possible that some people with a high salt preference developed hypertension that led to CVD during the follow-up period. Among the women, salt preference was associated with the incidence of CVD after age adjustment. After adjustment for smoking status, alcohol drinking status, BMI, HDL-C, and years of education, the risk of CVD was attenuated. Accordingly, the influence of common risk factors on CVD incidence was strong for women, and salt preference may reflect accumulation of confounding risk factors except for age. These common factors can be self-managed and self-controlled. People indicating a high salt preference in the detailed interview during health check-ups should be recommended to practice adequate health behavior for the prevention of CVD in daily life, especially for women.

Salt preference and food intake are affected by socioeconomic and psychophysiological factors such as recent dietary habit, culture, and income [22] [23]. Taste preferences are acquired early in life through the process of choosing foods and actual salt intake [24]. Lampure *et al.* reported that as a new pathway without a common route that leads to CVD, salt preference was associated with uncontrolled eating behavior [25], which is the tendency to lose control over eating when hungry or when exposed to external stimuli. A previous study showed that binge eating was associated with a higher incidence of a new diagnosis of dyslipidemia, any metabolic syndrome component (hypertension, dyslipidemia, or type 2 diabetes), and two or more components of metabolic syndrome after 5 years of follow-up [26]. Thus, eating disorders such as uncontrolled eating behavior can result in a relationship between salt preference and the occurrence of CVD.

In our study, salt preference tended to be inversely associated with the incidence of MI in the men. Our results are similar to those of a previous study [11] although the reason for this cannot be fully explained. The decreased risk of MI associated with high salt preference might reflect the beneficial cardiovascular effects of the intake of n − 3 polyunsaturated fatty acids and isoflavones in the inhibition of platelet aggregation, lowering of blood pressure, and modulation of the inflammatory system [27] [28]. For the men in the present study, the low incidence of MI and the high incidence of SAH were based on a small number of incident cases. Thus, there was wide range of 95% CIs for the point estimates.

For women, salt preference may reflect common risk factors that will cause CVD in the future and other unknown factors such as eating behavior in an earlier stage of life. Especially in women, early assessment of salt preference may be effective in reducing the incidence of CVD. For subjects with high salt preference, early intervention may be able to prevent excessive salt intake and uncontrolled eating behavior in the future.

Our study has several strengths. First, it was conducted as a large-scale multicenter cohort study. In addition, we investigated the incidence of not only CVD but also stroke subtypes as endpoints. However, there were several limitations. First, the follow-up period was shorter, and second, the numbers of subjects with an incidence of CVD were less than those of a previous study [11]. Third, estimated salt intake is not measured quantitatively. It is unclear whether the salt preference questionnaire reflects the responder's actual salt intake. Fourth, the participants were recruited through a mass screening program, and therefore, their concern for health may exceed that of the general population, which could result in differences in salt intake and other behavioral profiles. Finally, we were unable to control for other potential confounders such as nutrient factors and income.

5. Conclusion

We found that salt preference was positively associated with an increased risk of the incidence of SAH in men after multivariate adjustment and in CVD in women after adjustment for age. As with other common risk factors for CVD, assessing salt preference may lead to the prevention of CVD because such assessment may help to prevent excessive salt intake and uncontrolled eating behavior in the future. These tendencies may apply especially to women.

Acknowledgements

We are grateful to Mr. Yasuyuki Fujita and Mr. Tsuyoshi for the advice to this study. This study was supported by Grant-in-Aid from the Ministry of Education, Culture, Sports, Science and Technology, Japan, and grants from the Foundation for the Development of the Community, Tochigi, Japan.

References

[1]   World Health Organization (2015) Cardiovascular Diseases. http://www.who.int/mediacentre/factsheets/fs317/en/

[2]   He, F.J. and MacGregor, G.A. (2007) Salt, Blood Pressure and Cardiovascular Disease. *Current Opinion in Cardiology*, **22**, 298-305. http://dx.doi.org/10.1097/HCO.0b013e32814f1d8c

[3]   Gardener, H., Rundek, T., Wright, C.B., Elkind, M.S. and Sacco, R.L. (2012) Dietary Sodium and Risk of Stroke in the Northern Manhattan Study. *Stroke*, **43**, 1200-1205. http://dx.doi.org/10.1161/STROKEAHA.111.641043

[4]   Strazzullo, P., D'Elia, L., Kandala, N.B. and Cappuccio, F.P. (2009) Salt Intake, Stroke, and Cardiovascular Disease: Meta-Analysis of Prospective Studies. *BMJ*, **339**, b4567. http://dx.doi.org/10.1136/bmj.b4567

[5]   Tuomilehto, J., Jousilahti, P., Rastenyte, D., Moltchanov, V., Tanskanen, A., Pietinen, P. and Nissinen, A. (2001) Urinary Sodium Excretion and Cardiovascular Mortality in Finland: A Prospective Study. *Lancet*, **357**, 848-851. http://dx.doi.org/10.1016/S0140-6736(00)04199-4

[6]   Umesawa, M., Iso, H., Date, C., Yamamoto, A., Toyoshima, H., Watanabe, Y., Kikuchi, S., Koizumi, A., Kondo, T., Inaba, Y., Tanabe, N., Tamakoshi, A. and Group, J.S. (2008) Relations between Dietary Sodium and Potassium Intakes and Mortality from Cardiovascular Disease: The Japan Collaborative Cohort Study for Evaluation of Cancer Risks. *The American Journal of Clinical Nutrition*, **88**, 195-202.

[7]   Zhou, B.F., Stamler, J., Dennis, B., Moag-Stahlberg, A., Okuda, N., Robertson, C., Zhao, L., Chan, Q., Elliott, P. and Group, I.R. (2003) Nutrient Intakes of Middle-Aged Men and Women in China, Japan, United Kingdom, and United States in the Late 1990s: The INTERMAP Study. *Journal of Human Hypertension*, **17**, 623-630. http://dx.doi.org/10.1038/sj.jhh.1001605

[8]   Ministry of Health, of Health, Labour and Welfare (2013) National Health and Nutrition Survey Japan. (In Japanese). http://www.mhlw.go.jp/bunya/kenkou/eiyou/dl/h25-houkoku-04.pdf

[9]   Ministry of Health Labour and Welfare (2012) The Basic Policies for Comprehensive Public Health Promotion (Health Japan 21, 2nd Term). http://www.mhlw.go.jp/file/06-Seisakujouhou-10900000-Kenkoukyoku/0000047330.pdf

[10]   Bentley, B. (2006) A Review of Methods to Measure Dietary Sodium Intake. *The Journal of Cardiovascular Nursing*, **21**, 63-67. http://dx.doi.org/10.1097/00005082-200601000-00012

[11]   Ikehara, S., Iso, H., Date, C., Kikuchi, S., Watanabe, Y., Inaba, Y., Tamakoshi, A. and Group, J.S. (2012) Salt Preference and Mortality from Stroke and Coronary Heart Disease for Japanese Men and Women: The JACC Study. *Preventive Medicine*, **54**, 32-37. http://dx.doi.org/10.1016/j.ypmed.2011.10.013

[12]   Takamura, K., Okayama, M., Takeshima, T., Fujiwara, S., Harada, M., Murakami, J., Eto, M. and Kajii, E. (2014) Influence of Salty Food Preference on Daily Salt Intake in Primary Care. *International Journal of General Medicine*, **7**, 205-210.

[13]   Van der Veen, J.E., De Graaf, C., Van Dis, S.J. and Van Staveren, W.A. (1999) Determinants of Salt Use in Cooked Meals in The Netherlands: Attitudes and Practices of Food Preparers. *European Journal of Clinical Nutrition*, **53**, 388-394. http://dx.doi.org/10.1038/sj.ejcn.1600737

[14]   Ishikawa, S., Gotoh, T., Nago, N. and Kayaba, K. (2002) The Jichi Medical School (JMS) Cohort Study: Design, Baseline Data and Standardized Mortality Ratios. *Journal of Epidemiology/Japan Epidemiological Association*, **12**, 408-417. http://dx.doi.org/10.2188/jea.12.408

[15]   Adams Jr., H.P., Bendixen, B.H., Kappelle, L.J., Biller, J., Love, B.B., Gordon, D.L. and Marsh 3rd., E.E. (1993) Classification of Subtype of Acute Ischemic Stroke. Definitions for Use in a Multicenter Clinical Trial. TOAST. Trial of Org 10172 in Acute Stroke Treatment. *Stroke*, **24**, 35-41. http://dx.doi.org/10.1161/01.STR.24.1.35

[16]   World Health Organization (1988) The World Health Organization MONICA Project (Monitoring Trends and Determinants in Cardiovascular Disease): A Major International Collaboration. WHO MONICA Project Principal Investigators. *Journal of Clinical Epidemiology*, **41**, 105-114. http://dx.doi.org/10.1016/0895-4356(88)90084-4

[17]   Hashimoto, T., Yagami, F., Owada, M., Sugawara, T. and Kawamura, M. (2008) Salt Preference According to a Ques-

tionnaire vs. Dietary Salt Intake Estimated by a Spot Urine Method in Participants at a Health Check-Up Center. *Internal medicine*, **47**, 399-403. http://dx.doi.org/10.2169/internalmedicine.47.0622

[18] Takachi, R., Ishihara, J., Iwasaki, M., Ishii, Y. and Tsugane, S. (2014) Self-Reported Taste Preference Can Be a Proxy for Daily Sodium Intake in Middle-Aged Japanese Adults. *Journal of the Academy of Nutrition and Dietetics*, **114**, 781-787. http://dx.doi.org/10.1016/j.jand.2013.07.043

[19] Frohlich, E.D. and Varagic, J. (2004) The Role of Sodium in Hypertension Is More Complex than Simply Elevating Arterial Pressure. Nature Clinical Practice. *Cardiovascular Medicine*, **1**, 24-30.

[20] Meneton, P., Jeunemaitre, X., de Wardener, H.E. and MacGregor, G.A. (2005) Links between Dietary Salt Intake, Renal Salt Handling, Blood Pressure, and Cardiovascular Diseases. *Physiological Reviews*, **85**, 679-715. http://dx.doi.org/10.1152/physrev.00056.2003

[21] Simon, G. (2003) Experimental Evidence for Blood Pressure-Independent Vascular Effects of High Sodium Diet. *American journal of hypertension*, **16**, 1074-1078.

[22] Leshem, M. (2009) Biobehavior of the Human Love of Salt. *Neuroscience & Biobehavioral Reviews*, **33**, 1-17. http://dx.doi.org/doi:10.1016/j.neubiorev.2008.07.007

[23] Drewnowski, A. (1997) Taste Preferences and Food Intake. *Annual Review of Nutrition*, **17**, 237-253. http://dx.doi.org/doi:10.1146/annurev.nutr.17.1.237

[24] Birch, L.L. (1999) Development of Food Preferences. *Annual Review of Nutrition*, **19**, 41-62. http://dx.doi.org/doi:10.1146/annurev.nutr.19.1.41

[25] Lampure, A., Schlich, P., Deglaire, A., Castetbon, K., Peneau, S., Hercberg, S. and Mejean, C. (2015) Sociodemographic, Psychological, and Lifestyle Characteristics Are Associated with a Liking for Salty and Sweet Tastes in French Adults. *The Journal of Nutrition*, **145**, 587-594. http://dx.doi.org/doi:10.3945/jn.114.201269

[26] Hudson, J.I., Lalonde, J.K., Coit, C.E., Tsuang, M.T., McElroy, S.L., Crow, S.J., Bulik, C.M., Hudson, M.S., Yanovski, J.A., Rosenthal, N.R. and Pope Jr., H.G. (2010) Longitudinal Study of the Diagnosis of Components of the Metabolic Syndrome in Individuals with Binge-Eating Disorder. *The American Journal of Clinical Nutrition*, **91**, 1568-1573. http://dx.doi.org/doi:10.3945/ajcn.2010.29203

[27] Iso, H., Kobayashi, M., Ishihara, J., Sasaki, S., Okada, K., Kita, Y., Kokubo, Y., Tsugane, S. and Group, J.S. (2006) Intake of Fish and n3 Fatty Acids and Risk of Coronary Heart Disease among Japanese: The Japan Public Health Center-Based (JPHC) Study Cohort I. *Circulation*, **113**, 195-202. http://dx.doi.org/doi:10.1161/CIRCULATIONAHA.105.581355

[28] Kokubo, Y., Iso, H., Ishihara, J., Okada, K., Inoue, M., Tsugane, S. and Group, J.S. (2007) Association of Dietary Intake of Soy, Beans, and Isoflavones with Risk of Cerebral and Myocardial Infarctions in Japanese Populations: The Japan Public Health Center-Based (JPHC) Study Cohort I. *Circulation*, **116**, 2553-2562. http://dx.doi.org/doi:10.1161/CIRCULATIONAHA.106.683755

Appendix

The Jichi Medical School Cohort Study Group: Akizumi Tsutsumi (Occupational Health Training Center, University of Occupational and Environmental Health, Fukuoka), Atsushi Hashimoto (Aichi Prefectural Aichi Hospital, Aichi), EijiKajii (Department of Community and Family Medicine, Jichi Medical School, Tochigi), Hideki Miyamoto (former Department of Community and Family Medicine, Jichi Medical School, Tochigi), Hidetaka Akiyoshi (Department of Pediatrics, Fukuoka University School of Medicine), Hiroshi Yanagawa (Saitama Prefectural University, Saitama), Hitoshi Matsuo (Gifu Prefectural Gifu Hospital, Gifu), Jun Hiraoka (Tako Central Hospital, Chiba), Kaname Tsutsumi (Kyushu International University, Fukuoka), Kazunori Kayaba (Saitama Prefectural University), KazuomiKario (Department of Cardiology, Jichi Medical School, Tochigi), Kazuyuki Shimada (Department of Cardiology, Jichi Medical School, Tochigi), Kenichiro Sakai (Akaike Town Hospital, Fukuoka), Kishio Turuda (Takasu National Health Insurance Clinic, Gifu), Machi Sawada (Agawa Osaki National Health Insurance Clinic, Kochi), Makoto Furuse (Department of Radiology, Jichi Medical School, Tochigi), Manabu Yoshimura (Kuze Clinic, Gifu), Masahiko Hosoe (Gero Hot-Spring Hospital, Gifu), Masahiro Igarashi, Masafumi Mizooka (Kamagari National Health Insurance Clinic, Hiroshima), Naoki Nago (Tsukude Health Insurance Clinic, Aichi), Nobuya Kodama (Sakugi Clinic, Hiroshima), Noriko Hayashida (Tako Central Hospital, Chiba), Rika Yamaoka (Awaji-Hokudan Public Clinic, Hyogo), Seishi Yamada (Wara National Health Insurance Hospital, Gifu), Shinichi Muramatsu (Department Neurology, Jichi Medical School, Tochigi), Shinya Hayasaka, Shizukiyo Ishikawa (Department of Community and Family Medicine, Jichi Medical School, Tochigi), Shuzo Takuma (Akaike Town Hospital, Fukuoka), Tadao Gotoh (Wara National Health Insurance Hospital, Gifu), Takafumi Natsume (Oyama Municipal Hospital, Tochigi), Takashi Yamada (Kuze Clinic, Gifu), Takeshi Miyamoto (former Okawa Komatsu National Health Insurance Clinic, Kochi), Tomohiro Deguchi (Akaike Town Hospital, Fukuoka), Tomohiro Saegusa (Sakuma National Health Insurance Hospital, Shizuoka), Yoshihiro Shibano (Saiseikai Iwaizumi Hospital, Iwate) Yoshihisa Ito (Department of Laboratory Medicine, Asahikawa Medical College, Hokkaido), and Yosikazu Nakamura (Department of Public Health, Jichi Medical School).

Abbreviations

CVD: cardiovascular disease
JMS Cohort Study: Jichi Medical School Cohort Study
HDs: hazardratios
HR-all[*]: hazard ratios adjusted for age, smoking status and drinking status, history of hyperlipidemia, and education years
HR-all[†]: hazard ratios adjusted for age, smoking status and drinking status, BMI, HDL-cholesterol, and education years
BMI: body mass index
SBP: systolic blood pressure
DBP: diastolic blood pressure
HDL-C: high density lipoprotein cholesterol
MI: myocardial infarction
SAH: subarachnoid hemorrhage
MONICA Project: Multinational Monitoring of Trends and Determinants in Cardiovascular Disease Project
JACC study: the Japan Collaborative Cohort Study for Evaluation of Cancer Risk

8

Relationships between Demographic Variables and Breast Self-Examination among Women in a Rural Community South East of Nigeria

Ada C. Nwaneri[1], Eunice Ogonna Osuala[2*], Ijeoma Okoronkwo[1], Patricia Uzor Okpala[1], Anthonia Chidinma Emesowum[3]

[1]Department of Nursing, University of Nigeria, Enugu Campus, Nsukka, Nigeria
[2]Department of Nursing Science, Nnamdi Azikiwe University, Nnewi Campus, Awka, Nigeria
[3]Department of Nursing, Imo State University, Orlu Campus, Owerri, Nigeria
Email: *euniceosuala@yahoo.com

Abstract

This study examined the relationships between demographic variables of women in a rural community, South East of Nigeria and their practice of Breast Self-Examination (BSE). A descriptive survey design was adopted. The study population of 349 was drawn using system atichousehold sampling technique. Two research questions and three null hypotheses guided the study. The instruments used for data collection were validated structured questionnaire which was interview administered. Demographic information of the women such was also obtained for the study. The result indicated significant correlation between respondents' educational level and BSE. There was however no significance difference between age, parity and BSE. There was need for community health nurses to reinforce home visits in order to enhance the awareness of breast cancer and needed skill for BSE among the rural populace while liberal education irrespective of age should be instituted by the Government.

Keywords

Demographic Variables, Breast Self-Examination, Rural-Women

---

*Corresponding author.

1. Introduction

Breast cancer is the commonest cancer and remains the most lethal malignancy in women across the world [1]. It constitutes a major public health issue globally with over one million new cases diagnosed annually, resulting in over 400,000 annual deaths and about 4.4 million women living with the disease [2] [3]. In Nigeria, the number of women at risk of breast cancer increased steadily from approximately 24.5 million in 1900 to approximately 40 million in 2010 and is projected to rise to over 50 million by 2020 [4]. Statistics from the Ministry of Health Nigeria shows that breast cancer has risen at least four times over the decade and has accounted for 40 percent of women cancers [5]. In the present scenario, roughly 1 in 26 women is expected to be diagnosed with breast cancer in their life time, majority of cases occurring in pre-menopausal women [1]. Following hospital records in Nigeria, breast cancer is truly an epidemic among women as it is estimated that 211,000 new cases of invasive breast cancer are diagnosed in a year, and 43,000 patients died of the disease [6].

The high mortality reported on breast cancer is as a result of late presentation at advanced stage with poorer clinical and pathological prognostic outcome. With early detection, five year survival rate of over 85% is achieved whereas late detection decreases the survival rate to 5% (1: 4). The low survival rates of breast cancer in less developed countries can be attributed to lack of early detection as well as inadequate diagnosis and treatment facilities. Chiejina [7] notes that what is more worrisome in a country like Nigeria with over 140 million people is that the detection of the disease is usually late. For women to present early, they must be able to recognize symptoms of breast cancer through routine practice. BSE may be influenced by awareness of breast cancer, some demographic variables as age and parity as well as the skill for breast examination. Descriptive survey design with the aid of a questionnaire is served as an interview schedule for the study on 349 women in Umuowa, Orlu L.G.A of Imo State. The objective of this study is to find out if there exists relationships between age, educational level, parity of rural women and their practice of Breast Self-Examination. Findings will guide future intervention in scaling up BSE in the community. The study is guided by four research questions and three hypotheses.

2. Research Questions

- How do the women of Umuowa Orlu LGA practice BSE?
- How does demographic variable of age, academic attainment and parity of respondents relate to practice of BSE?

3. Hypotheses

- There is no significant relationship between the age of respondents and their BSE practice.
- There is no significant relationship between the educational attainment of respondents and their BSE practice.
- There is no significant relationship between the parity of respondents and their BSE practice.

4. Materials and Methods

4.1. Design and Sampling

This is a descriptive survey design conducted among 349 women (Ages 20-70) from a rural community in the South East of Nigeria from 3rd to 28th February 2015. The sample was drawn from a target population [8] of 3820 using Krejcie and Morgan [9] power analysis formular (S = X^2NP (1 − P)/d^2 (N − 1). Systematic sampling technique was used to pick the required households. The sampling interval was every 11th household. The women in each of the selected households that met the inclusion criteria (aged between 20 and 70, single or married, residing in the community for a minimum of one year) were included in the study based on their willingness.

5. Instrument

Instrument for data collection was a questionnaire formulated by researchers based on the objective of the study. Questionnaire was validated through experts in the field of Gynacology, Measurement and Evaluation and Community Health Nursing. Back translation from English to Igbo language was done by higher school teachers in English and Igbo (Local) languages respectively for congruency. The instrument consisted of two major sections A and B. Section A contains the demographic characteristics while section B had questions on practice. A pilot study on 40 women from another community with same characteristics was done. Coefficient correlation of 0.78 was computed on a test-retest of the instrument. Same was interview administered by three nurses. The exercise was on daily basis and the interview was on one on one lasting for 10 minutes per participant. The literate ones were interviewed in English while the non literate were interviewed in Igbo. Research question was answered using responses to questions 19 to 27 of the research instrument which extracted responses on frequency, procedure and observations made. The questionnaire which was interview administered was filled for every woman, in the 11th household, who is within the age limit and gave consent to participate, until the required sample was got. Data was collected after obtaining ethical approval from the ethical committee of the University of Nigeria Teaching Hospital, Enugu, Nigeria.

6. Data Analysis

Research questions were answered using responses to questions 19 to 27 of the research instrument which extracted information on breast self examination. The 4 questions on frequency and 1 on observation had a maximum score of 8 and 3 respectively while the 4 questions on procedure had a maximum score of 8. Composite score was computed after summation of scores per participant. The responses were scored over 19, and rated as follows:

Scores ≤ 6   -   Inadequate practice
Scores from 7 to 12   -   Moderately adequate practice
Scores from 13 to 19   -   Highly adequate practice

Descriptive and inferential analysis was carried out using Social Package for Social Sciences version 18. Mean score, standard deviation (SD) Pearson's Correlation Coefficient (R), and Spearman Rank Correlation Coefficient (rho) were used to answer the research questions while Chi-square, was adopted in testing the null hypotheses at 0.05 level of significance.

7. Results

7.1. Demographic Characteristics

The respondents that were within the age range of (20 - 30) constituted 30.1% while those that were within the ages 51 - 60 were the least in number 38 (10.5%). Mean age of respondents was 42 ± 10.7. Majority of the respondents, 183 (52.41%) were married while 88 (25.2%) were single. One hundred and twenty nine (37.0%) had tertiary education and only 15 (4.3%) had no formal education. Ninety-six (27.5%) were civil servants while 52 (14.9%), 46 (13.2%) and 39 (11.2%) were farmers, traders and business women. One hundred and two (29.2%) of the women are primigravida, 53 (15.2%) have one child each while 108 (31%), 52 (15%) and 34 (10 %) have 2 - 3, 4 - 5 and 6 or more children respectively (**Table 1**).

7.2. Practice of BSE

7.2.1. Frequency, Timing, Method and Barriers
Findings on practice showed that 50.1% of participants had inadequate level of practice, 33.5% moderately inadequate and 16.3% are highly adequate in practice. Responses on practice showed that one hundred and eighty one (51.9%) respondents have performed BSE while 168 (48.1%) respondents have not. Out of the 181 respondents that had performed BSE, 32 (17.7%) said they performed it once a month, 27 (16.0%) performed it once in two months, 19 (10.4%) performed it once in three months, 94 (51.9%) performed BSE anytime that was convenient while 9 (5.0%) respondents said they do not know how often they performed the examination. Concerning the timing of BSE, 24 (13.3%) respondents said they performed BSE 2nd to 3rd day after menstruation. 53 (27.3%) performed it 2nd to 3rd day before menstruation, 10 (5.5%) examined the breast during ovulation while 94 (51.9%) did not have any specific time for performing BSE. Reasons for not performing BSE were also sought. Out of the 168 respondents that have not performed BSE, 8 (4.4%) respondents gave their reason as lack of confidence on how to do it, 105 (62.4%) the respondents said it was because they were not sure of their ability to detect breast changes. 5 (3.0%) said it was because they found the process BSE difficult to remember. 40 (23.8%) respondents had no time while 10 (6.0%) respondents said it was because they had no family history of

breast cancer and do not see the need. None of respondents found BSE embarrassing, for BSE (**Table 1**). Assessment of the steps that the participants' follow when performing BSE showed that 36 (19.9%) respondents examined the breasts in front of a mirror with breast and chest (top) exposed, while 145 (80.1%) respondents did not. 35 (19.3%) respondents noted that they checked for dimpling, swelling, soreness, in all parts of the breast in front of the mirror while 146 (80.7%) did not. 45 (24.9%) respondents changed position to look at the different parts of the breast while 136 (75.1%) did not. 65 (35.9%) respondents said they looked for dimpling, swelling, soreness in all parts of the breast in the mirror with arm raised while 116 (64.1%) respondents deferred on this (**Table 2**).

Table 1. Demographic characteristics of respondents n = 349.

		Frequency	Percent (%)
Age	20 - 30	105	30.1
	31 - 40	67	19.2
	41 - 50	55	15.8
	51 - 60	38	10.9
	61 and above	84	24.1
	Total	349	100.0
Marital Status	Single	88	25.2
	Married	183	52.4
	Divorced	16	4.6
	Widowed	51	14.6
	Separated	11	3.2
	Total	349	100.0
Educational Qualification	No formal education	15	4.3
	Primary education	79	22.6
	Secondary education	121	34.7
	Tertiary education	129	37.0
	Others	5	1.4
	Total	349	100.0
Parity	None	102	29.2
	1 Only	53	15.2
	2 - 3	108	30.9
	4 - 5	52	14.9
	6 and above	34	9.7
	Total	349	100.0

Table 2. Frequency of practice of BSE n = 181.

Question	Options	Freq. (%)
Have you ever performed breast self examination?	Yes	181 (51.9)
	No	168 (48.1)
If yes, how often do you perform it? (n = 181)	Once a month	32 (17.7)
	Once in two months	27 (16.0)
	Once in three months	19 (10.0)
	Anytime is convenient	94 (51.9)
	Don't know how often	9 (17.7)
At what time do you perform breast self examination? (n = 181)	2nd-3rd day after menses	24 (13.3)
	2nd-3rd day before menses	53 (27.3)
	during menses	0 (0.0)
	during ovulation	10 (5.5)
	no specific time	94 (51.9)
If you don't, what are your reasons for not doing it? (n = 168)	Not confident on how to do it	8 (4.8)
	Not sure of ability to detect breast changes	105 (62.4)
	Find it difficult to remember	5 (3.0)
	Find it embarrassing	0 (0.0)
	Has no time	40 (23.8)
	Has no family history of breast cancer and do not see the need for it	10 (6.0)

7.2.2. Answers to Research Question on How the Demographic Variables Are Related to BSE Are Stated Below

Table 3, showed that 44 (41.9%) respondents aged 20 to 30, have inadequate practice of BSE while only 19 (18.1%) have high adequate practice. Respondents aged 31 to 40, 20 (29.9%), 24 (35.8%) and 23 (34.3%) inadequate, moderately adequate and highly adequate practice of BSE respectively. Respondents aged 41 to 50, 13 (23.6%), 30 (54.5%) and 12 (5.3%) inadequate, moderately adequate and highly adequate practice of BSE respectively. Those aged 51 to 60, 21 (53.3%), 15 (39.5%) and 2 (5.3%) inadequate, moderately adequate and highly adequate practice of BSE. While respondents aged 61 and above, 77 (91.75%), 6 (7.1%) and 1 (1.2%) had inadequate, moderately adequate and highly adequate practice of BSE. This showed respondents between 31 and 40 years old had more practice of BSE than the other age groups (as 34.3% of them had high BSE practice) and respondents from 61 years old above had the least practice. With a Pearson's Correlation Coefficient (R) of −0.234 and a Spearman's Rank Correlation Coefficient (R) of −0.232 and a p-value of $0.000 < 0.05$, a correlation between age and practice of BSE was established. With the correlation coefficient being negative, the result showed that with increase in age, the practice of BSE reduced and vice versa. Thus, there was a negative relationship between age and the practice of BSE.

The results in **Table 4** revealed that the 15 (100.0%) of respondents with no formal education rated inadequate practice in BSE and none was rated moderately adequate or highly adequate practice. 78 (98.7%) with primary education were rated inadequate practice of BSE, 1 (1.3%) moderately adequate and none for highly adequate practice. Those with secondary education had 94 (77.7%) for inadequate practice of BSE, 15 (12.4%) moderately adequate practice of BSE and 12 (9.9%) highly adequate practice of BSE. Respondents that had tertiary education had 48 (37.2%) for inadequate practice of BSE, 28 (21.75) moderately adequate practice of BSE and 53 (41.1%) highly adequate practice of BSE. Respondents with other qualifications had 1 (20.0%) for inadequate practice of BSE. 2 (40.0%) for both moderately adequate and highly adequate practice of BSE. Thus respondents with no formal education practiced BSE the least (as 100% of them had low practice of BSE) while respondents with tertiary education practiced BSE the most (as 41.1% of them had high practice of BSE). With a Pearson's Correlation Coefficient (R) of 0.550 and a Spearman's Rank Correlation Coefficient (R) of 0.516 and a p-value of $0.000 < 0.05$, a correlation between educational attainment and practice of BSE is established. With the correlation coefficients being positive, the result showed that with increase in educational qualification, the

Table 3. Practice of BSE in relation to age.

Age Group	Practice of Breast Self-examination			Total (%)
	Inadequate (%)	Moderately Adequate (%)	Highly Adequate (%)	
20 - 30	44 (41.9)	42 (40.0)	19 (18.1)	105 (100.0)
31 - 40	20 (29.9)	24 (35.8)	23 (34.3)	67 (100.0)
41 - 50	13 (23.6)	30 (54.5)	12 (21.8)	55 (100.0)
51 - 60	21 (55.3)	15 (39.5)	2 (5.3)	38 (100.0)
61 and above	77 (91.7)	6 (7.1)	1 (1.2)	84 (100.0)
Total	175 (50.1)	117 (33.5)	57 (16.3)	349 (100.0)

Table 4. Cross-tabulation between Educational attainment and practice of BSE.

Educational Qualification	Practice of BSE			Total (%)
	Inadequate (%)	Moderately Adequate (%)	Highly Adequate (%)	
No formal education	15 (100.0)	0 (0.0)	0 (0.0)	15 (100.0)
Primary education	78 (98.7)	1 (1.3)	0 (0.0)	79 (100.0)
Secondary education	94 (77.7)	15 (12.4)	12 (9.9)	121 (100.0)
Tertiary education	48 (37.2)	28 (21.7)	53 (41.1)	129 (100.0)
Others	1 (20.0)	2 (40.0)	2 (40.0)	5 (100.0)
Total	236 (67.6)	46 (13.2)	67 (19.2)	349 (100.0)

practice of BSE increases and *vice versa*. This showed that the practice of BSE can be associated with the level of education.

Table 5 revealed that respondents with no child had 65 (63.7%), 19 (18.6%) and 18 (17.6%) in adequate, moderately adequate and highly adequate practice of BSE respectively. Respondents with only one child had 33 (63.7%), 9 (17.0%) and 11 (20.85) inadequate, moderately adequate and highly adequate practice of BSE respectively. Those with 2 and three children had 69 (63.9%), 14 (13.0%) and 25 (23.1%) for inadequate, moderately adequate and highly adequate practice of BSE respectively. Respondents with 4 and 5 children had 38 (73.1%), 1 (1.9%) and 13 (25.0%) inadequate, moderately adequate and highly adequate practice of BSE respectively. This indicated that respondents with parity of 6 and above practiced BSE the least (as 91.2% of them had low practice of BSE) while respondents with parity of 4 to 5 practiced it the most (as 25% of them had high practice of BSE). Pearson's Correlation Coefficient (R) of −0.184 (*p*-value of 0.001 > 0.05) and a Spearman's Rank Correlation Coefficient (R) of −0.192 (*p*-value of 0.039 < 0.05) was established, showing that a correlation existed between parity and BSE practice. With the correlation coefficient being negative, the result showed that with increase in parity, the practice of BSE reduced and *vice versa*. Therefore, there was a negative relationship between parity and the practice of BSE.

8. Hypotheses

The three hypotheses on significant relationships between the demographic variables and BSE were computed using Chi-Square. For educational attainment Chi-Square value of 154.421 and *p*-value of 0.000 < 0.05 showed that there was a significant relationship between level of education and practice of BSE. There was no significant relationship between age, parity and BSE as their *p*-value were >0.05

9. Discussion

A little more than half of the respondents claimed to have performed BSE. Majority of the respondents who performed BSE did not follow the correct steps for BSE. Half of the respondents reported that they have no specific time when performing BSE. A significant proportion of the respondents do not follow any pattern while performing BSE. The major reason for not practicing BSE was lack of confidence in the ability to detect breast changes. Generally, the practice of BSE was inadequate for majority of the participants. These may likely be among the factors that contribute to late detection of breast cancer as noted by Chiejina [7] coupled with limited information which is characteristic of a rural community [10]. There was a negative relationship between age and practice of breast self examination. This implies that with increase in age, the practice of BSE reduced. This may be due to lack of confidence or ignorant of the fact that cancer of the breast knows no age limit. Training on BSE and constant practice may promote self care and efficacy, thus health promotion programmes on behavior change should target the older ones. There was a positive relationship between educational attainment and practice of breast self-examination as in the study by Subramanian [11]; this showed that with increased educational level, the practice of BSE increased. This portrays the importance of education in scaling up practice. There was a negative relationship between parity and practice of breast self examination; this implied that with increased parity, the practice of BSE reduced. Some mothers may have thought that because they are having babies and no history of breast cancer in the family, they are immuned to breast cancer hence the apathy in practice among them. This misconception need to be corrected through Health Education for BSE to be promoted.

Table 5. Cross-tabulation between parity and practice of BSE.

Parity	Practice of BSE			Total (%)
	Inadequate (%)	Moderately adequate (%)	Highly adequate (%)	
None	65 (63.7)	19 (18.6)	18 (17.6)	102 (100.0)
1 Only	33 (62.3)	9 (17.0)	11 (20.8)	53 (100.0)
2 - 3	69 (63.9)	14 (13.0)	25 (23.1)	108 (100.0)
4 - 5	38 (73.1)	1 (1.9)	13 (25.0)	52 (100.0)
6 and above	31 (91.2)	3 (8.8)	0 (0.0)	34 (100.0)
Total	236 (67.6)	46 (13.2)	67 (19.2)	349 (100.0)

10. Conclusion and Recommendation

Only about half of the respondents have performed BSE yet majority of them do not follow the correct steps for BSE. The elderly women among them seem not to have seen the need for the test. Educational attainment is found to be positively related to BSE. Education should be made free and accessible to all women in the community irrespective of age to boost the practice of BSE in order to promote early detection and prevent untimely death among women sequel to breast cancer.

References

[1]   Doshi, D., Reddy, B., Kulkarn, S. and Karunakar, P. (2010) Breast Self Examination. Knowledge, Attitude and Practice among Students in India. *Indian Journal of Palliative Care*, **1**, 66-67.

[2]   Globocan (2008) Cancer Incidence, Mortality and Prevalence. Worldwide. http://www.ncbi.nim.nih.gov\pub\21351561

[3]   Ganiyi, O. and Ganiyu, A. (2012) Epidemiology of Breast Cancer in Europe and Africa. *Journal of Cancer Epidermiology*, **2012**, Article ID: 915610. http://dx.doi.org/10.1155/2012/915610

[4]   Akarolo, S., Ogundiran, T. and Adebamowo, C. (2010) Emerging Breast Cancer Epidemic: Evidence from Africa. *Breast Cancer Research*, **20**, S8.

[5]   Adepeju, W. (2012) Are Cancer Cases Increasing in Nigeria? *Home Health*, **11**, 6.

[6]   Otunne, C. (2008) Breast Cancer: Causes and Therapies. CKC, Rex Press, Aba.

[7]   Chiejina, A. (2011) Experts Make Case for Cancer Care and Management in Nigeria. http://www.academia.edu/4510582/PROJECT_-_CHAPTERS_ONE_TO_FIVE

[8]   FRON (2007) Population Census. Federal Republic of Nigeria Official Gazette 24:94, Federal Government Printer (FGP 71/52007) 2500 24, B186, Lagos.

[9]   Krejice, R.V. and Morgan, D.W. (1970) Determining Sample Size for Research Activities, Educational and Psychological Measurement. *The NEA Research Bulletin*, **30**, 607-610.

[10]   Oluwatosin, O. (2010) Assessment of Women's Risk Factors for Breast Cancer and Predictors of the Practice of BSE in Two Rural Areas in Ibadan, Nigeria. *Cancer Epidemiology*, **34**, 425-428. http://dx.doi.org/10.1016/j.canep.2010.04.005

[11]   Subramanian, P., Oranye, N.O., Masri, A.M., Taib, N.A. and Ahmad, N. (2013) Breast Cancer Knowledge and Screening Behaviour among Women with a Positive History: A Cross Sectional Study. *Asian Pacific Journal of Cancer Prevention*, **14**, 6783-6790. http://www.ncbi.nilm.nih.gov/pubmed/24377606

9

The Effects of Aerobic Exercise Training on Basal Metabolism and Physical Fitness in Sedentary Women

Fatma Kizilay[1]*, Cengiz Arslan[2], Fatma İ. Kerkez[3], Aysegul Beykumul[1], Egemen Kizilay[4]

[1]PMR Department, Turgut Ozal Medical Center, Inonu University, Malatya, Turkey
[2]Faculty of Sports Science, Firat University, Elazığ, Turkey
[3]School of Physical Education and Sports, Mugla Sıtkı Kocman University, Mugla, Turkey
[4]PMR Clinic, Malatya State Hospital, Malatya, Turkey
Email: *fatmakizilay@hotmail.com.tr

Abstract

Objective: Aerobic exercises are the basic activity on fight against obesity. And obesity is related with metabolic rate. So our study is aimed to investigate the effects of 8 weeks aerobic exercise on basal metabolic rate and physical parameters. Methods: Sedentary women between the ages of 35 - 45 (n = 40) were randomized into control group (CG) (n = 20) and exercise group (EG) (n = 20). EG underwent 8 weeks of aerobic-run-walk exercise training: 3 days a week, 1 hour sessions. The CG was not trained. Basal metabolic rate (BMR), body mass index (BMI), waist-hip ratio (WHR), body fat percentage (BFP), body fat mass (FM) and lean body mass (LBM) were measured for all of the subjects before and after the training program. Results: Mean BMR decreased from 1386 ± 213.6 kcal to 1327 ± 253.7 in CG, and raised from 1308 ± 201.8 to 1409 ± 218.3 kcal in EG. While BMI raised from 31.39 ± 6.15 kg/m^2 to 31.51 ± 6.09 kg/m^2 in CG, it decreased from 29.62 ± 3.78 kg/m^2 to 28.47 ± 3.74 kg/m^2 in EG. There was also statistically significant difference in parameters of WHR, BFP, FM and LBM in favour of EG ($p < 0.05$). Conclusion: After 8 weeks aerobic exercise training program, there was a statistically significant difference in favour of EG in BMR, BMI, BFP, FM, LBM, WHR and weight parameters.

Keywords

Sedentary, Aerobic, Basal Metabolism, Physical Fitness

---

*Corresponding author.

1. Introduction

The importance of exercise in daily life has increased due to developing technology and studies focusing on this subject. Obesity which is closely associated with energy metabolism is a very common health problem in nearly all societies and becoming a global epidemic [1]. Obesity is common in the United States and is a major public health problem because of its association with considerable morbidity, including hypertension, diabetes mellitus, and coronary artery disease [2] [3]. Sedentary lifestyle is a major factor causing obesity. The appearance of increase in the risk of hypertension, metabolic syndrome and diabetes in adults if sedentary lifestyle becomes more widespread in the future, emphasizes the need of focus to health and coronary heart disease on society in terms of protection [4]. Lately though, as a result of the emphasis on this requirement, a partly awareness of sport has begun to occur. Due to this awakening, new sports options have been consisting. For example, the number of people who have been deailng with Pilates in the United States exceeded 5 million at this point [5]. Exercises which everyone will find easier and to do by one's own such as cycling, walking and running, maintain their own importance and popularity from the past to the present. Latey (2001) pointed out that this increase in people's demand on doing sports occured due to protection from injuries and wellness status [6]. Fundamental elements of being healthy are balanced body composition, physical fitness and to be able to keep it well [7]. Various techniques like BMI, skinfold, circumference measurements and bioelectrical impedance analysis (BIA) are used to determine physical fitness [8].

Metabolism and its speed are also effective factors on physical well-being. Anabolic and catabolic processes in the organism are always in equilibrium. Almost all the body's cells are renewed permanently, they are synthesized apart again. Also, metabolic activity can be described as generating new molecules from one to another [8]. Return of surplus proteins and carbonhydrates to fat in the organism is basically related with this metabolism [9] [10]. BMR, which is an important parameter of energy metabolism, is the lowest amount of energy, necessary for the vital functions of the person [11]. Basal metabolism comprises 60% to 75% of the daily energy expenditure [12]. Activities of the brain, heart, kidneys and other organs constitute a significant portion of BMR, the main cause of differences between people are amount of skeletal muscles, the fat mass and body size [13]. Therefore metabolic rate is lower in women compared with men [2]. In people whose LBM is more, their BMR is higher too. Between the ages of 20 - 40, for each m^2 of body surface area men spend 38 kcal, while women spend 35 kcal average [14] [15]. Metabolic activity of adipose tissue, and therefore energy consumption is lower than in the muscle tissue. The changes of body combine which occur in adulthood, so age-related increase in fat mass and decrease in lean mass explains the decrement of 2% - 3% of BMR in adult men and women decennially [12].

The effects of exercise on basal metabolism is the subject of researches for many years. Studies obtained different results are available on this topic [16]-[19]. There is no consensus regarding the long-term effects of regularly done physical activity on basal metabolism. This disagreement raises the necessity of new researches. Further studies are needed to define the role of energy metabolism on determining exercise approaches to treat obesity. Therefore the aim of this study is to examine the effect of 8-week aerobic exercise on basal metabolic rate and physical parameters in premenopausal sedentary women.

2. Materials and Methods

2.1. Participants

40 healthy female premenopausal volunteers between the ages of 35 - 45 with sedentary life style participated in the study. Volunteers were randomized into two groups; CG with 40.30 ± 4.47 mean age (n = 20) and EG with 41.05 ± 3.26 mean age (EG) (n = 20).

Individuals with a history of chronic disease, surgery, smoking, having or had on a diet or exercise program for last one year, or in a pregnancy or breastfeeding period were excluded. Individuals were selected by criteria on to be sedentary women in premenopausal period and between the ages of 35 - 45.

Before starting the research participants were informed about the content of the study, its purpose, application and the potential risks. Voluntary consent forms were distributed and were signed to all participants. Consent was obtained from "Malatya Clinical Research Ethics Committee" for this research (decision no: 2011-32). Subsequently, CG had not undergone exercise program; EG did aerobic-run-walk exercise 1 hour a day, 3 days a week for 8 weeks. BMR, BMI, WHR, BFP, FM and LBM were measured for all of the subjects before and after the training program.

2.2. Study Design

At the weeks before the beginning and immediately after the 8 weeks of aerobic exercise, volunteers were invited to the laboratory for measurements. BMR measurement which was to be done on resting condition and after 12 hours of fasting, performed between 8:00 to 10:00 am. According to the admission criteria, from the day of measurements subjects were required to avoid from smoking environment.

Temperature of room which measurements will be performed in, fixed with air conditioning to 22°C. Also necessary isolation provided for not to change of humidity, light and sound. Light dose was isolated to be slightly dark and quiet room. All measurements were performed by an experienced person using the same equipment for each subject.

The measurements were made in the following order:

- Height and weight values required for the BMR measurement was measured and recorded.
- For BMR measurement each participant was allowed to rest on supine position 30 minutes (min.) prior of measurement.
- BMR measurements performed for 30 min. after resting period.
- BMR measurement ending subjects were taken into BIA measurements.
- Subsequently circumference measurements were performed.

2.3. Experimental Protocol

2.3.1. Height and Weight Measurement

Height measurement is powered by a Soehnle brand gauge working with ultrasound method [20].

Tanita brand bioelectrical impedance analyzer "Tanita Body Composition Analyser BC-418" was used for weight measurement. Weight of subject's clothes were allowed to be deducted from the weight of subject. After all reading from the device's LCD screen values have been saved [20].

2.3.2. BMR Measurement

Fit Mate® BMR measurement device of Cosmed firm was used. The subjects was measured after 30 min. of rest in the supine position. Sensor mask of device was used separately for each participant. Subjects were measured while normal breathing for 30 min. Subjects warned about not to move during the measurement. At the end of measurement automatic output was received and the BMR value (kcal) recorded [21].

2.3.3. Bioelectrical Impedance Analysis (BIA)

"Tanita Body Composition Analyzer BC-418" was used for BIA analysis. Height (cm), age (years) and subject's clothes weigt (kg) values were entered to divice. With this device LBM, BFP, FM parameters were calculated and automatic output received. BMI value was calculated using the formula weight (kg)/height (m)^2 [22].

2.3.4. Circumference Measurements

Circumference measurements were performed using standard tape measure (Gullick strip). For determining of waist-to-hip ratio, 2 region of body measured (waist, hips). The measurement region of subjects was allowed to be naked. Circumference measurements were repeated three times to each point and taking the mean value of these three measurements was recorded.

Waist: waist measured at the narrowest area parallel to the ground during normal breathing. Hips: maximum protrusion of the buttocks muscle (gluteus maximus) were measured in parallel position over the place [8]. WHR value obtained by dividing waist circumference to hip circumference (WHR = waist circumference/hip circumference) [23].

2.4. 8 Weeks Exercise Protocol

Run-walk exercises are made in the 1700-meters jogging track located on the Inonu University campus. Heart rate was controlled with portable polar device during exercise. Exercise intensity was determined with Karvonen Method [24] and the number of heart beats were calculated for each subject separately [11]. Exercise group did run-walk exercises in the intensity of 60% target heart rate 1 hour a day, 3 days a week for 8 weeks. **Table 1** shows the training program.

Table 1. Applied training program.

Weeks	Exercise	Exercise Period (min)	Distance (km)	Frequency (day/week)
	Warm-up	10		
1 - 2	Training Period	45	4	3
	Cool-Down	5		
3 - 4	Same with first week	60	5	3
5 - 6	Same with first week	60	6	3
7 - 8	Same with firts week	60	6	3

Warm-up Period (10 min.):
- Light tempo 5 min. jog, direction-changing walks,
- Warm-up and stretching exercises for the muscle groups to be used in the exercise [25].

Training Period (45 min):
- Run-walk exercises at Inonu University jogging track with 60% of maximum heart rate of subjects determined with Karvonen method [24].

Cool-down Period (5 min):
- Light Tempo jogging,
- Minimal Stretching [25].

2.5. Statistical Analysis

Mann-Whitney U test was used to determine whether there are differences in age, height and weight parameters between exercise and control groups in this study. Normal distribution of data was examined by the Kolmogorov-Smirnov test. Two-way analysis of variance (ANOVA) was used for comparison of pre-test - post test results. All statistical analyzes were performed using SPSS program and the significance level was set at 0.05.

3. Results

After randomisation of 40 healthy female volunteers into two groups; control group (n = 20) and exercise group (n = 20) Mann-Whitney U test was used for comparison of age, height, weight, WHR, BMI, BFP, FM, LBM and BMR between two groups before the intervention. There was no statistically significant difference between CG and EG (p > 0.05).

Table 2. Descriptive statistics of circumference measurements.

VARIABLES	CG (n = 20)				EG (n = 20)				F	p
	Pre test		Post test		Pre test		Post test			
	$\overline{X}$	SD	$\overline{X}$	SD	$\overline{X}$	SD	$\overline{X}$	SD		
Waist (cm)	102.72	12.15	103.78	12.97	98.65	9.58	93.27	8.07	54.966	0.000*
Hip (cm)	115.47	10.45	116.42	11.02	111.17	7.41	107.65	7.00	83.452	0.000*
WHR (%)	0.88	0.04	0.89	0.05	0.88	0.05	0.86	0.06	6.464	0.015*

*There was a statistically significant difference (p < 0.05).

As shown in **Table 2** waist circumference values remained unchanged after the final test in the control group, a statistically significant reduction is detected in the exercise group (p < 0.05). While hip circumference increased in the control group, decrease was observed in the exercise group and the difference was statistically significant (p < 0.05). Waist-hip ratio remained unchanged in the control group, decreased in the exercise group and according to the latest test scores this difference was found statistically significant (p < 0.05).

Table 3. Change of the physical fitness parameters.

VARIABLES	CG (n = 20)				EG (n = 20)				F	p
	Pre test		Post test		Pre test		Post test			
	$\bar{X}$	SD	$\bar{X}$	SD	$\bar{X}$	SD	$\bar{X}$	SD		
Weight (kg)	81.17	15.15	81.43	15.15	74.81	11.68	72.03	11.68	69.372	0.000*
BMI (kg/m²)	31.39	6.15	31.51	6.09	29.62	3.78	28.47	3.74	7.957	0.000*
BFP (%)	36.64	6.28	35.53	6.32	37.10	4.47	34.59	4.47	12.340	0.001*
FM (kg)	30.54	10.52	29.06	9.64	28.12	7.46	25.47	7.46	7.037	0.012*
LBM (kg)	46.63	4.68	46.69	5.03	50.62	5.41	51.55	5.95	6.000	0.019*

*There was a statistically significant difference (p < 0.05).

While BMI raised from 31.39 ± 6.15 kg/m² to 31.51 ± 6.09 kg/m² (0.38%) in CG, it was decreased from 29.62 ± 3.78 kg/m² to 28.47 ± 3.74 kg/m² (3.11%) in EG. While LBM was raised from 46.63 ± 4.68 kg to 46.69 ± 5.03 in CG, it was increased from 50.62 ± 5.41 kg to 51.55 ± 5.95 kg in the exercise group. BFP was decreased 3.02% in the control group, 6.76% in the exercise group. FM was decreased 4.84% in the control group, 9.42% in the exercise group and there was a statistically significant difference between groups according to the last test results (p < 0.05).

Table 4. Change of BMR values.

VARIABLE	CG (n = 20)				EG (n = 20)				F	p
	Pre test		Post test		Pre test		Post test			
	$\bar{X}$	SD	$\bar{X}$	SD	$\bar{X}$	SD	$\bar{X}$	SD		
BMR (kcal)	1386	213.6	1327	253.7	1308	201.8	1409	218.3	5.41	0.025*

*There was a statistically significant difference (p < 0.05).

BMR value remained unchanged in the control group, increased in the exercise group and according to the test scores this difference was found statistically significant (p < 0.05). **Figure 1** presents the change of BMR value in CG and EG.

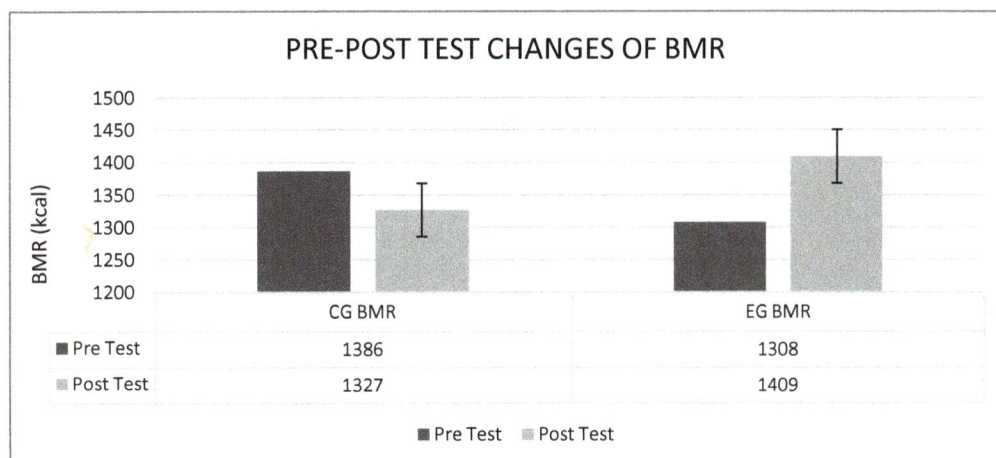

Figure 1. Change of BMR in EG and CG.

4. Discussion

There are several studies about the aerobic exercises and their effects. Our study has been focused on aerobic exercise too and carried out to investigate the effects of 8 weeks of aerobic-run-walk exercise training on BMR and physical fitness parameters in sedentary women between the ages of 35 - 45. After 8 weeks aerobic run-walk exercise program there was a statistically significant difference between CG and EG in the parameters of BMR, BMI, BFP, FM, LBM, WHR and weight ($p < 0.05$) (**Table 3**). In this respect, Amano *et al.* have reported that obese men and women who underwent aerobic exercise training for 30 minutes, three times a week, over 12 weeks had significant reduction in body weight, BMI, BFP, FM and LBM in their study [1]. Again like that as, William *et al.* were randomly assigned sedentary women to one of three groups that either 1) performed 25 min. of step aerobic exercise only; 2) performed a combination of 25 min. of step aerobic exercise and a multiple-set upper and lower body resistance exercise program; 3) performed 40 min of step aerobic exercise only to investigate the effects of different exercise groups to physical and physiologic performance parameters and observed significant reduction in BFP (5% - 6%) in all training groups after training [26].

In a randomized controlled trial, 60 patients were randomly divided into 3 groups: control group, group with aerobic exercise, and group with resistance exercise in a study. After 12 weeks of exercise, statistically significant decreases in BMI and FM were noted in groups with aerobic and resistance exercises [27]. Struggling with obesity gained further importance nowadays and thus easily accessible and inexpensive methods like exercise and results of the studies about the exercise gained importance [17] [27]-[29].

Our study showed that positive effects can be achieved with only an 8-week aerobic exercise program. The results of the study are valuable in the fight against obesity. The role of aerobic exercise in increasing basal metabolism is trying to be identified with studies. At this point, the results obtained from our study appears to provide a significant contribution.

In a randomized controlled intervention trial, Geliebter *et al.* assigned sixty-five (25 men and 40 women) moderately obese subjects (aged 19 - 48 y) to one of three groups: diet plus strength training, diet plus aerobic training, or diet only. Statistically significant differences were found in BMR in all of the groups [30]. Douglas and Poehlman investigated 82 young women who separated into three groups: sedentary (n = 48), aerobically trained (n = 21), and resistance trained (n = 13); only aerobic exercise group had statistically significant difference in BMR than the other two groups [31]. These studies show aerobic exercises are more effective on the basal metabolism when compared to resistance exercise but our study provides answers to the questions of how often, with how much load and how long these exercises should be done. In our study, BMR was found to decrease from 1386 ± 213.6 kcal to 1327 ± 253.7 in CG, raised from 1308 ± 201.8 to 1409 ± 218.3 kcal in EG and there was a statistically significant difference between EG and CG ($p < 0.05$) (**Table 4**). After 8 weeks of aerobic-run-walk exercise training: 3 days a week, 1 hour sessions there was a statistically significant BMR difference in our study.

Studies concerning how metabolic activity is influenced by exercise in obese, gain more importance day by day. In our study, 40 subjects with the mean BMI 31.45 and defined as obese according to obesity index by the WHO were evaluated and effects of the exercise on obesity parameters were investigated [22]. This study's limitation was to be worked with a small number of objects. So there is need of new studies including large number of subjects to define the role of aerobic exercise on basal metabolism and physical fitness.

5. Conclusion

BMR value increased significantly in the exercise group and patients with "obesity" status got in the "overweight" category. Consequently, 8 weeks of aerobic exercise is effective in increasing basal metabolic rate and normalising physical fitness in sedentary women due to our study results.

Note

This study was presented as a poster presentation at the International Gender and Sports Symposium, Ankara-2014.

References

[1]   Amano, M., Kanda, T. and Maritani, T. (2001) Exercise Training and Autonomic Nervous System Activity in Obese
        Individuals. *Medicine & Science in Sports & Exercise*, **33**, 1287-1291.
        http://dx.doi.org/10.1097/00005768-200108000-00007

[2]   US Department of Health and Human Services (1987) Anthropometric Reference Data and Prevalence of Overweight. DHHS Publication, USA.

[3]   Lew, E.A. and Garfinkel, L. (1979) Variations in Mortality by Weight among 750,000 Men and Women. *Journal of Chronic Diseases*, **32**, 563-576. http://dx.doi.org/10.1016/0021-9681(79)90119-X

[4]   Onat, A. (2007) Fiziksel Etkinlik, Metabolik Bozukluklardan Korunma ve Koroner Mortalite. Türk Halkının Kalp Sağlığı, Argos-Cortex, İstanbul.

[5]   Segal, N.A., Hein, J. and Basford, J.R. (2004) The Effects of Pilates Training on Flexibility and Body Composition: An Observational Study. *Archives of Physical Medicine and Rehabilitation*, **85**, 1977-1981. http://dx.doi.org/10.1016/j.apmr.2004.01.036

[6]   Latey, P. (2001) The Pilates Method: History and Philosophy. *Journal of Bodywork and Movement Therapies*, **5**, 275-282. http://dx.doi.org/10.1054/jbmt.2001.0237

[7]   Fox, E.L., Bowers, R.W. and Foss, M.L. (1989) The Physiological Basis of Physical Education and Athletics. William C Brown Publication, Philadelphia.

[8]   Günay, M., Tamer, K. and Cicioğlu, İ. (2010) Spor Fizyolojisi ve Performans Ölçümü. Gazi Kitabevi, Ankara.

[9]   Baysal, A. (2000) Genel Beslenme. Hatipoğlu Yayınları, Ankara.

[10]   Ersoy, G.K. (1986) Spor ve beslenme. Mili Eğitim, Gençlik ve Spor Bakanlığı Yayınları, Ankara.

[11]   Ganong, W.F. and Barrett, K.E. (2005) Review of Medical Physiology. McGraw-Hill Medical Publication, New York.

[12]   McArdle, W.B., Katch, F.I. and Katch, V.L. (2001) Exercise Physiology-Energy, Nutritionand Human Performance. Lippincott Williams and Wilkins, Philadelphia.

[13]   Guyton, A.C. and Hall, J.E. (2006) Tıbbi Fizyoloji (Çev. Ed. Çavuşoğlu H.). Nobel TıpKitabevleri, İstanbul, 297-421.

[14]   Petra, M.L., Herbert, B.M. and Neuh, M. (2001) Effects of Fat Mass and Body Fat Distribution on Resting Metabolic Rate in the Elderly. *Metabolism*, **50**, 972-975.

[15]   Heyward, V. (1997) Advanced Fitness Assessment Exercise Prescription. Human Kinetics, Champaign.

[16]   Bingham, S.A., Goldberg, G.R., Coward, W.A., Prentice, A.M. and Cummings, J.H. (1989) The Effect of Exercise and Improved Physical Fitness on Basal Metabolic Rate. *British Journal of Nutrition*, **61**, 155-173. http://dx.doi.org/10.1079/BJN19890106

[17]   Çolakoğlu, F.F. and ve Karacan, S. (2006) Genç Bayanlar ile Orta Yaş Bayanlarda Aerobik Egzersizin Bazı Fizyolojik Parametrelere Etkisi. *Kastamonu Eğitim Dergisi*, **14**, 277-284.

[18]   Lennon, D., Nagle, F., Stratman, F., Shrago, E. and Dennis, S. (1985) Diet and Exercise Training Effects on Resting Metabolic Rate. *International Journal of Obesity*, **9**, 39-47.

[19]   Lovlin, R., Cottle, W., Pyke, I., Kavanagh, M. and Belcastro, A.N. (1987) Are Indices of Free Radical Damage Related to Exercise Intensity. *European Journal of Applied Physiology*, **56**, 313-316. http://dx.doi.org/10.1007/bf00690898

[20]   Baumgartner, R.N., Cameron, C. and Roche, A.F. (1998) Bioelectrical Impedance for Body Composition. *American Journal of Clinical Nutrition*, **48**, 16-25.

[21]   Nieman, D.C., Trone, G.A. and Austin, M.D. (2003) A New Handheld Device for Measuring Resting Metabolic Rate and Oxygen Consumption. *Journal of the American Dietetic Association*, **103**, 588-593. http://dx.doi.org/10.1053/jada.2003.50116

[22]   World Health Organization (1995) Expert Committee on Physical Status: The Useand Interpretation of Anthropometry. WHO, Geneva.

[23]   American College of Sports Medicine, Ed. (2013) ACSM's Health-Related Physical Fitness Assessment Manual. Lippincott Williams & Wilkins, Philadelphia.

[24]   Fox, E.L., Bowers, R.W. and Foss, M.L. (1993) The Physiological Basis For Exercise and Sport. 5th Edition, Brown & Benchmark, New York.

[25]   Güllü, A. and Güllü, E. (2001) Genel Antrenman Bilgisi. Umut Matbaacılık, İstanbul.

[26]   William, J.K., Monica, K., Nicholas, A.R., Jeff, S.V., Mathew, M., Jill, A.B., Bradley, C.N., Scoott, A.G., Scoott, A.M., Robert, U.N., Ana, L.G., Robbin, B.W., Martyn, R.R. and Keijo, H. (2001) Resistance Training Combined with Bench-Step Aerobics Enhances Woman's Health Profile. *Medicine & Science in Sports & Exercise*, **33**, 259-269.

[27]   Fenkci, S., Sarsan, A., Rota, S. and Ardic, F. (2006) Effects of Resistance or Aerobic Exercises on Metabolic Parameters in Obese Women Who Are Not on a Diet. *Advances in Therapy*, **23**, 404-413. http://dx.doi.org/10.1007/BF02850161

[28]   Mensink, G.B., Ziese, T. and Kok, F.J. (1999) Benefits of Leisure-Time Physical Activity on the Cardiovascular Risk Profile at Older Age. *International Journal of Epidemiology*, **28**, 659-666. http://dx.doi.org/10.1093/ije/28.4.659

[29] Stasiulis, A., Mockiene, A., Vizbaraite, D. and Mockus, P. (2009) Aerobic Exercise-Induced Changes in Body Composition and Blood Lipids in Young Women. *Medicina*, **46**, 129-134.

[30] Geliebter, A., Maher, M.M., Gerace, L., Gutin, B., Heymsfield, S.B. and Hashim, S.A. (1997) Effects of Strength or Aerobic Training on Body Composition, Resting Metabolic Rate and Peak Oxygen Consumption in Obese Dieting Subjects. *The American Journal of Clinical Nutrition*, **66**, 557-563.

[31] Ballor, D.L. and Poehlman, E.T. (1992) Resting Metabolic Rate and Coronary-Heart-Disease Risk Factors in Aerobically and Resistance-Trained Women. *The American Journal of Clinical Nutrition*, **56**, 968-974. http://dx.doi.org/10.1249/00005768-199205001-00303

10

The Influence of Exercise and Caffeine on Cognitive Function in College Students

Rachel J. Shulder, Eric E. Hall, Paul C. Miller

Department of Exercise Science, Elon University, Elon, USA
Email: ehall@elon.edu

Abstract

Exercise has widely been shown to improve cognition, potentially by making individuals more receptive to sensory stimulation or inhibiting irrelevant information. Caffeine, one of the world's most widely used stimulants, seems to have similar effects. It seems that both exercise and caffeine improve cognitive function separately, but little research has been done examining their combined effects. The purpose of this study was to examine the impact of caffeine and exercise, independently and combined, on cognitive function. 20 healthy college students completed the study. These participants were low caffeine consumers. Each participant came to the lab 5 times. During the first session, they completed a graded exercise test on a cycle ergometer to determine ventilatory threshold (VT). The following four sessions were test sessions involving supplementation and exercise. During these, each participant engaged in 30 minutes of cycling (at 90% VT) or 30 minutes of quiet reading after consuming either caffeine (at 4 mg/kg body weight) or a placebo. The Contingent Continuous Performance Task (CPT) and Wisconsin Card Sorting Task were used to measure cognitive function and were completed 5 minutes and 20 minutes after exercise or quiet reading. There were no significant differences found for any variables tested, for condition effect, time effect or condition*time interaction, except for a significant time effect on false alarms on the Contingent CPT ($p = 0.017$). This study may have been limited by multiple variables including the population, executive function measures, caffeine dosage, or exercise prescription. These findings point to the need for future research to understand the changes in cognition from exercise and caffeine in combination. Future research may include looking at exercise at different intensities, different dosages of caffeine, or looking at the long-term cognitive effects.

Keywords

Exercise, Caffeine, Cognitive Function, Executive Function

1. Introduction

Exercise has widely been shown to improve cognition by making individuals more receptive to sensory stimulation or inhibiting irrelevant information. Changes include increased long-term and short-term memory, increased executive function and decreased reaction time [1] [2]. Moderate steady-state exercise increases central nervous system arousal, which may make the individual more receptive to stimulation and increasing motor process speeds [2]. It is also possible that with limited resources (oxygen, neurotransmitters, etc.), resources are directed only to important brain centers, allowing us to focus on those tasks [3]. Pontifex, Hillman, Fernhall, Thompson, and Valentini [4] studied the effect of a 30-minute bout of running (at 60% - 70% VO$_2$max) on working memory, an aspect of executive control, in 21 young adults. Reaction time and accuracy were measured, and the results indicated shorter reaction time both immediately after exercise and 30 minutes after completion of exercise. Reaction time was fastest after exercise during the tasks requiring increased working memory capacity. These results are consistent with a recent meta-analysis of the effect of acute exercise on cognitive performance [5].

In addition to exercise, caffeine is suggested to have positive effects on multiple aspects of cognition including vigilance, mental alertness, reaction time, visual selective attention, task switching, conflict monitoring and response inhibition [6]-[8]. Caffeine is thought to cause these improvements by antagonizing adenosine receptors; it blocks the action of this inhibitory neurotransmitter by directly acting on both pre- and postsynaptic receptors [8]. Caffeine antagonizes the adenosine receptors in dopamine-rich brain areas, resulting in increased wakefulness and motor activity. Childs and de Wit [7] investigated the effects of 0, 50, 150 or 450 mg caffeine on light, nondependent caffeine users (to rule out the possibility of caffeine's effects being due to reversal of withdrawal). Forty minutes after ingestion, allowing time for plasma levels of caffeine to peak, participants completed tasks including attention, short-term memory and inhibition. Participants consuming caffeine increased the number of correct response and decreased reaction time, though memory was impaired. The researchers concluded caffeine has psychoactive effects, enhancing performance in consumers, dependent on dose and nature of the task.

Hogervorst and colleagues [9] provide one of the few studies which examined the combined effects of exercise and caffeine on measures of cognitive function. In this study, fifteen young male athletes were given a water placebo, a carbohydrate-electrolyte placebo, or carbohydrate-electrolyte solutions containing 150 mg, 225 mg or 320 mg caffeine. A cognitive battery, including attention, psychomotor speed, visual detection, and long-term memory tasks; was completed before and immediately after a 1-hour cycling bout. After exercise, all cognitive functions were improved in the participants who had consumed the beverages with 150 mg and 225 mg caffeine. This novel finding, showing the effects of caffeine on cognitive performance after exercise, demonstrated an improvement in complex cognitive functions, dependent on dose. A follow-up study showed similar improvement: better concentration, faster response speed and detection and improved scores on RVIP, Stroop and Visual Search tasks after caffeine ingestion and an exercise bout compared to placebo ingestion [10].

It seems that both exercise and caffeine improve cognitive function separately, but little research has been done examining their combined effects. The purpose of this research is to determine the effect that caffeine and aerobic exercise have on executive function in young adults. More specifically, this study looked at the effects of exercise + caffeine, exercise + no caffeine, no exercise + caffeine, no exercise + no caffeine on executive function. Based on previous research, it was hypothesized that performance would be the best during the exercise + caffeine session, and performance would be worst during the no exercise + no caffeine session.

2. Methods

2.1. Participants

Twenty healthy undergraduate college students (16 females, 4 males) were recruited for this study. Recruitment of participants occurred through a posting on the university's website as well as flyers posted in classrooms at the university. All participants reported they were in good health and free of any medical conditions or injuries that may be contraindications of aerobic exercise. All participants completed a caffeine intake log and a written informed consent form which was approved by the university's Institutional Review Board. Participants were compensated with a $25 gift-card. See **Table 1** for participant descriptive information.

2.2. Measures

The modified Wisconsin Card Sort Task (WCST) and Contingent Continuous Performance Task (CPT) were

Table 1. Participant characteristics (Means ± SD).

	Males	Females
Age (years)	19.3 ± 0.5	19.9 ± 1.2
Height (in)	71.4 ± 1.9	64.1 ± 2.8
Weight (lbs)	150.4 ± 12.1	143.6 ± 22.5
Body Fat (percent)	13.9 ± 2.6	27.5 ± 5.2
BMI (kg/m^2)	20.7 ± 0.9	24.7 ± 4.4
VO$_2$peak (mL O$_2$/kg·min)	39.7 ± 8.5	29. 4 ± 6.3
Caffeine Intake (mg/day)	42.5 ± 79.1	114.4 ± 88.6

administered using Neuroscan's STIM2 software (Compumedics Limited; Australia). The tests were projected onto a 17" computer screen in front of the participant. A 4-buttoned Compumedics Neuroscan-Stim System Switch Response Pad (Compumedics Limited; Australia) was used to record participant responses for each of the tasks.

A modified version of the Wisconsin Card Sort Task (WCST) was used in the present study. The WCST was designed to test abstract behavior and shift of set. It has been shown to be an effective measure of executive function, assessing multiple dimensions of cognition including cognitive processing speed, concept formation, inhibition capacity and cognitive flexibility [11].

The task consists of 64 stimulus cards and 4 base cards. The four base cards were always one red triangle, two yellow stars, three green crosses and four blue circles, displayed from left to right at the top of the screen. Each stimulus card had one of the four shapes (triangle, star, cross, or circle), colors (red, yellow, green, or blue) and number of objects (one, two, three, or four). The stimulus cards were displayed in the bottom right corner of the screen. The participant was told by the researcher to match the stimulus card to one of the four base cards by color, shape or number. Feedback was given as to whether the card matching was correct by a tone and the appearance of the word "CORRECT" or "INCORRECT" at the top of the screen. Participants were unaware, but the computer changed the rule after ten cumulative correct placements of the cards. The test was completed after the participant successfully sorted 60 cards. The participants were allowed as long as was necessary to finish the task. Total errors from each trial were recorded as a measure of executive control. Total errors were calculated as the number of times a card was matched incorrectly based on the currently applicable rule.

The Contingent Continuous Performance Task (CPT) is an attentional task involving executive control components. To successfully complete the CPT task, inhibitory control, a part of executive control processes, must prevent mistakes [12]. The participant was presented with a series of letters flashed in the middle of the screen for 200 ms, with 1000 ms in between each letter. The instructions were to press the first button on the response pad when the target letter "T" was shown. The letter "S" always preceded the letter "T" but the display of "S" did not mean that the target letter "T" would necessarily follow. A lure occurred when the letter "S" was shown and the letter "T" did not follow. Twenty target letters and ten lures were presented in each trial of the task. Average reaction time (RT) to each target letter was recorded. A false alarm (FA) was recorded anytime the participant pressed the button and the target letter "T" was not shown.

2.3. Procedures

All participants came into the lab for five sessions. The participants completed 1 session per day with a minimum of 48 hours between sessions. All sessions took place at the same time of day. During the first session, participants completed the informed consent form and height and weight were assessed. The participant was fitted with a Polar Target heart rate monitor and a V2 mask and headstrap (Hans Rudolph, Inc; USA). The participants were seated on a Corival Lode recumbent bike (Lode B.V. Technology; Groningen, The Netherlands) and a breathing mask was attached to record expired oxygen and carbon dioxide levels using a Parvo Medics True One Metabolic System. After a 60 second warm-up at 0 W, the exercise test began with two minutes at 50 W and increased 25 W every two minutes until volitional exhaustion. Heart rate, VO$_2$ and Respiratory Exchange Ratio (RER) were constantly recorded throughout the trial and participants were verbally encouraged to go as long as possible. At the end of the trial, the breathing mask was taken off and the participant was told to continue biking at 0 W. Expired gas data was used to determine VO_2 peak and ventilatory threshold (VT). VT was determined in order to set individualized exercise intensity for each participant in the following sessions. VT is the point during graded exercise when ventilation rate increases exponentially while workload continues to increase linearly.

Sessions two through five measured cognitive function after one of four conditions: exercise + caffeine, exercise + no caffeine, no exercise + caffeine, no exercise + no caffeine. The order of sessions were randomly assigned and counterbalanced so each participant took part in each of the conditions, and each session lasted eighty to ninety minutes total. Participants were told after the first session to arrive for each following session dressed in workout clothes and sneakers, ready to exercise if necessary, and ready with reading material of their choice if not asked to exercise. Participants were also asked to abstain from both caffeine and exercise for a minimum of 12 hours before testing sessions. Immediately on arriving to the lab for sessions two through five, the participant was given a colored capsule containing anhydrous caffeine (4 mg/kg body weight; NutraBio Pharmaceutical Grade Caffeine) or placebo (Arrowhead Mills Organic Brown Rice Powder). This study was double blind so the participants and first author were unaware of the contents of the capsules consumed. The capsules content was revealed upon completion of the study. Upon arriving to the laboratory for the second session, or first cognitive testing session, participants were introduced to the cognitive tests and allowed to practice one trial each of WCST and CPT. Body composition (BMI and percentage body fat) was measured at the second session by bioelectrical impedance using a OMRON Fat Loss Monitor (OMRON Healthcare Inc; Bannockburn, Illinois).

After consuming the capsule at the start of each session, the participant was fitted with a heart rate monitor and was told to sit quietly for thirty minutes. They were allowed to read, or use a computer or other technology, but not allowed to leave the laboratory. Resting HR was recorded at the end of the thirty-minute delay. During sessions with exercise, the participant was seated on a SciFit recumbent bike (SCIFIT Systems Inc.; Tulsa, OK) and told to start pedaling. After a minute of warm-up at self-determined power, the power was increased to elicit 90%VT of the participant. Ten minutes into exercise, twenty minutes and thirty minutes (immediately before the end of exercise), HR was recorded to validate the participant was exercising at the proper intenisty. Water was offered every ten minutes but participants could choose whether or not they wanted to drink. After the exercise bout, the participant was told to dismount, offered additional water, and waited five minutes to complete the WCST and CPT. The WCST was always performed first, followed by the CPT. The participants then waited another fifteen minutes (for a total of twenty minutes post-exercise) and completed the WCST and CPT again.

During sessions with no exercise, the participants completed the same protocol, but instead of cycling for thirty minutes, they were simply asked to stay seated on the SciFit recumbent bike and quietly read for thirty minutes. The reading material was the participant's choice. No music or technology was allowed during this thirty-minute session. After completing the thirty minutes, participants waited five minutes and completed the cognitive test battery. They then waited until twenty minutes post-exercise and completed the second round of the cognitive tests.

2.4. Statistical Analyses

To determine if there was a significant difference between the different conditions and over time for the dependent variables (cognitive function), a 4 (Condition: caffeine + exercise, caffeine + no exercise, exercise + no caffeine, no caffeine + no exercise) by 2 (Time: 5 min post, 20 min post) Repeated Measures General Linear Model (RM GLM) was performed. Separate RM GLM analyses were run for reaction time and false alarms from the Contingent CPT as well as for total errors from the WCST. A p value of <0.05 was used to determine if the condition, time or condition by time interaction were significant.

3. Results

The 4 (Condition: caffeine + exercise, caffeine + no exercise, exercise + no caffeine, no caffeine + no exercise) by 2 (Time: post 5, post 20) RM GLM did not reveal a significant condition effect [$F(3,17) = 2.80$, $p = 0.071$], time effect [$F(1,19) = 2.47$, $p = 0.133$] or condition*time interaction [$F(3,17) = 2.36$, $p = 0.108$] for reaction time on the Contingent CPT. These results indicate that there was no differences between conditions or over time for reaction time (See **Figure 1**).

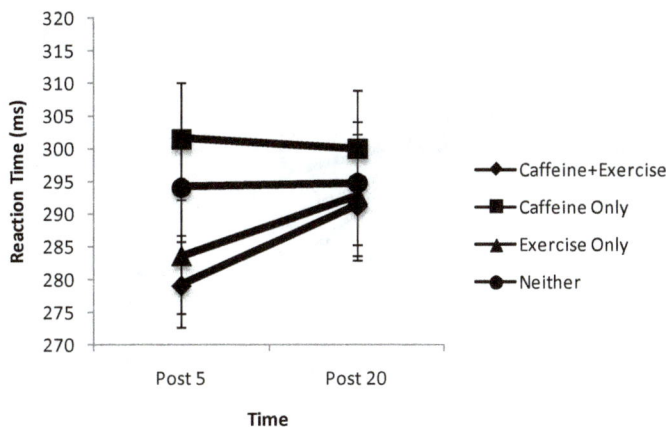

Figure 1. Reaction time for contingent CPT by condition∗time.

For false alarms on the Contingent CPT a 4 (Condition) by 2 (Time) RM GLM did not reveal a significant condition effect [$F(3,17) = 1.85$, p = 0.176] or condition∗time interaction [$F(3,17) = 1.69$, p = 0.206] but did reveal a significant time effect [$F(1,19) = 6.83$, p = 0.017]. This suggests that on the second administration of the test (20 minutes post condition) participants performed better as indicated by fewer false alarms on the Contingent CPT (See **Figure 2**).

The RM GLM for total errors on the WCST did not show a significant condition [$F(3,17) = 0.41$, p = 0.752], time [$F(1,19) = 2.25$, p = 0.150] or condition∗time interaction [$F(3,17) = 1.09$, p = 0.380]. These results demonstrate that there were no statistical differences in performance across the different conditions or over time on total errors of the WCST (See **Figure 3**).

4. Discussion

The purpose of this study was to examine the effect of caffeine and aerobic exercise, together and separately on executive function. The current study failed to show significant differences between the four groups on any of the measures of cognitive function.

The current study showed no significant differences between conditions' reaction times, in contrast to most research, which has shown that reaction time is faster after caffeine consumption or a bout of aerobic exercise. Previous studies have found reaction time to be faster following exercise Davranche and McMorris [1] [4] [13]-[15] and caffeine consumption [7] [11] [16] [17]. Crowe, Leicht, and Spinks [18] examined the effects of caffeine consumption and anaerobic exercise, and found no differences in reaction time between groups which is consistent with the findings of the current study.

For the false alarms portion of the Contingent CPT, there was a significant time effect, but not an effect for condition. All conditions decreased from 5 minutes after exercise or quiet reading to 20 minutes after exercise or quiet reading, displaying a possible learning curve. The measurement of false alarms is a measure of selective inhibition because irrelevant stimuli must be inhibited in order to decrease the false alarms score. The lack of a condition effect in the current study is similar to other previous research which showed no differences in measures of selective inhibition [13] [19] In contrast to the results from the current study, several studies have shown an improvement between conditions after exercise [9] [20] [21] and Childs and de Wit [7] also saw an improvement in inhibition following the consumption of caffeine. Hogervorst et al. [10] also found greater inhibition in a group that received a combination of caffeine and exercise.

Once again this study showed differences by condition or time on performance of the WCST as measured by total errors. The WCST is used to measure of executive function, specifically planning, set shifting, working memory and goal directed behavior [11]. In contrast to the findings of the current study, previous research has found improvements in executive function following exercise [4] [22] and caffeine consumption [7] [17]. However, the findings of the current study are consistent with other studies which have not found a difference after caffeine consumption [11] [16].

The current study does have some limitations. The findings of the current study were based on a small number of participants, potentially influencing the non-significant findings. Though the number of participants in the

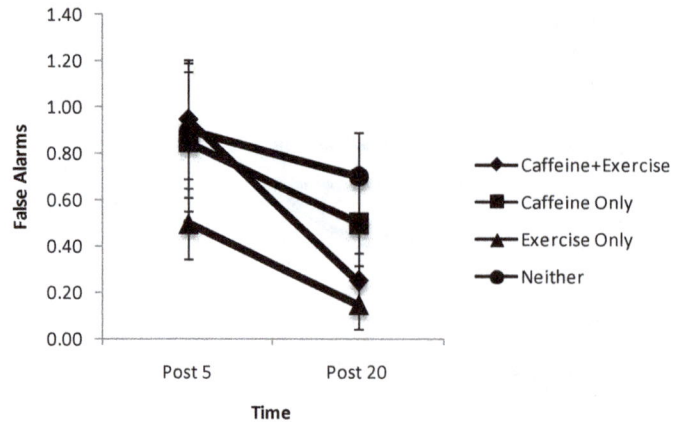

Figure 2. False alarms for contingent CPT by condition*time.

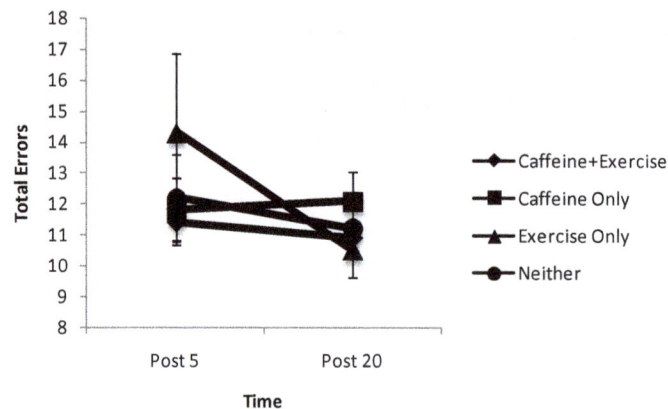

Figure 3. Total errors for Wisconsin card sort task by condition*time.

current study is similar to many of the previous research studies, it is possible that some of the results in the current study would have been statistically significant with a larger sample size. Another limitation may have come been the dosages of caffeine and exercise that were prescribed to the participants. Previous research has used a wide variety of intensities of exercise and dosages of caffeine. This study attempted to normalize caffeine and exercise based on the individual, but a lower intensity of exercise or higher dose of caffeine may have been better to show the differences hypothesized. A final limitation may have been the measures of cognitive function utilized in the present study. While the Contingent CPT and WCST are valid and reliable tests of cognitive function, other measures of cognitive function might be more sensitive to the influence of exercise and caffeine.

5. Conclusion

In this current study, there were no significant differences found for the three variables tested-total errors on the WCST, and reaction time and false alarms on the Contingent CPT, for condition effect, time effect or condition*time interaction, except for a significant time effect on false alarms on the Contingent CPT. There are many variables that may account for the variability in results seen in research studying at the effects of caffeine and exercise, individually and combined, on cognitive function. The lack of consistency points to the need for more research.

Acknowledgements

The authors would like to thank the Elon University Honors Program and Undergraduate Research Program for support which included funding for a Summer Undergraduate Research Experience.

References

[1] Davranche, K. and McMorris, T. (2009) Specific Effects of Acute Moderate Exercise on Cognitive Control. *Brain and Cognition*, **69**, 565-570. http://dx.doi.org/10.1016/j.bandc.2008.12.001

[2] Lambourne, K., Audiffren, M. and Tomporowski, P.D. (2010) Effects of Acute Exercise on Sensory and Executive Processing Tasks. *Medicine & Science in Sports & Exercise*, **42**, 1396-1402. http://dx.doi.org/10.1249/mss.0b013e3181cbee11

[3] Tomporowski, P.D. (2003) Effects of Acute Bouts of Exercise on Cognition. *Acta Psychologica*, **112**, 297-324. http://dx.doi.org/10.1016/s0001-6918(02)00134-8

[4] Pontifex, M.B., Hillman, C.H., Fernhall, B., Thompson, K.M. and Valentini, T.A. (2009) The Effect of Acute Aerobic and Resistance Exercise on Working Memory. *Medicine & Science in Sports & Exercise*, **41**, 927-934. http://dx.doi.org/10.1249/MSS.0b013e3181907d69

[5] Chang, Y.K., Labban, J.D., Gapin, J.I. and Etnier, J.L. (2012) The Effects of Acute Exercise on Cognitive Performance: A Meta-Analytic Review. *Brain Research*, **1453**, 87-101. http://dx.doi.org/10.1016/j.brainres.2012.02.068

[6] Brunyé, T.T., Mahoney, C.R., Lieberman, H.R. and Taylor, H.A. (2010) Caffeine Modulates Attention Network Function. *Brain and Cognition*, **72**, 181-188. http://dx.doi.org/10.1016/j.bandc.2009.07.013

[7] Childs, E. and De Wit, H. (2006) Subjective, Behavioral, and Physiological Effects of Acute Caffeine in Light, Non-dependent Caffeine Users. *Psychopharmacology*, **185**, 514-523. http://dx.doi.org/10.1007/s00213-006-0341-3

[8] Fine, B.J., Kobrick, J.L., Lieberman, H.R., Marlowe, B., Riley, R.H. and Tharion, W.J. (1994) Effects of Caffeine or Diphenhydramine on Visual Vigilance. *Psychopharmacology*, **114**, 233-238. http://dx.doi.org/10.1007/BF02244842

[9] Hogervorst, E.E., Riedel, W.J., Kovacs, E.E., Brouns, F.F. and Jolles, J.J. (1999) Caffeine Improves Cognitive Performance after Strenuous Physical Exercise. *International Journal of Sports Medicine*, **20**, 354-361. http://dx.doi.org/10.1055/s-2007-971144

[10] Hogervorst, E., Bandelow, S., Schmitt, J., Jentjens, R., Oliveira, M., Allgrove, J., Carter, T. and Gleeson, M. (2008) Caffeine Improves Physical and Cognitive Performance during Exhaustive Exercise. *Medicine & Science in Sports & Exercise*, **40**, 1841-1851. http://dx.doi.org/10.1249/MSS.0b013e31817bb8b7

[11] Adan, A. and Serra-Grabulosa, J.M. (2010) Effects of Caffeine and Glucose, Alone and Combined, on Cognitive Performance. *Human Psychopharmacology*, **25**, 310-317. http://dx.doi.org/10.1002/hup.1115

[12] Smid, H.G., de Witte, M.R., Homminga, I. and van den Bosch, R.J. (2006) Sustained and Transient Attention in the Continuous Performance Test. *Journal of Clinical and Experimental Neuropsychology*, **28**, 859-883. http://dx.doi.org/10.1080/13803390591001025

[13] Davranche, K., Hall, B. and McMorris, T. (2009) Effect of Acute Exercise on Cognitive Control Required during an Eriksen Flanker Task. *Journal of Sport & Exercise Psychology*, **31**, 628-639.

[14] Pesce, C., Capranica, L., Tessitore, A. and Figura, F. (2002) Focusing of Visual Attention under Submaximal Physical Load. *International Journal of Sport Psychology*, **1**, 275-292. http://dx.doi.org/10.1080/1612197X.2003.9671719

[15] Pesce, C., Tessitore, A., Casella, R. and Capranica, L. (2007) Focusing of Visual Attention at Rest and during Physical Exercise in Soccer Players. *Journal of Sports Sciences*, **25**, 1259-1270. http://dx.doi.org/10.1080/02640410601040085

[16] Durlach, P.J. (1998) The Effects of a Low Dose of Caffeine on Cognitive Performance. *Psychopharmacology*, **140**, 116-119. http://dx.doi.org/10.1007/s002130050746

[17] Giles, G.E., Mahoney, C.R., Brunyé, T.T., Gardony, A.L., Taylor, H.A. and Kanarek, R.B. (2012) Differential Cognitive Effects of Energy Drink Ingredients: Caffeine, Taurine and Glucose. *Pharmacology Biochemistry and Behavior*, **102**, 569-577. http://dx.doi.org/10.1016/j.pbb.2012.07.004

[18] Crowe, M.J., Leicht, A.S. and Spinks, W.L. (2006) Physiological and Cognitive Responses to Caffeine during Repeated, High-Intensity Exercise. *International Journal of Sport Nutrition and Exercise Metabolism*, **16**, 528-544.

[19] Hillman, C.H., Snook, E.M. and Jerome, G.J. (2003) Acute Cardiovascular Exercise and Executive Control Function. *International Journal of Psychophysiology*, **48**, 307-314. http://dx.doi.org/10.1016/s0167-8760(03)00080-1

[20] Lichtman, S. and Poser, E.G. (1983) The Effects of Exercise on Mood and Cognitive Functioning. *Journal of Psychosomatic Research*, **27**, 43-52. http://dx.doi.org/10.1016/0022-3999(83)90108-3

[21] Sibley, B.A., Etnier, J.L. and Le Masurier, G.C. (2006) Effects of an Acute Bout of Exercise on Cognitive Aspects of Stroop Performance. *Journal of Sport & Exercise Psychology*, **28**, 285-299.

[22] Tomporowski, P.D., Cureton, K., Armstrong, L.E., Kane, G.M., Sparling, P.B. and Millard-Stafford, M. (2005) Short-Term Effects of Aerobic Exercise on Executive Processes and Emotional Reactivity. *International Journal of Sport and Exercise Psychology*, **3**, 131-146. http://dx.doi.org/10.1080/1612197X.2005.9671763

11

Search of Biomarker in the Oral Rehabilitation

Masakazu Azuma[1,2], Senichi Suzuki[1,2], Masaki Sawa[2], Tomoko Yoshizawa[2], Ailing Hu[3], Takuji Yamaguchi[3], Hiroyuki Kobayashi[2,3]

[1]Lion Implant Center, Ebina-shi, Japan
[2]Department of Hospital Administration, Juntendo University Graduate School of Medicine, Bunkyo-ku, Japan
[3]Center of Advanced Kampo Medicine and Clinical Research, Juntendo Graduate School of Medicine, Bunkyo-ku, Japan
Email: azuma-dental@nifty.com

Abstract

Are there any ways to analyze objectively if any good changes happen to the bodies for the patients with acquired edentulous by getting a treatment to recover occlusion? In this study, we focused on interleukin 6 (IL-6) as inflammatory cytokine, cortisol known as a stress related substance and secretory immune globulin A (SIgA) related to immune reaction, and chose 14 patients who had occlusion reconstructed by the immediately loaded dental implants because occlusion contact with maxillary and mandibular dentition was lost caused by edentulous jaws or maxillary and mandibular teeth crossing each other and their jaw position and central occlusion position could not settle, and verified the relationship with changes of patients' physical and mental states during the 6 months of the treatment and the effect of the immediately loaded implants treatment by using saliva which was non-invasive and easy to sample in biomarkers in saliva. Moreover for female subjects, the changes of facial color tones were measured by using Robo Skin Analyzer®, a digital image analyzer, to measure the condition of their skin. In conclusion, the positive correlation between the amount of IL-6 and cortisol was not admitted. However, it was admitted that IL-6 tended to increase when a systemic change which interrupted curing such as the interruption of fusion of the implant and the bone was observed even though the patient did not notice any particular symptoms and cortisol tended to increase when the patient noticed discomfort and mentioned any events under stress on his or her medical record. Moreover with the skin color analysis by Robo Skin Analyzer®, the possibility that the occlusion treatment by the immediate implant had an effect on physical and psychological health promotion through the acquisition of the masticatory function and the aesthetic recovery was indicated.

Keywords

Occlusion, Immediate Load Dental Implants, IL-6, Cortisol, Skin Condition

1. Introduction

Recently, in the choices of prosthesis treatments for patients with edentulous to recover the masticatory function and the sensuousness, the recovery of occlusional function (oral rehabilitation) applying dental implant is becoming common besides the treatment with removal dentures which has been the mainstay for a long time. The reconstruction of occlusion with implant fixture which made it possible to recover the function disorder caused by the deficit of a tooth and a jawbone and the morphological disorder which were once considered difficult to do with a removal denture because it loaded the oral mucosa absorbability instantly became the focus of the research and the development as a new trend of dental care, and grew to the reliable treatment method keeping its technical stability. On the other hand, there are several problems regarding patients' physical and psychological burdens, such as costs and surgical stress, and especially to shorten the duration of treatment which is required until the occlusion function recovers has been expected. It makes the immediately loaded implants by All-on-4 reality to meet the patients' desire [1], "I want occlusion get recovered immediately". The concept of the immediate load dental implants [2] and All-on-4 taking full advantage of its characteristic feature is not to regenerate the lost paradentium biologically but to fix strongly the implant superstructure consists of the artificial tooth and the artificial substitute for paradentium, and the supporter composed of 4 implants fixtures implanted in the jawbone to the residual ridge after the tooth loss through the attachment of screws. After the tooth loss, only four implant bodies are placed to the staunch part on the remaining jawbone keeping the ideal depth by making an angle to the implant direction to gain stronger fusion. Furthermore, geometric resistance can be obtained by arranging the four placed implant fixtures evenly like making a horseshoe arch from occlusal surface.

This resistance does not only avoid the each patient's unique habitual lateral movement of jaw causing fibrous healing which blocks the fusion of the implant fixtures and the bone and the tiny movement caused by traumatic occlusal force, but also obtains the strength against occlusion. This uniqueness of All-on-4 makes the immediate functional loading which reconstructs occlusion by dentition with 12 artificial teeth for both upper and low jaws possible for edentulous patients just after the dental implant surgery.

In this study, we targeted patients with a provisional bridge which was the therapeutic upper structure applied for six months until the final form of the implant super structure was completed, focused on interleukin 6 (IL-6), cortisol and SIgA in saliva and verified the relationship with the effect of obtaining the occlusional function and the changes of patients' physical and psychological states during the immediate load dental implant treatment. Moreover for female subjects, their skin colors were measured with the color information from the digital image of the skin taken by a CCD camera using Robo Skin Analyzer®, a digital image analyzer, and measured the changes of their facial skin tones.

2. Material and Method

2.1. Subject

The subjects were 14 patients (64.1 ± 5.8 years), 7 males (68.7 ± 4.5 years) and 7 females (59.4 ± 2.1 years), who visited Ebina Lion Implant Center with complaints that the contact with the maxillary and mandibular dentition was lost because of edentulous jaws or maxillary and mandibular teeth crossing each other and their mandibular positions could not settle and requested for occlusion recovery with immediate load dental implants to July 2014 from January 2013. The subjects were obtained consent by a purpose of this study and this research was performed according to the ethic official regulation that nonprofit foundation Japanese Society of Oral Implantology to belong to of the Ebina Lion Implant Center established.

Patients who received a diagnosis when in condition not to be able to take the centric occlusion for completely losing occlusal contact were chosen as a subject. After obtaining consent by a purpose of this study, they started taking saliva before and right after the implant placement surgery and at the monthly follow-ups after the surgery. The subjects were placed a provisional bridge as the upper structure right after the implant placement surgery, and occlusion of the upper and lower jaws were recovered. Replace Select Tapered RP® (Nobel Biocare Japan K.K.) was used as the implant fixture, and tightening torque over 35 N cm for all of the placed implant fixtures were confirmed. The temporary bridge was composed with the resin artificial tooth and dental polymerized resin, and Temporary Cylinder Plastic® (DCA468-0) and Prosthetic Screw® (29285) (Nobel Biocare Japan K.K.) were used as its connector.

2.2. The Method for Collecting Saliva

As for collecting saliva for the test, the duration was determined for six months which was required for ISQ, the bone fusion indicator that implant prosthetics recommend, to get over 70 until paradentium stabilized and the provisional bridge transited to the final prosthesis [3] [4]. Interleukin 6 (IL-6) as inflammatory cytokine, cortisol known as a stress related substance and secretory immune globulin A (SIgA) were measured.

After putting bland and innocuous Salimetrics Oral Swab (Salimetrics, USA) into the subject's mouth for 5 minutes in a sitting posture, it was collected and the saliva was taken by centrifugation (1500 rpm × 40 minutes, 4°C). The saliva was stored at −20°C until the measurement. The time of collection was determined from 11:30 to 17:30 at which the value of cortisol stabilizes in consideration of the circadian variation of cortisol value [5] [6].

2.3. The Measurement Method of Salivary Components

SALIVARY IL-6 ELISA KIT (Salimetrics, USA) for the amount of IL-6, High Sensitivity SALIVARY CORTISOL ENZYME IMMUNOASSAY KIT (Salimetrics, USA) for the amount of cortisol, and Salivary Secretory IgA Indirect Enzyme Immuoassay kit (Salimetrics, USA) for the amount of SIgA were used for the measurement.

2.4. The Measurement of Skin Color

For seven female subjects, skin color was measured using Robo Skin Analyzer® (MM & NiiC Co., Ltd.) besides collecting saliva at the monthly follow-ups from before the implant surgery and to six months after the surgery. Robo Skin Analyzer® is a measurement device for skin color with images taken by a CCD camera, and expresses the colors of skin as three attributions of hue, brightness, and intensity by measuring skin reflectivity [7] [8].

As the measurement conditions, after the subject washed her face to take her makeup off, three facial images (right 45°-front-left 45°) were taken with the built-in CCD camera keeping the distance from the object and the camera constant by fixing the forehead and the jaw in the box of Robo Skin Analyzer® which was blocked the surrounding environmental colors and kept the shooting condition constant.

(The correlation between the amount of IL-6, cortisol and SIgA and the facial color tones were discussed.)

2.5. Statistical Analysis

All the data are presented as mean ± SEM. The data were analyzed by the Wilcoxon Rank Sum Test to evaluate the difference between pre-surgery and post-surgery. p values of < 0.05 were defined as statistically significant.

3. Results

3.1. The Change in Salivary Components

The transition of the amount of IL-6 in saliva for six months was shown in **Figure 1**.

IL-6 increased rapidly after the treatment and kept high value repeating the increase and the decrease. However, it presented the comparable value as the one before the treatment at the measurement after six months when it changed to the final prosthesis. Comparing the changes in males to females, for males it remained high value after the treatment and presented the comparable value as the one before the treatment after six months when it changed to the final prosthesis (**Figure 2(a)**). For females on the other hand, it remained high value one month after the treatment, however, it transited at the comparable value as the one before the treatment after two months (**Figure 2(b)**).

The transition of the amount of cortisol in saliva for six months was shown in **Figure 3**. As for cortisol, it presented high value before the treatment, however it started decreasing after the treatment and it decreased significantly after six months when it changed to the final prosthesis. Comparing the changes in male and female, it presented the same transition patters and gender differences could not been observed (**Figure 4**). No correlation was shown between then although the correlation about the amount of IL-6 and cortisol in saliva was considered coefficient value at 0.2528 and p value at $p < 0.001$ (**Figure 5**).

As for SIgA, no change was shown during the six month treatment (**Figure 6**).

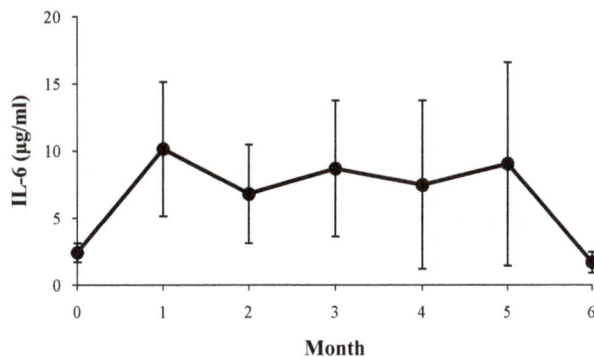

Figure 1. Temporal change of the salivary IL-6 levels (Mean ± S.E, n = 14).

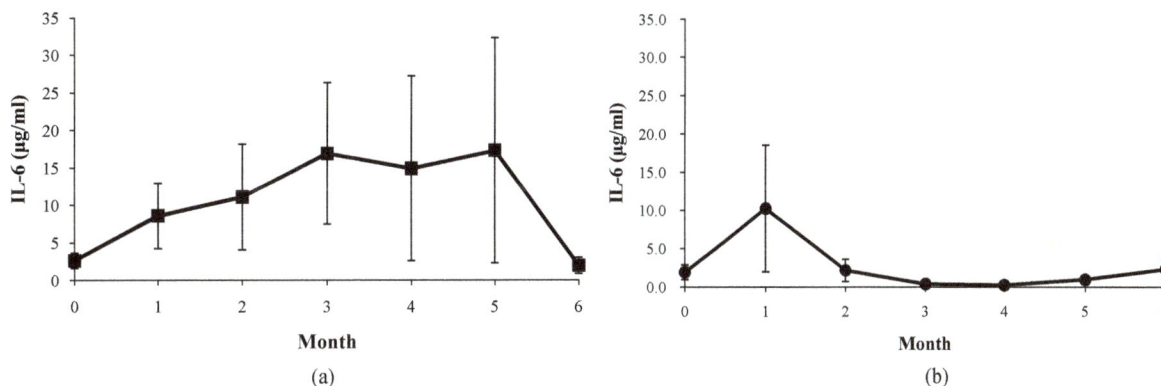

(a)

(b)

Figure 2. Temporal change of the salivary IL-6 levels (a) male (Mean ± S.E, n = 7); (b) female (Mean ± S.E, n = 7).

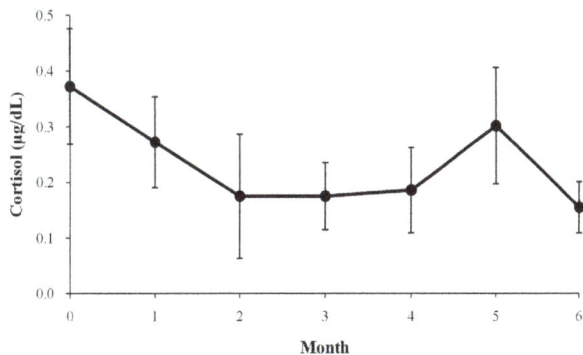

Figure 3. Temporal change of the salivary cortisol levels (Mean ± S.E, n = 14), $^*p < 0.05$ vs. 0.

3.2. The Change in Skin Color

The transition of three components of colors, hue, brightness, and intensity of seven female patients in six month was measured and its change was shown in **Figure 7**. The three components representing facial skin tones generally increased in ascension curve after the treatment. The hue increased significantly after six months compared to the one before the treatment.

4. Discussion

The clinical application of All-on-4 initiated in Japan from 2005, however, quite a lot of dental implant specialists inside and outside the country had objections to its innovation at the beginning. The goal of the oral implant

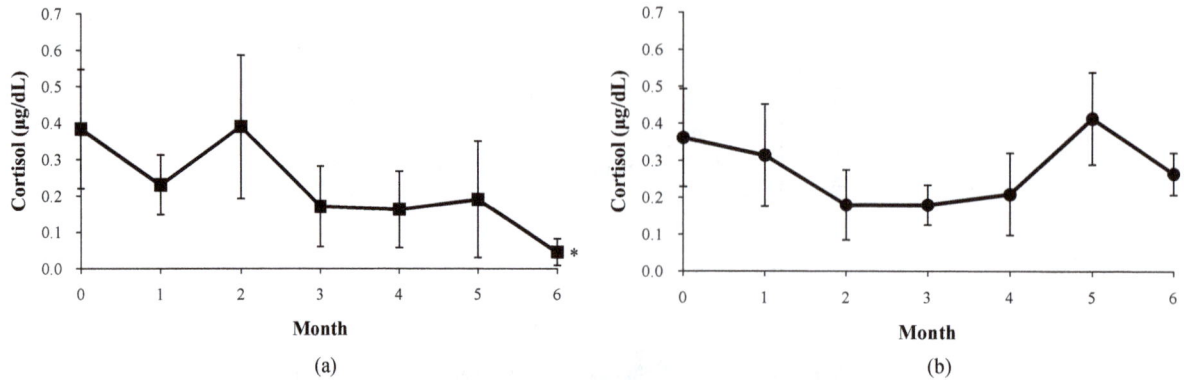

(a)   (b)

Figure 4. Temporal change of the salivary cortisol levels (a) male (Mean ± S.E, n = 7); (b) female (Mean ± S.E, n = 7), *p < 0.05 vs. 0.

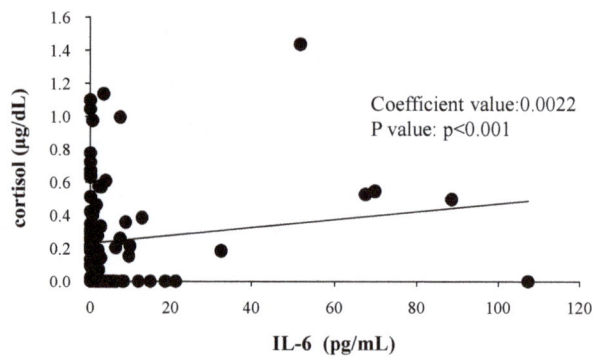

Figure 5. Correlation of salivary IL-6 and cortisol.

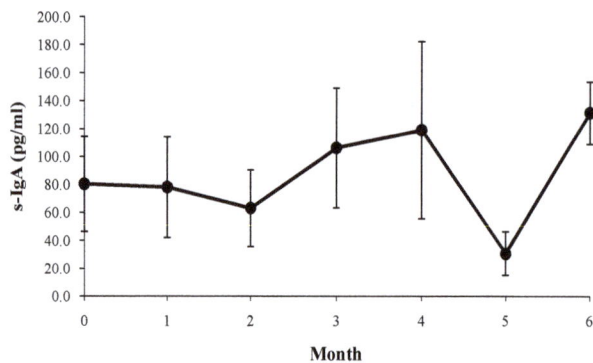

Figure 6. Temporal change of the salivary Ig-A (Mean ± S.E, n = 14).

technology before All-on-4 was just to replace the lost natural tooth with the artificial dental root as a substitute and to make it work. It is so to speak the biomimetics which is faithful to anatomical science [9]. Under the current dental implant situation, the success criteria are mostly about the connection of the bone and the implant fixture [10] [11], and the objective judgment criteria about obtaining masticatory movement and sensuousness which is the original goal for the occlusion function recovery are not required. The way to measure success and failure of the clinical implant is to examine the connection condition of the implant fixture and the bone, such as measurement of disturbance by the x-ray image diagnosis [12], the resonance frequency analysis [13], the measurement of the torque value and the Periotest [14] [15], and we only have to wait for the patient's complaint to notice the defect of the implant superstructure in the present circumstances. It is the beginning of this study to determine objectively if the immediate load dental implants which became close to us and the reconstruction of

(a)

(b)

(c)

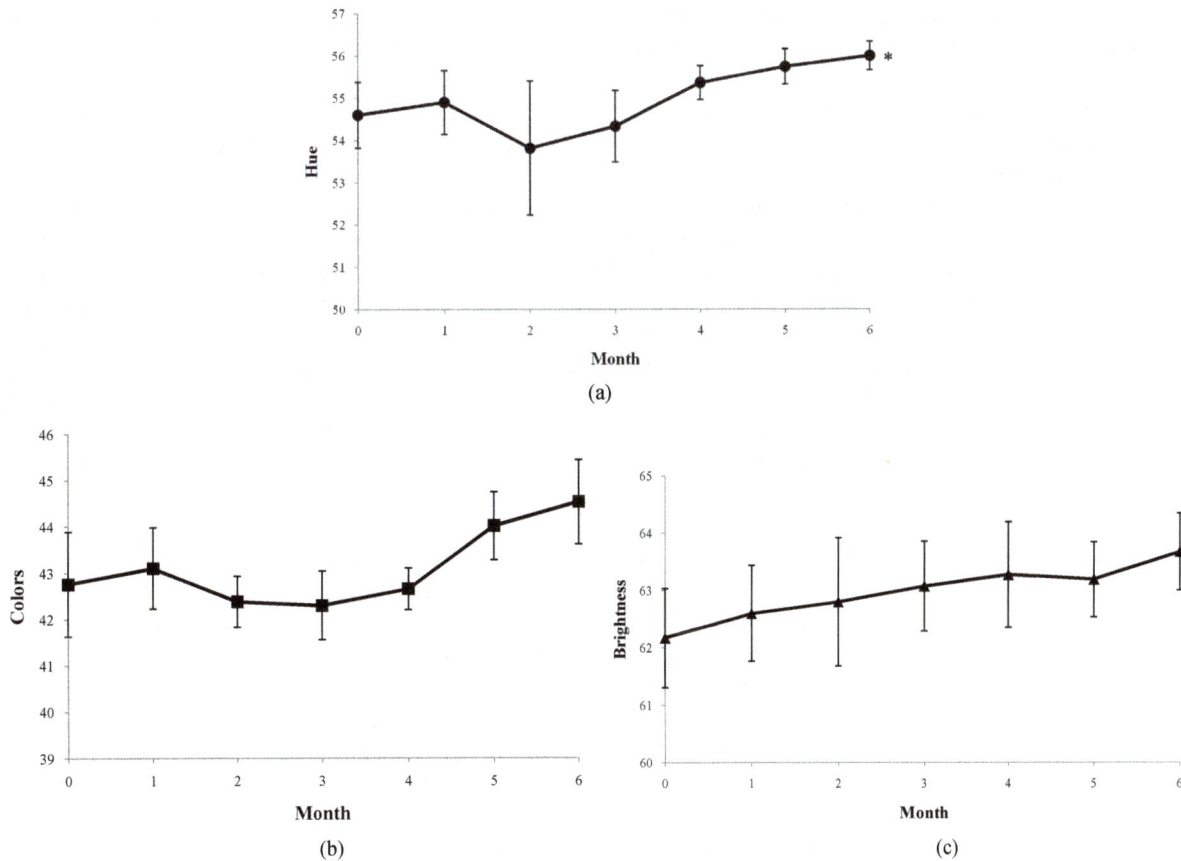

Figure 7. Temporal change of the skin-colored on the female patient after the implant operation (a) hue; (b) colors; (c) brightness (Mean ± S.E, n = 7), *p < 0.05 vs. 0.

occlusion using the system really make the patients happy. For example, how the patient's mind and body who had replaced his or her teeth with artificial substitutes in a large ratio will change right after the implant surgery? What kinds of reactions will happen to the patient with the adjusting provisional bridge during the six months until the final prosthesis is completed? The patients' physical and psychological changes before and right after the implant surgery and during the six months of the treatment were examined through the correlation of the secretion concentration of the stress related substances in saliva.

In this study, the correlation between IL-6 in saliva and inflammation caused by surgical stress was proven as the amount of the measured value of IL-6 as inflammatory cytokine always increased remarkably after surgery and decreased to the comparative level of the one before surgery one month after the surgery although the difference of the values between the one before surgery and after surgery was concerned at first (**Figure 1**) [16]-[18].

The results of the present study demonstrated the correlation between IL-6 and surgical stress [19]-[22], or IL-6 and the inflammatory reaction caused by periodontitis [23]-[28]. The amount of IL-6 rapidly increased after surgery and remain high value almost all the time to the final prosthesis in six months, even though a little of the increase and the decrease was admitted in the middle, and the value became comparative to the one before surgery. The provisional bridge guides the mandibular position to the occlusion point where there are no tension on temporomandibular joint and masticatory muscle, and recovers occlusion at the central occlusion position where the occlusional surface between the upper and lower jaws connects at the maximum area and is considered as the most balanced jaw position in clinical dentistry [29].

On the other hand, as the performance needed for therapeutic dentures until it gets to the final prosthesis, the provisional bridge is recommended to be designed to avoid excessive occlusal pressure such as biting something hard. Differences among individuals reflected to the change of the graph in some degree, however the amount of IL-6 originated the process to infuse the implant body and the bone. It is reported that the implant stability decreased for a while after surgery and recovered six months later by the research of the remodeling process of the implant fixture immediately loaded and the bone right after the placement to the molar area on the upper jaw [30], before surgery and every month after surgery using the resonance frequency analysis. The graph showing the implant stability during remodeling the early bone and the measurement graph showing the amount of IL-6 flipped vertically and were orbited symmetrically. This suggests that the amount of IL-6 is affected by the systematic changes around the implant.

The amount of cortisol did not indicate the extreme increase after surgery (**Figure 3**). The transition of the amount of cortisol basically tended to decrease gradually repeating the increase and the decrease from before the treatment to the final prosthesis transition in 6 months. Cortisol is secreted in response to the stress which is also the physical and psychological events causing distortion to homeostasis as a mechanism to keep the physiological situation in a body constant [31]. As both of stress caused by the physical and the psychological events stimulates ACTH (andreno-corticotorpic hormone) from hypothalamic-anterior pituitary and secretes cortisol from adrenal cortex [32], it is able to figure out whether the person is stressed or not by measuring cortisol [33]-[35]. As for the transition of cortisol, a patient's unique significant change of the amount of cortisol was observed as well as the change of IL-6, and the rapid shift of the increase and the decrease was observed at the different timing from IL-6. In reviewing medical records about the events happened to each patient at the observation point of the increase of the amount of cortisol, the patients complained about the adoption of the provisional bridge in their months in most of the situation, and it found out that the provisional bridge form was adjusted meticulously or repaired to fit in their mouths at the chair-side on demand from the patients in each case. As cortisol is the biomarker related to stress, it seemed that the patients removed stress associated with edentulous gradually, not right after the surgery when their occlusion was recovered. In particular, it seems that the process of the fusion of the implant fixture and the bone getting smooth and the process of the treatment that the provisional bridge form gradually got refined and adjusted in the patients' mouths on demand from patients at the monthly clinic visits was expected. In general, the graph gently decreasing formed a specific peak at the point of five months and it showed the increase of the amount of cortisol, however, the increase of the amount of cortisol was observed for two patients at this time of saliva measurement, and the amount of cortisol constantly transited with high value for one patient from before the treatment and during the treatment. This was the case that the only two mandibular molar teeth on the right side were compensated with the implants and the untreated remaining teeth were mixed although All-on-4 was applied to the upper jaw, and the crown prosthesis on bicuspid tooth on the right side which was the implant adjacent tooth was taken off at the time of this measurement. The body of the provisional bridge was fractured for the other patient. For each case, the increased amount of cortisol decreased at the next month's measurement after duplicating the prosthesis and repairing the provisional bridge. It was expected that there would be the positive correlation between the amount of IL-6 and cortisol as both of IL-6 and cortisol increased in respond to some events, however the correlation between the two was not observed. Moreover IL-6 increased when a systematic change which caused the damages to the implant fixture and the fusion of the implant fixture around the gum and the bones like preventing to promote healing was observed even though the patients did not notice any symptoms. Cortisol increased when the patient noticed discomfort and mentioned any events under stress on his or her medical record.

In this study, IL-6 indicated that systemic abnormalities about the jawbones which built the basic part to support artificially reconstructed occlusion, implant fixture, and the surrounding tissue, and cortisol could be considered as something to alert the mechanical problems about the implant superstructure which played a role of a fixed over denture with implant fixtures and screws. The information is extracted from two aspects, periodontological and prosthesis by using both for the measurement. By evaluating this data and the implant stability obtained from clinical x-ray images or by resonance frequency analysis, there is a possibility that it will help modifying the provisional bridge more accurately, designing the final prosthesis and for the post operational management. Moreover, as the amount of IL-6 and cortisol both indicated the lowest value in six months, the clinically recommended guide that the timing to transit to the final prosthesis was six months after the implant replacement when the bone fusion stabilized was confirmed.

For the female subjects, it was measured by using Robo Skin Analyzer® how it affected to the skin condition by recovering the occlusional function. The anti-aging theory that recovering occlusion can gain their youth is commonly known. The measuring intention here, however is to discuss how the occlusion recovery spills over to the rejuvenation effect not only around the mouth and the lips but also on physical appearance of a whole body by measuring freshness and moisture of women's skin condition with the image analysis and by comparing the amount of IL-6 as inflammatory cytokine, cortisol as a stress related biomarker, and SIgA related to immune competence. Three components of colors, hue, brightness, and intensity, were measured as an indicator by Robo Skin Analyzer®. All of hue, brightness and intensity gently increased in six months after surgery and the improvement of skin tone color was observed. In conclusion, statically, the provisional restoration recovered maxillary and mandibular occlusion at first, set the jaw position to the central occlusion point, and counterbalanced and stabilized the mandibular position by masseter muscle, temporal muscle and internal and external pterygoid muscle, which organized the back and forth and lateral movement on lower jaw, keeping moderate load. It also maintained moderate stress on the mimic muscle group gathered in a lip and a mouth, consists of orbicularis oris muscle, cheek muscle, laughing muscle, mentalis muscle, musculus levator anguli oris, depressor anguli oris muscle, greater zygomatic muscle, lesser zygomatic muscle, elevator muscle of upper lip, depressor muscle of lower lip, etc., by compensating the lost dentition and alveolar part artificially. Dynamically, moreover, the movement of the masseter muscle group promoted as the masticatory function became active. As for the effect of esthetic recovery, the actions with positive expression, such as smiling with teeth, became diverse. Therefore it promoted the movement of the mimic muscle group which spread to the whole face, such as frontalis muscle, orbicularis oculi muscle and corrugator muscle leading from the mimic muscle of a mouth, and stimulated lymphatic circulation. It is considered that these results were reflected to the skin condition. Furthermore, it is expected that daily stress will be relived if the irritation on eating and the frustration with the physical appearance are removed. However regarding the correlation of the graph of the amount of cortisol for the subjected seven female patients, their facial hue, brightness, and intensity increased in contradiction to the amount of cortisol gradually decreased every time at the follow-ups after surgery. The decrease of the amount of cortisol and the improvement of their facial color tone observed six months after the surgery suggested the possibility that the recovery of the occlusion function by the immediate load dental implants did not only make the patients expressive for their physical appearance health but also brought their skin firmness and moisture by making their "feeling" balanced and affected deeply to the physical and psychological health promotion through the acquisition of masticatory function and the aesthetic recovery.

It is a purpose to measure how an effect of the oral rehabilitation applied immediate loading implant system affects the body as for this study, but, about the physical influence except the oral area, does not lecture in particular. The consideration about the influence that the physical factor except the oral area caused by health condition and the psychology situation of the subject and a lifestyle affects measurement data is a future research.

Facing an aging society, the demand for the treatment applying the immediate load dental implants will grow. Along with it, however, the situations that patients who take the dental implant treatment would visit other branches or they would need a long-term hospitalization are concerned as well. Originally strict and periodic maintenances by professionals are necessary to maintain the restructured occlusion with the implant treatment [36]. However, if stress reactant materials which can be measured by the non-invasive and simple saliva collection can be applied to the diagnosis as the biomarker [37], it may be contributory to find out oral functional problems in the future medical front.

Moreover, the decrease of stress reactant hormones and the improvement of skin color tones obtained from the analysis by Robo Skin Analyzer® indicated that the occlusion recovery released the patients from physical and psychological stress, such as the decrease of masticatory function and aesthetical complex, and enriched their "feeling". It is expected that the restructure of occlusion by the immediate load dental implants brings the patients smile back and recuperates their sociability and positive attitude, and enhances their quality of life.

References

[1]   Maló, P., Rangert, B. and Nobre, M. (2003) "All-on-Four" Immediate-Function Concept with Brånemark System Implants for Completely Edentulous Mandibles: A Retrospective Clinical Study. *Clinical Implant Dentistry and Related Research*, **5**, 2-9.

[2]   Tarnow, D.P., Emtiaz, S. and Classi, A. (1997) Immediate Loading of Threaded Implants at Stage 1 Surgery in Edentulous Arches: Ten Consecutive Case Reports with 1- to 5-Year Data. *The International Journal of Oral & Maxillofacial Implant*, **12**, 319-24.

[3]   Garg, A.K. (2007) Osstell Mentor: Measuring Dental Implant Stability at Placement, before Loading, and after Loading. *Dent Implantol Update*, **18**, 49-53.

[4]   Kim, H., Kashiwagi, K. and Kawazoe, T. (2009) Measurement Errors for the Primary Stability of Implants Using a Wireless Resonance Frequency Analyzer. *The Journal of the Osaka Odontological Society*, **72**, 69-76.

[5] Hucklebridge, F., Clow, A. and Evans, P. (1998) The Relationship between Salivary Secretory Immunoglobulin A and Cortisol: Neuroendocrine Response to Awakening and the Diurnal Cycle. *International Journal of Psychophysiology*, **31**, 69-76. http://dx.doi.org/10.1016/S0167-8760(98)00042-7

[6] Knutsson, U., Dahlgren, J., Marcus, C., Rosberg, S., Brönnegård, M., Stierna, P. and Albertsson-Wikland, K. (1997) Circadian Cortisol Rhythms in Healthy Boys and Girls: Relationship with Age, Growth, Body Composition, and Pubertal Development. *The Journal of Clinical Endocrinology & Metabolism*, **82**, 536-403.

[7] Akimoto, M., Miyazaki, M., Lee, H.-H., Nishimura, T., Tamura, M. and Miyakawa, M. (2009) Using Fuzzy Reasoning to Support System of Diagnosis of the Skin Disease. *Bioimages*, **17**, 11-20.

[8] Takiwaki, H. (1998) Measurement of Skin Color Using Reflectance Instruments and Image Analysis of the Skin. Cosmetic Stage. *The Journal of Medical Investigation*, **44**, 121-126.

[9] Misch, C.E. and Degidi, M. (2003) Five-Year Prospective Study of Immediate Early Loading of Fixed Prostheses in Completely Edentulous Jaws with a Bone Quality-Based Implant System. *Clinical Implant Dentistry and Related Research*, **5**, 17-28. http://dx.doi.org/10.1111/j.1708-8208.2003.tb00178.x

[10] Albrektsson, T. and Sennerby, L. (1991) State of the Art in Oral Implants. *Journal of Clinical Periodontology*, **18**, 474-481. http://dx.doi.org/10.1111/j.1600-051X.1991.tb02319.x

[11] Zarb, G.A. and Albrektsson, T. (1998) Consensus Report: Towards Optimized Treatment Outcomes for Dental Implants. *Journal of Prosthetic Dentistry*, **80**, 641.

[12] Lindh, C., Petersson, A. and Rohlin, M. (1996) Assessment of the Trabecular Pattern before Endosseous Implant Treatment: Diagnostic Outcome of Periapical Radiography in the Mandible. *Oral Surgery, Oral Medicine, Oral Pathology, Oral Radiology, and Endodontology*, **82**, 335-343. http://dx.doi.org/10.1016/S1079-2104(96)80363-5

[13] Meredith, N., Alleyne, D. and Cawley, P. (1996) Quantitative Determination of the Stability of the Implant-Tissue Interface Using Resonance Frequency Analysis. *Clinical Oral Implants Reseach*, **7**, 261-267. http://dx.doi.org/10.1034/j.1600-0501.1996.070308.x

[14] Johansson, P. and Strid, K.G. (1994) Assessment of Bone Quality from Placement Resistance during Implant Surgery. *The International Journal of Oral & Maxillofacial Implant*, **9**, 279-288.

[15] Olivé, J. and Aparicio, C. (1990) Periotest Method as a Measure of Osseointegrated Oral Implant Stability. *The International Journal of Oral & Maxillofacial Implant*, **5**, 390-400

[16] Kishimoto, T. (2005) Interleukin-6: From Basic Science to Medicine—40 Years in Immunology. *Annual Review of Immunology*, **23**, 1-21. http://dx.doi.org/10.1146/annurev.immunol.23.021704.115806

[17] Hirano, T., Akira, S., Taga, T. and Kishimoto, T. (1990) Biological and Clinical Aspects of Interleukin 6. *Immunol Today*, **11**, 443-449. http://dx.doi.org/10.1016/0167-5699(90)90173-7

[18] Ohzato, H., Yoshizaki, K., Nishimoto, N., Ogata, A., Tagoh, H., Monden, M., Gotoh, M., Kishimoto, T. and Mori, T. (1992) Interleukin-6 as a New Indicator of Inflammatory Status: Detection of Serum Levels of Interleukin-6 and C-Reactive Protein after Surgery. *Surgery*, **111**, 201-209.

[19] Gabay, C. and Kushner, I. (1999) Acute-Phase Proteins and Other Systemic Responses to Inflammation. *The New England of Journal Medicine*, **340**, 448-454.

[20] Douglas, R.G. and Shaw, J.H. (1989) Metabolic Response to Sepsis and Trauma. *British Journal of Surgery*, **76**, 115-122.

[21] Levine, S.J., Larivée, P., Logun, C., Angus, C.W. and Shelhamer, J.H. (1993) Corticosteroids Differentially Regulate Secretion of IL-6, IL-8, and G-CSF by a Human Bronchial Epithelial Cell Line. *American Journal of Physiology*, **265**, 360-368.

[22] Kato, M., Suzuki, H., Murakami, M., Akama, M., Matsukawa, S. and Hashimoto, Y. (1997) Elevated Plasma Levels of Interleukin-6, Interleukin-8, and Granulocyte Colony-Stimulating Factor during and after Major Abdominal Surgery. *Journal of Clinical Anesthesia*, **9**, 293-298. http://dx.doi.org/10.1016/S0952-8180(97)00006-8

[23] Kamagata, Y., Miyasaka, N., Inoue, H., Hashimoto, J. and Iida, M. (1989) Cytokine Production in Inflamed Human Gingival Tissues—Interleukin-6. *Journal of Japanese Society of Periodontology*, **31**, 843-848. http://dx.doi.org/10.2329/perio.31.843

[24] Sugano, N. (1992) Study of Interleukin-6 Expression in Periodontitis. *Journal of Japanese Society of Periodontology*, **34**, 277-285. http://dx.doi.org/10.2329/perio.34.277

[25] Takahashi, K. (1992) Assessment of Interleukin-6 in the Progression of Disease. *Journal of Japanese Society of Periodontology*, **34**, 286-300. http://dx.doi.org/10.2329/perio.34.286

[26] Takigawa, M. (1992) Study of Interleukin-6 Produced from Human Gingival Fibroblasts. *Journal of Japanese Society of Periodontology*, **34**, 301-314. http://dx.doi.org/10.2329/perio.34.301

[27] Ito, H., Takata, T., Miyauchi, M., Ogawa, I. and Nikai, H. (1994) Immunohistochemical Localization of Interleu-

kin-1α,Interleukin-1β and Interleukin-6 in Human Gingival Tissue. *Journal of Japanese Society of Periodontology*, **36**, 545-551. http://dx.doi.org/10.2329/perio.36.545

[28] Yamaguchi, T. (2009) Enamel Protein Suppress Inflammatory Reaction. *Journal of Japanese Society of Periodontology*, **51**, 38-50. http://dx.doi.org/10.2329/perio.51.038

[29] Hobo, S. (1984) A Kinematic Investigation of Mandibular Border Movement. *Journal of Prosthetic Dentistry*, **51**, 642-646. http://dx.doi.org/10.1016/0022-3913(84)90409-8

[30] Glauser, R., Portmann, M., Ruhstaller, P., Lundgren, A.K., Hammerie, C.H. and Gottlow, J. (2001) Stability Measurements of Immediately Loaded Machined and Oxidized Implants in the Posterior Maxilla. A Comparative Clinical Study Using Response Frequency Analysis. *Applied Osseointegration Research*, **2**, 27-29.

[31] Cannon, W.B. (1914) The Emergency Function of the Adrenal Medulla in Pain and the Major Emotions. *American Journal of Physiology*, **33**, 356-372.

[32] Selye, H. (1936) A Syndrome Produced by Diverse Nocuous Agents. *Nature*, **138**, 32. http://dx.doi.org/10.1038/138032a0

[33] Izawa, S. and Suzuki, K. (2007) The Comparison of Salivary Cortisol Immunoassay Kits: Correlations between Salivary and Plasma Cortisol Concentrations and Comparison of Immunoassay Methods. *Japanese Journal of Complementary and Alternative Medicine*, **4**, 113-118. http://dx.doi.org/10.1625/jcam.4.113

[34] Ozawa, H. (2008) Neuronal Network for Regulation System of Stress, Feeding and Sexual Behavior. *The Medical Association of Nippon Medical School*, **4**, 25-31. http://dx.doi.org/10.1272/manms.4.25

[35] tatsuo, M., Mitsunori, U., Hajime, I. and Masakazu, K. (2009) Stress Evaluation by the Stress Response Material in the Saliva and Effect by Bruxism. *The Journal of Gifu dental Society*, **36**, 135-148.

[36] Mori, K. and Akiyoshi, M. (1967) Marginal Periodontitis: A Histological Study of Incipient Stage. *Journal of Periodontology*, **38**, 45-52. http://dx.doi.org/10.1902/jop.1967.38.1.45

[37] Vining, R.F., McGinley, R.A., Maksvytis, J.J. and Ho, K.Y. (1983) Salivary Cortisol: A Better Measure of Adrenal Cortical Function than Serum Cortisol. *Annals of Clinical Biochemistry*, **20**, 329-335. http://dx.doi.org/10.1177/000456328302000601

12

LDL-Related Intolerance to Glucose, Diastolic Hypertension and Additive Effects of Smoking Were Found with Three Female Study Groups

Ruth-Maria Korth

Practice and Research in General Medicine FiDA, Munich, Germany
Email: r.korth@fidaderm.com

Abstract

Initial prodiabetic risk profiles were invented here with three female study groups consisting of primarily healthy women (A1: 1990-1999, n = 160; A2: 2009, n = 88; A: n = 248, 36 ± 14 years; B: 2014: n = 65, aged 37± 11 years). Significantly higher blood pressure was found comparing intolerance versus tolerance to glucose ($p < 0.05$, IGTT, 22 of 68). High LDL-cholesterol (LDL-C) showed additive effects as LDL-related intolerance was further related with rise of blood pressure ($p < 0.05$), of triglycerides ($p = 0.02$), of fasting blood glucose ($p = 0.07$) and of urine pathology ($p = 0.07$). High LDL-C of women who reported smoking at baseline was correlated with diastolic hypertension whereby alcohol problems overlapped ($p = 0.036$, A). Unhealthy combinations were found consisting of LDL-related intolerance to glucose, LDL-related smoking, of alcohol-related hypertriglyceridemia or of combined drinking and smoking testing urine pathology over the course of time. Obese women were at direct risk for hypertension in the presence of high LDL-C and submaximal ratio of serum albumin to triglycerides (Alb/Trig). Obese women reacted highly sensitive to critical alcohol consumption showing then macroalbuminuria. Current participants who disowned daily alcohol consumption showed healthy morning urines and normal fasting blood glucose. Mild decrease of HDL-C was observed during heavy smoking of relatively young women who had normal biomarkers. Women with intolerance to glucose were at direct risk for hypertension whereby high LDL-C and/or smoking triggered prodiabetic risk profiles. Obese women had elevated LDL-C during hypertension and reacted highly sensitive to alcohol-related proteinuria and/or hematuria.

Keywords

Combined Telemedical Care: Women's Health, Obesity, LDL-Intolerance to Glucose, Diastolic

Hypertension, Ratio of Serum Albumin to Triglycerides (Alb/Trig), Albuminuria

1. Introduction

Individual and combined risk factors characterized here middle aged women selected out of three consecutive study groups. Coded biomarkers were enrolled using equivalent criterions to determine initial risk factors of non-diabetic women over indicated time periods since 1990. Intolerance to glucose was compared to controls and dependable risk factors characterized then risk profiles for diastolic hypertension and critical glucose profiles. High LDL-C and/or self-reported smoking were evaluated with blood pressure, metabolic profiles and morning urines of primairily healthy women.

Several local study groups have provided evidence before that men and/or women with LDL-related hypertriglyceridemia have significantly higher blood pressure compared to normolipidemic persons [1]-[3]. Critical alcohol consumption of hyperlipidemic persons aggravates the risk for diastolic hypertension, significant rise of LDL/HDL, lowering of HDL-cholesterol (HDL-C) and rise of urine pathology compared to hyperlipidemic women reporting healthy lifestyle [1]. Obesity, hypertriglyceridemia and critical alcohol consumption were related with significantly lower serum albumin to triglycerides ratio (Alb/Trig) compared to appropriate controls [1]-[4]. Proteinuria or hematuria were not directly related with smoking or with rise of blood pressure perhaps because evaluated women were relatively young and the majority showed normal biomarkers [1].

The clinical study program was originally based on recognized pathways of alcohol-related phosphocholines as those specifically activate human cells [4]-[6]. Chemically defined alkyl-acyl-(long-chain)-phosphocholines (AAGPC, LA-paf) are released from cells together with apoprotein B [7]-[9]. Apoprotein B and related lipoproteins carry lipophilic phosphocholines to explain at least in part why LDL- or VLDL-particles upregulate human cells and make human endothelial cells sticky [7]-[9]. Phospholipases on outer membranes of human endothelial cells trigger release deacylated phosphocholines (lysopaf) and serum albumin incorporates lysopaf to some degree [9]-[12]. Functional serum albumin was invented here based on opposite relationships between serum albumin and triglycerides (Alb/Trig). Endogenous transcytosis of albumin-bound lysopaf across dysfunctional endothelium barriers has been shown before with cerebrospinal fluids (CSF) whereby upregulatory potency of lysopaf is clinically shown with significant increase of psychotic symptoms [13] [14].

Purified serum albumin protects human cells and completes specific antagonists of phosphocholines, so-called Ginkgoloides [9] [15]-[18]. Pure serum albumin further protects human cells against unhealthy formation and release of acetylhydrolases, phospholipases A2 (PLA2) [13]. Opposite unfavourable effects of human LDL-particles trigger accelerated formation of phospholipases to be then expressed on outer membranes of human endothelial cells, monocytic cells and platelets [10] [12] [13]. Receptor-dependent transcytosis of paf-like phosphocholines is confirmed with immune histology of large endosomal compartments showing that paf receptors are expressed in/on endothelial cells [19]. Early animal models show transcytosis of labeled serum albumin or of LDL-particles across endothelium of isolated organs [20].

Clinical studies correlate thickening of arterial intima media during insulin resistance, mild hypertension and increased plasma levels of antibodies against lipoprotein-associated phospholipids (LA-paf) [21]. Biomedical reports support migration of smooth muscle cells into the arterial intima whereby combined signalling of neighbouring cells is based on several growth factors such as insulin-like growth factor, vascular endothelial growth factor and/or angiotensin II [22] [23].

Tobacco-related rise of urine pathology has been found with morning urines of men but alcohol consumption overlapped [2] [3]. Reviews summarize various tobacco-related aldehydes suggesting conjugation of proteins whereby radicals in arterial plaques impair lipoprotein-associated phospholipases during late arterial disorders [24]-[28]. High prevalence of smoking is correlated with type 2 diabetes of elderly persons in a Finnish study suggesting that smoking impairs regeneration of pancreatic betacells [29]. Impaired filtration of renal endothelium is shown with insulin, thyroid hormones and angiotensinogen in urinary compartments of diabetic persons [30].

Clinical observations show enhanced exsudation of labeled albumin into tissues during obesity and insulin resistance of men while no relevant exsudation of labeled albumin has been found of persons during isolated hypertension [31]. Clinical follow-up studies establish the predictory values of persistent albuminuria/proteinuria showing high prevalence of sustainable hypertension, stroke and/or cardiovascular disorders among elderly US persons [32]. Hypertension and proteinuria predict renal failure as shown with a 24 year follow up study of 1462 women in Sweden [33]. The present study invented critical glucose profiles and mild hypertension at baseline of middle-aged women who often reported smoking at baseline.

Physicians know that persistent hypertension needs pharmacotherapy in the presence of additive risk factors and that sustainable hypertension needs early antihypertensive pharmacotherapy with diuretics and/or antagonists against adrenergic receptors, angiotensins or elevated aldosterone ($\geq 150/\geq 100$ mmHg). Dietary supplements are adapted to complete antihypertensive pharmacotherapy and benefit is shown with treated hypertension of abstinent former alcohol abusers [6] [17].

Next, hyperlipidemic persons are at risk for hypertension and react highly sensitive to critical alcohol consumption [1]-[3]. Alcohol-free liquids are developed to replace alcohol use and to reduce uptake of cholesterol, saturated fat, sugar alcohol, adverse carbohydrates, sodium, transformed phospholipids to neutralize lipid-related problems [17]. Skilled persons know that transformed food components contain unhealthy transformed fatty acids and that some dairy products contain unfavourable glycated albumin so that only certified low fat dairy products and certified oils from ecologically grown plants were recommended as healthy supplements [17] [34] [35]. Lipid lowering strategies aim to reduce high triglycerides and balance insulin-related uptake of glucose. Biomedical pathways of high triglycerides are shown with cells as triglycerides trigger insulin resistance, translocation of glucose transporters and activation of proteinkinases [36].

Physicians know that abdominal fat of younger persons triggers insulin resistance and that metabolic syndromes predict arterial lesions at 21 to 39 years of age [37]. Rise of childhood obesity over the past 30 years leads to higher quality of school lunch, improves dietary education of children and skills healthy food early in life [38]. Dietary strategies recommend obese persons to reduce uptake of salty food, of saturated fat and of adverse carbohydrates to neutralize insulin resistance [39].

Higher risk of obese women for thrombotic events must be considered during oral uptake of contraceptives as obese families often show endothelial-derived thrombotic risk factors [40] [41]. Obese women are at higher risk for antiphospholipid syndromes based on endogenous formation of antibodies against adverse carrier proteins initiating then a dramatic inflammatory cross talk between endothelium and smooth muscle cells with accelerated risk for thrombotic events [42] [43].

Classical antihypertensive diets recommend low fat dairy products and fresh vegetables to reduce uptake of sodium, fat and sugar [44]. These recommendations are originally based on animal models teaching that high glucose of aging rats impairs endothelium-related glycoprotein matrix leading to disturbed filtration [45]. In addition, perfusion of the aortic cannula of rats with high doses of lysophospholipids triggers arrythmia during accelerated excretion of lysophospholipids into the cardial tissue [46]. Moderate intensity of exercising lowers expression of voltage-dependent calcium channels whereby these voltage-gated channels sensitize rats to adverse renal responses during intake of high sodium [47]. Insulin resistance and higher sensitivity to hypertension might share vulnerable regions of chromosome 4 at least of rats [48]. Recent dietary strategies monitor 24 h urines to reach healthy relationships of urinary sodium and potassium and recommend to reduce uptake of sodium and to increase uptake of potassium e.g. with vegetables [49]-[51].

Local internet presentations of the practice provide comprehensible stategies in good time against alcohol-related hypertriglyceridemia and related albuminuria (www.fida-aha.com). Telemedical informations are combined here with personal counseling and physical examinations recommend healthy food, lifestyle and exercising (www.fidabus.com) [1]-[6]. Coded case reports motivated as abstinent former alcohol abusers overcome hypertension during treatment with antihypertensive pharmacotherapy and healing of hematuria during complementary treatment with purified extracts from Ginkgo biloba [6] [17] [52]. Elderly hypercholesterolemic women who report heavy smoking overcome mild diabetes and hematuria during long lasting cessation of smoking providing prescriptions to lower cholesterol combined with Ginkgoloides to repair renal endothelium barriers [17] [53]-[55]. Low fat dairy products were supplemented with low doses of vitamin D considering that high doses of steroid derivatives can enhance the risk for hypertension [17] [56]. Plasmatic potassium, thyroidea hormones, C-reactive proteins, uric acids and glomerular filtration rates were tested and normal values widely excluded here hormonal, disorders, renal hypertension and silent kidney disorders at baseline [56]-[58].

The present study invented here the defense potency of opposite plasma compartments (LDL/HDL, Alb/Trig) testing blood pressure and morning urines. Combined monitoring aimed to improve self assessment of lifestyle problems as critical alcohol cosumption was often reported. Intolerance to glucose of non-pregnant women was invented here as independent risk factor of middle-aged women using two statistical methods. Interrelationships of dependable variants were then characterized to be neutralized. Isolated or combined risk factors can be neutralized to protect against progression of hypertension, prodiabetic risk profiles or disturbed renal endothelium barriers.

2. Subjects and Methods

Three female study groups were enrolled based on equivalent criterions using medical standard procedures as shown before [1]-[3]. The local ethical authority has approved the study program with self control documents and informed written consent of participants (BLÄK-EK No. 02088). The study was conducted with coded biomarkers of primairily healthy women who initially attended the practice of General Medicine since 1990 (Fi-DA-practice).

Participants did not suffer of known disorders as women were not included who had at least one of the below mentioned disorders at baseline (A: n = 923, B: n = 73). Complete blood counting excluded hematological disorders at baseline. Women with primairily known diabetes mellitus were not included (HBA1 ≤ 6%). Unexpected diabetes was treated at baseline and were not evaluated here. Patients with known inflammatory, urological, cerebral or neoplastic disorders were not included. Women with hepatitis or liver cirrhosis were excluded. Women using pharmaceutical treatment such as lipid-lowering and/or antidiabetic were not included. Sustainable systolic hypertension had to be treated at baseline (>160 mmHg, not shown here) and treated persons were not included. Women attending the practice only for vaccination were not included. Urine testing was not performed during menstruation. Women with known pregnancy were not included here.

Coded biomarkers were divided into three study groups enrolled over the course of time. First/early (A1: 1990-1999: n = 160, aged 30 ± 10 years) and second/recent study groups (A2-2009: n = 88, aged 37 ± 16 years) were compared. Equivalent risk factors were indicated and/or pooled (A1 & A2, n = 248 (A), aged 36 ± 14 years). Currently scored women were also characterized with coded biomarkers (B: 2010-2014, n = 65, aged 37 ± 11 years).

Age, personal history, intake of oral contraceptives, daily exercising and family disorders were initially documented. Self-reported risky/critical alcohol consumption was stated (≥20 g ethanol/day) in accordance with the Official German alcohol guidelines [59]. The number of daily cigarettes was confidentially documented as well. Physical examinations were provided at baseline in the practice of General Medicine (hereinafter Fida-practice) whereby body weight, blood pressure and morning urines were enrolled. Body mass index classified normal weight (BMIn: <25 kg/m^2), overweight (BMI1: ≥25 kg/m^2) or obesity (BMI2: ≥29 kg/m^2). Blood pressure was determined during initial examination after 10 min resting. Hypertension was stated with systolic or diastolic blood pressure (140 - 160 or ≥90 mmHg, stage 1). Pro-hypertension (135 - 139/85 - 89 mmHg) or normal blood pressure (<135/<85 mmHg) were indicated.

Venous blood was initially taken after 12 h fasting and metabolic profiles were determined at baseline. Clinical chemistry was performed using medical standard procedures. C-reactive proteins (CRP < 0.5 mg/dl), thyroid stimulating hormones (normal TSH: 0.3 - 3.5 μU/ml), serum potassium (normal 3.5 - 5.0 mmol/l) and liver values were indicated. Normal plasma creatinine (<1.3 mg/dl) and healthy glomerular filtration rates (GFR/MDRD-formula) were indicated excluding here silent kidney disorders (101 ± 19 > 90 ml/min/1.7 m^2) [60]. Uric acids were in the normal range (4.4 ± 1.0 < 6 mg/dl). Lipases were in the normal range as well (40 ± 12 < 60 U/l).

Fasting blood glucose values were fully enrolled. Critical fasting and postprandial blood glucose were invented here as "prodiabetic risk profiles" (FG: 90-119 mg/dl, 21% of A (n = 53); 14% of B (n = 9)). Normal (LDL-C < 150) or elevated LDL-C (≥150 mg/dl) classified fasting and postprandial blood glucose (1 h pp). Tolerance to glucose was tested one hour after oral uptake of 100 g glucose to compare intolerance versus normal tolerance to glucose (C out of A1 & A2 & B, n = 68). Intolerance to glucose (IGTT: 1 hpp 172 ± 40, 2 hpp 138 ± 22 mg/dl, 22 out of 68, aged 41 ± 15 years) or normal tolerance were found (NormGTT: 1 hpp < 140 mg/dl, 46 out of 68, aged 38 ± 19 years). Two of these women with intolerance to glucose showed elevated HBA1c (6% - 6.5%) and one case with diabetes was found (FG: 345 mg/dl, HbA1c: 12.5%). These women were treated and not evaluated here.

Direct comparison of mild intolerance versus tolerance of glucose was performed in the presence of critical (FG 90-119 mg/dl, D) or normal fasting blood glucose (FG < 90 mg/dl, E). Intolerance to glucose was characterized during high LDL-C and so-called "LDL-related intolerance to glucose" was evaluated using multivariate analysis. Smoking and high LDL-C further characterized intolerance to glucose (A5: IGTT & NIC, n = 13, LDL-C: 146 ± 25 mg/dl, aged 41 ± 21 years) compared to nomal LDL-C (A6: IGTT & NIC, LDL-C < 150 mg/dl: 135 ± 4 mg/dl, n = 3). Blood pressure of non-smoking IGTT women with high LDL-C was also tested (A7: NoNic-IGTT, LDL-C: 167 ± 47 mg/dl, n = 10).

High LDL-cholesterol characterized previously and currently scored biomarkers (LDL-C ≥ 150 mg/dl, 11% of 248 (A), aged 35 ± 15 years; 17% out of 65 (B), aged 49 ± 6 years). High triglycerides and high cholesterol were related (p = 0.06, Trig ≥ 170 mg/dl, 15% of A, aged 41 ± 16 years, chol ≥ 200 mg/dl, 17% of A, aged 40±19 year). Mixed hyperlipidemia and higher blood pressure were correlated before (p < 0.05, LDL + Trig: 10% of A, aged 35 ± 15 years versus normolipidemia 18% of A, aged 31 ± 11 years) [1]. Current participants were characterized with LDL-C, with high triglycerides (B: Trig ≥ 160 mg/dl: 9% of 65, aged 51 ± 11 years) or with normolipidemia (n = 54 out of B, 83% of 65, aged 33 ± 10 years).

Divisions of heavy or moderate smoking were previously observed testing adverse cholesterol distribution (LDL/HDL ≥ 3; ≥20 cig: 62% of 60 or <20 cig/day: 38% of 60 (A)). HDL-C currently characterized self-reported smoking (≥20 cig: 12% or <20 cig: 23% of B). Submaximal ratio of serum albumin to triglycerides (Alb/Trig < 40: 22% of B, aged 48 ± 16 years) or low HDL-C (HDL-C < 50 mg/dl: 23% of 65 (B), aged 38 ± 12 years) determined dyslipidemic risk profiles of currently scored women.

2.1. Urine Testing

Morning urines were fully screened over the course of time and urine pathology was tested as described [1]. Test strips were initially used to determine proteinuria and/or hematuria and to exclude leukocyturia (Combur of Roche). Women with leukocyturia were initially excluded. Urinary albumin and urinary creatinine were tested using first morning urines (Microalbustix from Bayer, Germany). Proteinuria, hematuria or albuminuria were confirmed in a collaborative laboratory (Synlab Munich). Urine microscopy confirmed intact red cells and excluded pathological casts. Proteinuria and albuminuria were confirmed using protein analysis to exclude pathological proteins. Normal glomerular filtration rates excluded silent kidney disorders [60]. Total urinary calcium in morning urines (n = 26, mmol/l) was tested with Arsenazo III method [61] in the collaborative laboratory (Olympus, photometric Calcium Arsenazo, normal value 1.5 - 6 mmol/l).

2.2. Statistical Methods

Medical data were coded and indicated here with means ± standard deviations. Blinded biomarkers were divided into time-related study groups. Intolerance and tolerance to glucose were compared (C: n = 68). It is noted that only one case of intolerance to glucose was currently found (B). Dependable variants were tested with multivariate ranking to classify biomarkers with critical fasting blood glucose, rise of blood pressure, hypertriglyceridemia, serum albumin, urine pathology, high LDL-C or self-reported drinking and/or smoking (**Table 1**). Alcohol-related urine pathology and triglyceride-related hypertension have been evaluated before using two statistical methods [1].

Direct comparison of blinded cohorts were evaluated by statistical experts using Tukey's tests for pairwise comparisons, controlling type I error rate from a generalized linear model (GLM, SAS-V8.2, PROC GLM, estimates, Augsburg, Germany). The multiple logistic regression evaluated related symptoms (SAS V8.2, PROC LOGIST "multivariate analysis").

2.3. Combined Telemedical Monitoring

Self control documentations were initially offered in the practice and women provided informed, written consent to initiate combined monitoring. Home testing of body weight, blood pressure, morning urines was combined with medical examinations [1]-[3]. Telemedical informations improved self assessment to overcome adverse alcohol consumption and to improve the quality of food and lifestyle. Healthy exercising was recommended, for example to walk at least 30 minutes per day. Healthy prescriptions were provided (www.fidabus.com, webstart 05/01/2001, www.fida-aha.com, webstart 10/31/2002), Germany). Non-pregnant participants were motivated

Table 1. Three female study groups had overlapping risk profiles, Alcohol use and hyperlipidemia (AHA, A) were related with hypertension (<0.05). High LDL-C, obesity, LDL-related hypertriglyceridemia and diastolic were also currently found (B).

Time periods	A1: 1990-1999	A2: 2000-2009	B: 2010-2014
Female study groups:	Fist study group, n = 160	Second study group, n = 88	Current study group, n = 65
Age, years	30 ± 10 years	37 ± 16 years	36 ± 14 years, % of 65
Diastolic hypertension RR ≥ 90 mmHg:	35 ± 14 years (33% of 160)	37%, 95 ± 7 mmHg, 41 ± 14 years	15%, 97 ± 11 mmHg, 42 ± 15 years
Fasting glucose (FG 90 - 119 mg/dl)	36 ± 14 years (23% of 160)	30%, 98 ± 8 mg/dl, 41 ± 18 years	14%, 98 ± 6 mg/dl, 48 ± 16 years
Figure 1: Self-reported smoking	30 ± 10 years (13% of 160)	47%, 17 ± 9 cig, 35 ± 13 years	35%, 13 ± 8, 28 ± 10 years
AHA: intake of ≥20 g ethanol/day	35 ± 10 years, 13%:45 ± 34 g	16%, 39 ± 17 g, 42 ± 11 years	6%, 16 ± 9 g, 48 ± 11 years
Hypertriglyceridemia ≥ 150 mg/dl	15 of 53 (28%), 30 ± 10 years	29% of 58, 257 ± 12, 41 ± 6 years	9%, 193 ± 48 mg/dl, 51 ± 11 years
Adiposity, BMI2 ≥ 29 kg/m²	35 ± 15 years (10% of 160)	36 ± 11 years (11% of 88)	45 ± 10 years (10% of 65)
High LDL-cholesterol ≥ 150 mg/dl	47 ± 18 years (13% of 160)	11%, 180 ± 30, 35 ± 14 years (11%)	17%, 169 ± 19, 49 ± 6 years
Low HDL-cholesterol < 50 mg/dl	35 ± 13 years, 15 of 53 (28%)	10% of years 41, 47 ± 9, 50 ± 21 years	12%, 45 ± 2 mg/dl, 43 ± 13
Albumin/triglycerides (Alb/Trig) < 40	not screened	11 of 22: 27 ± 5, 34 ± 8 years	22%, 29 ± 18, 48 ± 16 years
Figure 2: Urine pathology	31 ± 10 years (13% of 160)	40 ± 8 years (26% of 88)	39 ± 12 years, n = 6
Figure 2: Hematuria	16 of 160 (10%)	13 of 88 (15%)	N = 1
Albuminuria, proteinuria	5 of 160 (3%)	6 of 88 (7%)	n = 5 (30 ± 9 mg/l U-albumin)
AHA and gamma-GT ≥ 18U/l	35 ± 23 U/l	32 ± 21 U/l	17 ± 3 U/l

Drinking, smoking and hyperlipidemia overlapped and were related with diastolic hypertension ($p < 0.05$, A1&A2) and with urine pathology ($p = 0.005$) compared to hyperlipidemic women reporting healthy lifestyle [1]. Alcohol-relate dyslipidemia triggered hematuria and hypertension (122 ± 20/94 ± 5 mmHg; Alb/Trig 35±12, HDL: 46 ± 9; 6 out of A2). Alcoholic mixed hyperlipidemia (AHA) was correlated with diastolic hypertension ($p = 0.04$) and with high LDL/HDL (3.6 ± 1, $p = 0.001$). The second study group (A2 was at highest risk for hematuria. Current benefit was based on lower alcohol use (14% (A), 6% (B). Values are means ± 1 S.D.

with coded case reports reporting benefit of healthy lifestyle. For example, pregnant women initiated and continued cessation of smoking and overcome mild intolerance to glucose without hypertension (www.fidabus.com). Consenting women continued medical monitoring combined with home testing of blood pressure, body weight, morning urines (not shown here).

Non-pregnant women with proteinuria and/or hematuria were treated with diluted purified extracts from Ginkgo biloba to repair renal endothelium during settled cessation periods as shown before [6] [9] [10] [15]-[17]. Benefit and safety of the specifically adapted Fida-compositions have been shown before with longitudinal studies over five years in follow (not shown here) [17].

3. Results

Individual risk factors overlapped at baseline and three study groups were characterized over the course of time in **Table 1**. Better rates of critical fasting blood glucose and of diastolic hypertension were found and currently scored women showed better risk profiles as the majority disowned daily alcohol consumption (**Figure 1**). Better rates of diastolic hypertension were paralleled with decrease of LDL-related smoking as women with high LDL-C currently more often reported healthy lifestyle behaviour (**Figure 1**). In addition, better rates of urine pathology were paralleled with decreased rates of combined drinking and smoking, with better rates of hypertriglyceridemia or with better cholesterol distribution (LDL/HDL in **Figure 2**). Healthy morning urines confirmed benefit of abstinent periods in a reliable manner.

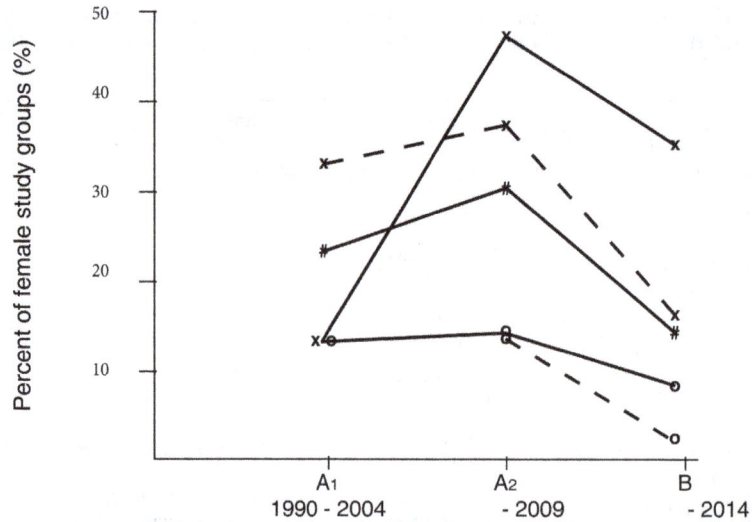

Figure 1. Female cohorts were characterized (A1: n = 160; A2: n = 88; B: n = 65). Better rates of diastolic hypertension (x- - -x, ≥90 mmHg); of critical fasting blood glucose (#   #, 90-119 mg/dl), of alcohol consumption (O   0, ≥20 g ethanol/day) or of LDL-related smoking (o- - -o) were found with current participants (out of B, aged 37 ± 11 years). Self-reported smoking (X__X) failed relevant benefit. The characteristics of three study groups were shown here in the methods section and in **Table 1**.

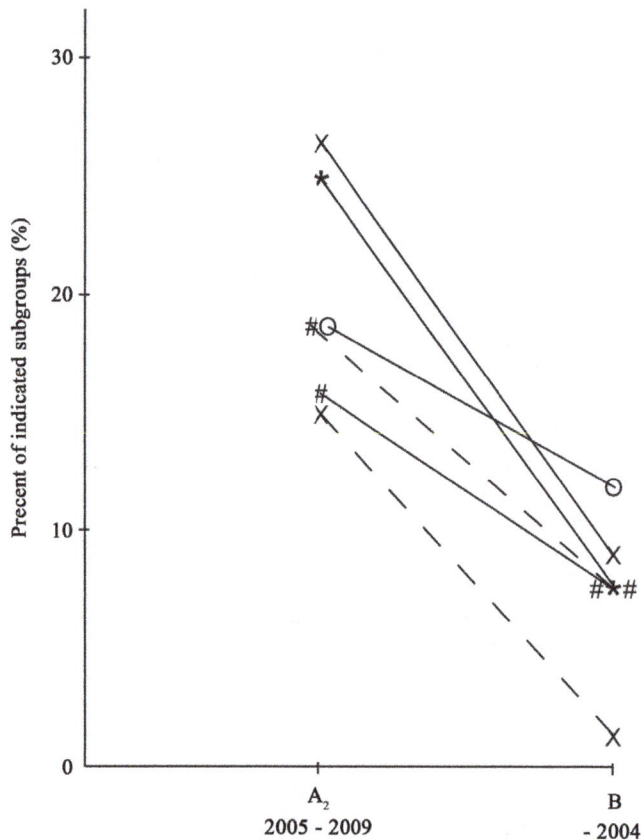

Figure 2. Better rates of urine pathology (X—X, A2: 26% of 88 (A2), B: 9% of 65 (B)) were paralleled with better cholesterol distribution (LDL/HDL≥3, *___*, 25% of A2:, 8% of B) and with decrease of   hypertriglyceridemia (O—O). Better rates of self-reported alcohol problems (#—#, ≥20 g/day, 16% of A2, 6 % of B) and of combined drinking and smoking (#- - -#, 19% of A2, 6% of B) were paralleled with decrease of hematuria (x- - - x, 15% of A2, n = 1 in B). Characteristics and urine pathology of three study groups were shown in **Table 1**.

Rates of self-reported smoking were high and self-assessment of smoking was reliable (**Figure 1**). Additive effects of self-reported smoking were invented here testing glucose profiles, blood pressure and morning urines (**Table 2** and **Table 3**).

The first and second study groups showed equivalent proportions of high LDL-cholesterol and/or obesity while underlying risk profiles changed over the course of time (**Table 3** and **Table 4**). Critical family history indicated age-related rise of vascular disorders, hypertension and diabetes (19% of A or B).

The current study group tended to normal glucose profiles, normal triglycerides and better rates of dependable variants evaluating here indicated risk profiles of non-pregnant women who often reported smoking.

3.1. Critical Glucose Profiles and Hypertension

Rates of critical glucose profiles currently decreased and rates of diastolic hypertension decreased as well (**Figure 1**, **Table 1**). Better rates of critical fasting blood glucose were currently found of women at higher age and these women often reported smoking (**Table 2**). Normal blood pressure was found with women having normal tolerance to glucose (**Table 2**).

Critical fasting and postprandial blood glucose overlapped with obesity, high triglycerides and mild increase of cholesterol overlapped with critical fasting blood glucose (**Figure 3**). LDL-related intolerance to glucose was then evaluated to overcome high variances of indicated prodiabetic risk profiles (**Figure 3**).

The direct comparison of intolerance versus tolerance to glucose determined raised blood pressure as major dependable variant (**Figure 4**, **Table 2**). Indeed, intolerance versus tolerance to glucose showed significantly

Table 2. Intolerance versus tolerance to glucose showed higher blood pressure (IGTT vs. NormGTT, $p < 0.05^{**}$, C out of A + B).

	Smoking or high LDL-C aggravated then hypertension. Alcohol-related obesity, hypertension and albuminuria overlapped (AHA).							
Targets:	A-FG: 90 - 119	B:FG 90 - 119	C: IGTT	C: Norm. GTT	C:IGTT & NIC	No NIC I GTT	Norm GTT-NIC	AHA-B
Cohort A out of 248	53 of 248, 21%	9 of 65, 14%	22 of 248, 9%	46 of 68, 68%	12 of 22, 55%	10 of 22, 45%	6 of 46, 13%	4 of 65, 6%
Age, years	36 ± 14	48 ± 16	41 ± 15	38 ± 19	41 ± 21	41 ± 15	31 ± 10	37 ± 24
Syst. RR mmHg	129 ± 20	122 ± 18	$135 \pm 29^{**}$	117 ± 12	$146 \pm 25^{**}$	129 ± 13	122 ± 15	136 ± 20
Diast. RR mmHg	86 ± 12	81 ± 8	$89 \pm 16^{**}$	78 ± 10	$98 \pm 6^{**}$	85 ± 15	85 ± 11	94 ± 19
Cholesterol mg/dl	212 ± 41	233 ± 22	221 ± 56	214 ± 15	249 ± 41	227 ± 43	201 ± 46	234 ± 26
LDL-C mg/dl	141 ± 38	130 ± 22	167 ± 54	122 ± 23	161 ± 47	167 ± 42	122 ± 23	137 ± 35
HDL-C mg/dl	60 ± 18	60 ± 12	50 ± 16	64 ± 9	48 ± 27	46 ± 11	62 ± 15	61 ± 11
LDL/HDL	2.9 ± 1.9	2.3 ± 0.6	2.6 ± 2.3	2.2 ± 0.9	2.6 ± 0.4	1.7 ± 0.5	1.7 ± 0.5	2.5 ± 1.1
TArlibgulymcienr i/dTersig mg/dl	137 ± 73	$143 \pm 68\%$	$238 \pm 125^{**}$	131 ± 80	$230 \pm 131^{**}$	230 ± 103	106 ± 25	125 ± 53
FG mg/dl	elected: 98 ± 8	elect. 98 ± 6	$95 \pm 6^{*}\%$	83 ± 19	$97 \pm 18^{*}$	93 ± 10	81 ± 13	89 ± 11
P-Creatinine mg/dl	0.8 ± 0.1	0.8 ± 0.1	0.8 ± 0.1	0.8 ± 0.2	0.8 ± 0.2	0.8 ± 0.1	0.7 ± 0.2	0.8 ± 0.2
CRP mg/dl	0.6 ± 0.4	0.4 ± 0.2	0.5 ± 0.4	0.4 ± 0.2	0.4 ± 0.2	0.5 ± 0.4	0.4 ± 0.2	0.5 ± 0.2
AHA ≥ 20 g/day	16 of 46, 22%	n = 1	n = 2, 1%	7 of 46, 15%	n = 2	n = 2	n = 2	elect 28 ± 5 g
BMI kg/m^2	25 ± 6	25 ± 4	28 ± 4	26 ± 6	28 ± 4	24 ± 4	25 ± 7	30 ± 4
Urine pathology	8 of 46, 17%	n = 1	2 of 22, 9%	6 of 46, 13%	3 of 12, 25%	n = 1	n = 2	n = 3
Smoking (cig/day)	19 of 46, 41%	3 of 9, 33%	8 of 22, 36%	6 of 68, 9%	elect. (18 ± 8)	elect No NIC	elected NIC	n = 1

Risky fasting blood glucose (FG) or intolerance to glucose were sensitive to higher age or smoking (IGTT, 1 hpp: 172 ± 40 mg/dl). Smoking or high LDL-C during IGTT triggered hypertension of women with overweight and high triglycerides overlapped. Alcohol use and obesity triggered hypertension and albuminuria (AHA: Alb/Trig: 31 ± 8, 28 ± 5g ethanol/day, 75 ± 3 mg/l U-albumin). One case of diabetes with hematuria was found among obese women during alcohol-related hyperlipidemia (see result section). Values are means $\pm$ 1 S.D.

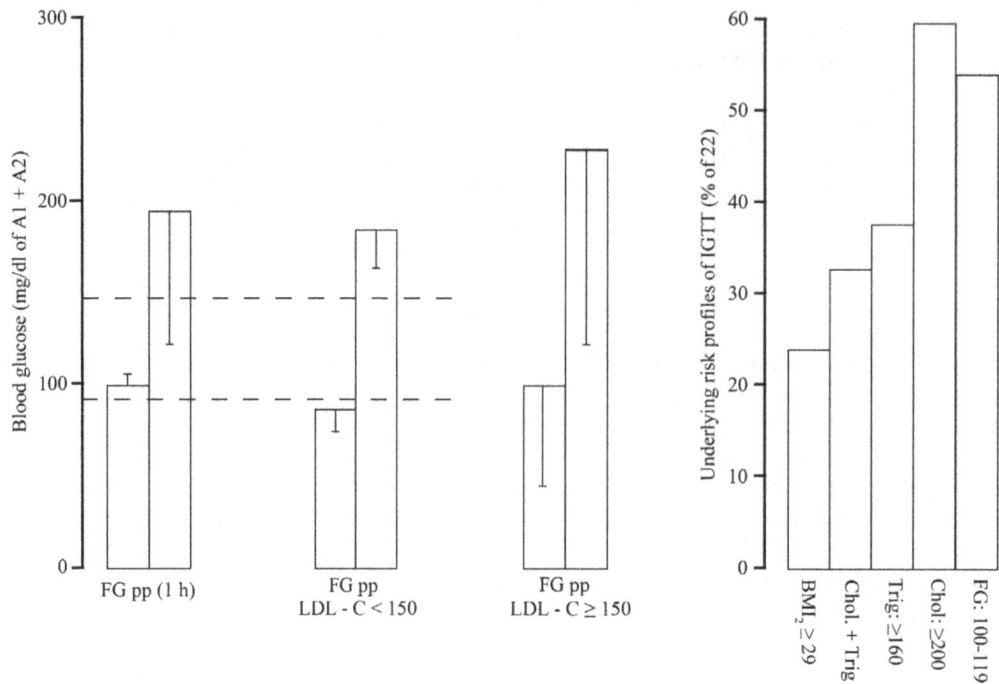

Figure 3. Critical fasting (FG) and postprandial (1 h pp) blood glucose were characterized with normal LDL-C (<150135 ± 4 mg/dl, n = 3) or high LDL-C (≥150 mg/dl; n = 13). High variances indicated inhomogenous cohorts as obesity (BMI2: ≥29 kg/m²), hyperlipidemia (Chol + Trig), moderate increase of cholesterol (≥200 mg/dl) overlapped with critical fasting blood glucose (FG). Characteristics of women with indicated glucose profiles were shown in **Table 2**. Values are means ± 1 S.D.

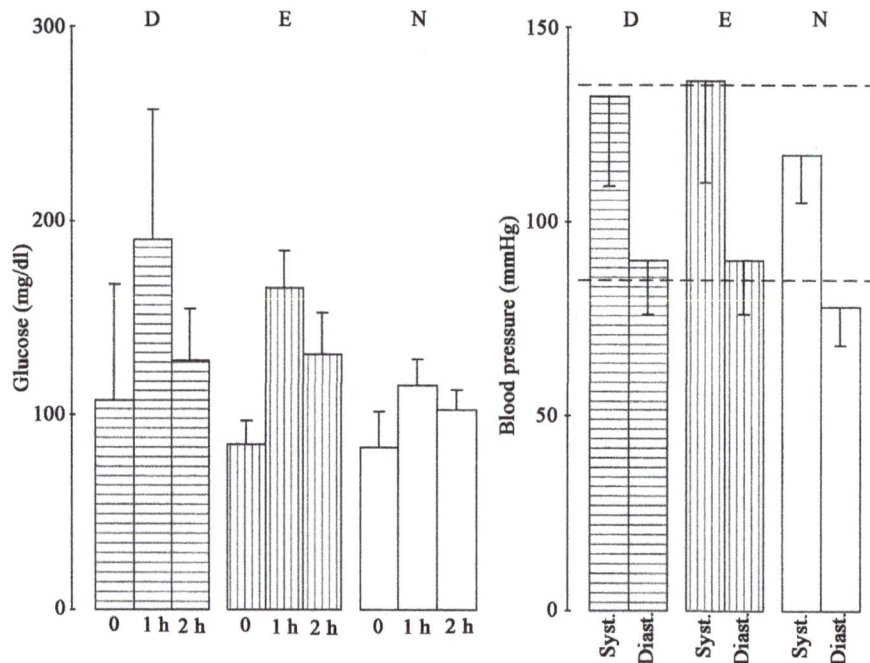

Figure 4. Blood glucose was determined preprandial or 1 h, 2 h after oral uptake of 100 g glucose and rise of blood pressure was found comparing women with intolerance versus normal tolerance to glucose (*p* < 0.05). Women with intolerance to glucose (IGTT) showed significantly higher blood pressure in the presence of critical (D, FG: 90 - 119 mg/dl, 1hpp: 191 ± 67 mg/dl, n = 10) or normal fasting blood glucose (E, FG < 90 mg/dl, 1hpp: 172 ± 40 mg/dl, n = 12) compared to normal glucose tolerance testing (N < 140 mg/dl, n = 46 of 68). Characteristics of indicated glucose profiles were shown in **Table 2**. Values are means ± 1 S.D.

Table 3. Diastolic hypertension of recent (A2) and current (B) groups showed high LDL-C, obesity and/or mixed hyperlipidemia and often reported smoking while the amount of reported alcohol consumption currently decreased (16 ± 9 g ethanol/day).

Targets:	A2: Diast RR ≥ 90	A2: Alb/Trig < 40	B: Diast RR ≥ 90	B:LDL & Trig	B: Alb/Trig < 40	B: HDL-C ≤ 50	B: LDL ≥ 150 mg
Cases of A2 or B	32 of 88, 37%	11 of 88, 13%	10 of 65, 15%	5 of 65, 8%	14 of 65, 22%	15 of 65, 23%	11 of 65, 17%
Systol. mmHg	139 ± 24	136 ± 17	144 ± 17	130 ± 20	138 ± 18	126 ± 24	138 ± 18
Diastol. mmHg	elect.95 ± 7	92 ± 10	elect. 97 ± 11	92 ± 17	90 ± 16	77 ± 13	90 ± 16
Age, years	36 ± 12	42 ± 15	42 ± 15	44 ± 16	48 ± 16	38 ± 12	48 ± 16
Cholesterol mg/dl	214 ± 43	222 ± 44	219 ± 32	236 ± 30	222 ± 33	185 ± 60	250 ± 15
LDL-C mg/dl	150 ± 46	162 ± 51	151 ± 22	elect. 150 ± 26	127 ± 33	115 ± 51	169 ± 19
HDL-C mg/dl	53 ± 15	61 ± 15	66 ± 20	56 ± 16	63 ± 17	elect. 45 ± 2	61 ± 15
LDL/HDL	4 ± 2.5	3 ± 0.6	2.5 ± 1	4 ± 0.09	2.2 ± 1.0	2.5 ± 1.1	3.3 ± 0.8
Triglycerides	194 ± 123	162 ± 46	135 ± 33	Elect. 193 ± 48	142 ± 25	112 ± 52	138 ± 80
Alb/Trig	28 ± 8	elect.29 ± 8	39 ± 20	23 ± 6	elect. 29 ± 18	44 ± 20	31 ± 13
Fast.Glucose, FG	86 ± 13	89 ± 10	84 ± 6	96 ± 8	86 ± 5	76 ± 20	83 ± 8
Pl-Creatinine	0.8 ± 0.2	0.9 ± 0.05	0.9 ± 0.05	0.9 ± 0.1	0.8 ± 0.2	0.7 ± 0.2	0.8 ± 0.2
TSH U/l	0.3 - 2.5	1.5 ± 0.9	1.5 ± 0.9	1.7 ± 0.8	1.5 ± 0.9	2 ± 2	1.3 ± 0.7
CRP mg/dl	0.7 ± 0.8	0.6 ± 0.4	0.6 ± 0.4	0.4 ± 0.2	0.4 ± 0.3	0.5 ± 0.6	0.4 ± 0.2
AHA ≥ 20 g ethanol	5 of 32, 16%	4 of 11, 36%	3 of 10,30%	2 of 5, 40%	4 of 14, 29%	n = 1	non
BMI kg/m²	26 ± 6	29 ± 6	29 ± 4	27 ± 6	26 ± 4	25 ± 4	27 ± 5
Urine pathology	9 of 32, 28%	4 of 11, 36%	2 of 10, 20%	2 of 5, 40%	5 of 14, 36%	non	non
Smoking %	10 of 32, 32%	7 of 11, 64%	3 of 10, 30%	non	4 of 14, 29%	5 of 9, 56%	2 of 11, 18%
PL-Albumin g/dl	4.1 ± 0.04	4 ± 0.1	4.2 ± 0.3	4.2 ± 0.07	4.0 ± 0.4	4.1 ± 0.2	4.1 ± 0.3

LDL-related hypertriglyceridemia versus normolipidemia showed here again higher blood pressure (LDL & Trig, $p \leq 0.05$, [1]). Currently scored diastolic hypertension was paralleled with LDL-related obesity or with LDL-related hypertriglyceridemia. HDL-C was lower during heavy smoking (HDL-C: 48 ± 2 mg/dl, 22 ± 8 cig/day: 6 of B) showig normal biomarkers. Low Alb/Trig and hypertension were currently paralleled (Alb/Trig 31 ± 8, 136 ± 12/98 ± 18 mmHg, n = 4, 29 ± 4 kg/m²). Normal serum potassium (B: 4.4. ± 0.1 mmol/l) and heal t h y glomerular filtration rates (101 ± 19 ml/min/1.7m²) were found.

Table 4. Obesity, high LDL-C, hypertension, low Alb/Trig and high sensitivity to alcohol consumption were found. Women with normal weight often smoked (BMIn), with overweight (BMI1) showed progress while obese women showed indicated risk profiles.

Targets	A: BMIn	B: BMIn	A: BMI1	B: BMI 1	A2: BMI 2	B: BMI 2	A-Smoking	B-Smoking
Cohorts: A: A1, A2, B	n = 191	n = 46	n = 31	n = 15	n = 10	n = 6	n = 60	n = 22
% out of cohort	77% of 28	71 % of 65	13% of 248	23 % of 65	11% of 88	10% of 65	24% of 248	34% of 65
Smoking (%)	19 of 19 (10%)	16 of 46 (35%)	9 of 31 (29%)	5 of 15 (30%)	3 of 10 (30%)	non	elected	elected
Age, years	36 ± 9	33 ± 10	40 ± 18	44 ± 13	36 ± 11	46 ± 11	37 ± 15	38 ± 10
BMI, kg/m²	21 ± 4	22 ± 2	27 ± 1	26 ± 2	33 ± 2	32 ± 1.2	24 ± 5	23 ± 4
Cholesterol mg/dl	206 ± 44	176 ± 37	206 ± 44	200 ± 27	213 ± 39	240 ± 32	205 ± 45	186 ± 43
LDL-C mg/dl	131 ± 43	100 ± 32	155 ± 53	118 ± 27	151 ± 65	154 ± 23	141 ± 43	115 ± 39
HDL-C mg/dl	65 ± 19	65 ± 14	56 ± 16	62 ± 13	68 ± 15	58 ± 15	64 ± 17	62 ± 14

Continued

LDL/HDL	1.8 ± 0.6	1.6 ± 0.6	2.5 ± 0.7	1.7 ± 0.6	2.4 ± 1.8	2.9 ± 0.8	2.4 ± 1.1	2.2 ± 1.1
Triglycerides mg/dl	110 ± 57	77 ± 27	145 ± 88	112 ± 37	145 ± 61	163 ± 77	140 ± 76	102 ± 57
Alb/Trig	52 ± 15	63 ± 21	37 ± 9	44 ± 19	32 ± 17	33 ± 21	36 ± 14	55 ± 24
Fast. Glucose	83 ± 12	78 ± 14	86 ± 11	89 ± 13	85 ± 11	85 ± 3.6	84 ± 8	78 ± 15
≥20 g ethanol/day	10 of 191 (5%)	n = 2	9 of 31 (29%)	n = 1	non	3 of 6 (50%)	13 of 60 (22%)	3 of 22
Urine pathology	15 of 191 (8%)	n = 2	12 of (39%)	n = 1	non	3 of 6 (50%)	21 of 60 (35%)	2 of 22
Systolic RR mmHg	117 ± 17	109 ± 4	132 ± 21	115 ± 17	133 ± 20	138 ± 20	122 ± 17	115 ± 7
Diastolic RR mmHg	82 ± 9	77 ± 9	86 ± 11	83 ± 9	91 ± 16*	97 ± 16	84 ± 8	82 ± 3
smoking	10% of 191 [1]	17 of 46, 41%	26% of 31 [1]	19% of 26	4 of 10, 40%	non	elected	elected
cigarettes/day	17 ± 9 [1]	14 ± 14	17 ± 9 [1]	12 ± 7	14 ± 8	non	17 ± 9 [1]	13 ± 8
Pl-Albumin	4.4 ± 0.6	4.3 ± 0.3	4.4 ± 0.3	4.1 ± 0.3	4.2 ± 0.3	4.1 ± 0.3	4.5 ± 0.5	4.3 ± 0.3

Obese women reacted highly sensitive to alcohol problems showing then macrolbuminuria, high LDL-C, low ratio of serum albumin to triglycerides (Alb/Trig 25 ± 5 < 30, Trig: 176 ± 49 mg/dl, Alb: 3.96 ± 0.24 ≤ 4 g, GammaGT: 16 ± 11 U/l, CRP-BMI2: 0.46 ± 0.2 mg/dl). Moderate smoking failed relevant effects while heavy smoking lowers HDL-C (n = 8 ≥ 20 cig vs n = 15 < 20 cig/day of B). Values are means ± 1 S.D.

higher systolic and diastolic blood pressure comparing intolerance versus tolerance to glucose in the presence of critical fasting blood glucose (**Figure 4**, IGTT-D: FG: 100-119 mg/dl, p=0.0029, p=0.002). Intolerance versus tolerance to glucose showed significantly higher blood pressure also in the presence of normal fasting blood glucose (**Figure 4**, IGTT-E: $p = 0.0146$, $p = 0.0007$). Intolerance to glucose showed a moderate relationship with critical fasting blood glucose ($p = 0.07$) and with diastolic hypertension using multivariate analysis ($p = 0.07$).

LDL-related intolerance to glucose was then more directly related with diastolic blood pressure ($p = 0.047$) and with high triglycerides ($p = 0.02$). Urine pathology ($p = 0.07$) was related with alcohol problems ($p < 0.05$) and then with critical fasting blood glucose of women with LDL-related intolerance to glucose ($p = 0.07$, **Table 1**).

Next, women with intolerance to glucose often reported smoking and a weak relationship was confirmed between intolerance to glucose and smoking using multivariate analysis ($p = 0.09$, **Table 2**). Smoking women with IGTT showed systolic and diastolic hypertension (**Figure 5(A5)**, **Table 2**). Smoking IGTT-women with normal LDL-C also showed systolic and diastolic hypertension (**Figure 5(A6)**, **Table 2**). The motivating message was that non-smoking women with intolerance to glucose had normal blood pressure even in presence of high LDL-C (**Figure 5(A7)**, **Table 2**). Thus, smoking more than high LDL-C aggravated systolic and diastolic hypertension during intolerance to glucose (IGTT & NIC: **Table 2**).

Altogether, intolerance to glucose was a direct risk factor for diastolic hypertension and smoking and/or high LDL-C were major additive risk factors for hypertension or critical fasting blood glucose. Overall, women with LDL-related intolerance to glucose who smoked had to perceive that smoking during LDL-related intolerance to glucose placed them into an even higher risk class for sustainable hypertension whereby alcohol problesm further triggered urine pathology and critical fasting blood glucose. These data implicated cessation of smoking and drinking to overcome moderate intolerance to glucose with healthy food and lifestyle.

3.2. Diastolic Hypertension and LDL-Cholesterol

Better rates of diastolic hypertension were paralleled here with decrease of LDL-related smoking keeping in mind that the pooled cohort (A1 & A2) with LDL-related hypertriglyceridemia was correlated with diastolic hypertension [1]. The recently scored women with diastolic hypertension showed imbalance of plasma compartments (LDL/HDL ≥ 3, Alb/Trig < 40) while HDL-C was in the normal range (A2 in **Table 3**).

Currently scored women with diastolic hypertension and/or with high LDL-C showed equivalent risk factors at higher age (B, **Table 3**). Hypertriglyceridemia currently decreased of women who were about ten years older (**Table 1**). Half of the currently scored women with diastolic hypertension showed obesity and high LDL-C and

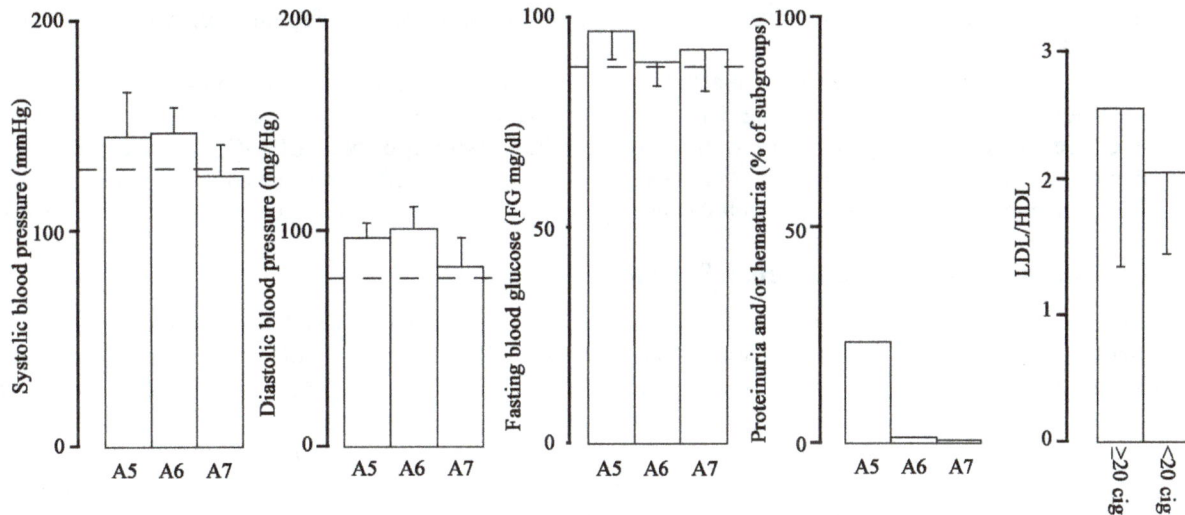

Figure 5. Systolic and diastolic blood pressure or urine pathology were found during intolerance to glucose (A5: IGTT & NIC n = 13, LDL: 146 ± 25 mg/dl). Three smoking IGTT-women with normal LDL-C showed hypertension as well (A6: IGTT & NIC, LDL: 135 ± 4 mg/dl, n = 3). Non-smoking women with IGTT showed normal blood pressure and normal morning urines in the presence of high LDL-C (A7: NoNIC-IGTT, n = 10, LDL: 167 ± 47, n = 10). Urine pathology was not found with IGTT-women who disowned alcohol consumption (A6, A7). Heavy smoking impaired cholesterol distribution (LDL/HDL) with high variances. Characteristics of indicated glucose profiles were shown in **Table 2**. Values were means ± 1 S.D.

the other half had LDL-related hypertriglyceridemia and often reported alcohol problems and smoking (LDL & Trig, **Table 3**).

Women with submaximal ratio of serum albumin to triglycerides (Alb/Trig < 40) recently and currently showed diastolic hypertension, often reported drinking and smoking and often showed urine pathology (**Table 3**). Low ALB/Trig was paralleled with hypertension of women with overweight or obesity whereby high triglycerides rather than low serum albumin triggered hypertension as serum albumin was still in the normal range (**Table 3**).

Smoking and high LDL-C previously overlapped with alcohol consumption forming then a higher-risk combination for diastolic hypertension (p = 0.036) and for critical morning urines (p = 0.06). Better rates of diastolic hypertension were currently found as women with high LDL-C disowned smoking and drinking (**Table 3**). Isolated smoking or isolated rise of LDL-C of abstinent women failed direct relationships with urine pathology using multivariate analysis (p > 0.1, **Table 4**).

Obese women previously and currently showed significantly higher blood pressure compared to women with normal weight (p ≤ 0.05, **Table 1**). Currently scored obese women with diastolic hypertension had high LDL-C with submaximal ratio of serum albumin (**Table 4**). Half of the currently scored obese women reported alcohol problems showing then macroalbuminuria (**Table 1** and **Table 4**).

Obese women often reported different lifestyle problems so that obesity cohorts were not pooled here (**Table 4**). It was clinically observed that half of the currently scored obese women reported alcohol consumption showing then macroalbuminuria and hypertension (**Table 4**). The recent obesity cohort often reported smoking without alcohol problems showing then diastolic hypertension with normal morning urines (**Table 4**). The first obesity cohort often reported alcohol use and showed hypertension with proteinuria and/or hematuria (**Table 1**).

Next, oral contraceptives did not modulate blood pressure as shown with multivariate analysis (p > 0.1, 20% of A). Obese women who reported uptake of oral contraceptives showed hypertension with normal morning urines (140 ± 20/95 ± 15 mmHg, n = 3 of A). The majority of the current participants had normal blood pressure and normal LDL-cholesterol during oral uptake of contraceptives (27 ± 7 years, LDL-C: 127 ± 36 mg/dl, 117 ± 13/82 ± 9 mmHg, 22 ± 4 kg/m^2 of A).

The motivating message was that women at risk were currently about ten years older (**Tables 1-4**). The currently scored women with overweight often reported healthy lifestyle and tended to normal lipid profiles, normal blood pressure and healthy morning urines (BMI1 **Table 4**). The majority of the participants had normal weight and normal biomarkers while relatively young women with normal weight currently often reported smoking (BMIn, **Table 4**).

Women with obesity or overweight reacted highly sensitive to hypertension in the presence of LDL-related hypertriglyceridemia whereby smoking during critical alcohol consumption aggravated urine pathology (**Table 3**). Obese women currently showed the major risk profile consisting of high LDL-C, diastolic hypertension, submaximal Alb/Trig and albuminuria (**Table 4**). Obese women reacted highly sensitive to alcohol-related albuminuria implicating to cede daily alcohol consumption and/or to prepare antihypertensive pharmacotherapy.

3.3. HDL-Related Female Defense System and Smoking

Better rates of LDL/HDL were paralleled with reduced alcohol consumption and healthy morning urines were often found (**Figure 2**). Alcohol consumption decreased while proportions of smoking remained relevant (**Figure 1**). Normolipidemic women who reported drinking and/or smoking had normal HDL-C compared to normolipidemic women with healthy lifestyle ($p > 0.1$).

Significant increase of smoking was found comparing the first versus second study groups (A2 vs A1, $p = 0.003$, **Figure 1**) but no effects were found with LDL/HDL or with HDL-C comparing the first and second study groups ($p > 0.1$). Multivariate analysis further argued against direct relationhships of isolated smoking and HDL-C ($p > 0.1$). Nevertheless, it was observed that heavy smoking previously triggered high variances of LDL/HDL (**Figure 5**).

Current participants who reported heavy smoking showed a mild decrease of HDL-C here for the first time. Heavy smoking in the presence of low HDL-C further decreased HDL-C (HDL-C: $48 \pm 2 < 50$ mg/dl, 23 ± 1 kg/m^2, 22 ± 8 cig./day, n = 5 out of **Table 3**). Moderate smoking showed normal HDL-C and normal biomarkers (n = 6, HDL-C: 62 ± 15 mg/dl, 7 ± 4 cig/day). In short, self-reporting smoking failed significancy testing isolated smoking among relatively young women but might impair cholesterol efflux to some degree.

Altogether, mild decrease of HDL-C was observed during heavy smoking of current participants in the presence of normal blood pressure and normal morning urines. These data implicated to cede smoking and to repair cholesterol efflux during settled cessation periods with healthy alcohol free liquids comprising supplements obtained from ecologically grown food such as appropriate vitamins, minerals and appropriate constituents.

3.4. Hematuria, Proteinuria, Albuminuria, Urinary Calcium Excretion

Better morning urines were currently paralleled with normal LDL/HDL and rates of initially reported alcohol problems also decreased (**Figure 2**). Healthy morning urines and better rates of urine pathology were paralleled here with decrease of combined drinking and smoking (**Figure 2**). In short, rates and amount of daily alcohol consumption currently decreased (6% of B: 16 ± 9 g/day ethanol (B), **Table 1**).

The recent study group showed the highest rate of alcohol-mediated hematuria and/or proteinuria during mixed hyperlipidemia with high LDL/HDL and low ratio of albumin to triglycerides (LDL/HDL: 3.6 ± 1, Alb/Trig 26 ± 8). Hematuria overlapped with drinking and smoking and LDL-related mixed hyperlipidemia triggered hypertension and adverse outcome of alcohol-related dyslipidemia was shown with recently and currently scored women as alcohol problems of hyperlipidemic women were again paralleled with urine pathology (**Table 3**).

Urine pathology was not directly related with hypertension using multivariate analysis ($p > 0.1$). However, alcohol consumption of hyperlipidemic women was related with urine pathology ($p = 0.07$). Thus, low HDL-C indicated degradation of HDL-particles in the presence of activated renal endothelium (LDL & Trig in **Table 3**). It has been shown before that alcohol use mediated urine pathology ($p = 0.04$) and that smoking aggravated alcohol-related urine pathology of hyperlipidemic women ($p = 0.001$, A [1]).

Reliable benefit was currently reached with women who disowned alcohol use showing then better morning urines (**Figure 2**). Alcohol-related hypertriglyceridemia currently decreased and better rates of morning urines were currently found (**Table 1**).

Obese women were currently at higher risk as half of these women reported critical alcohol consumption and showed macroalbuminuria (75 ± 23 mg/l U-albumin, **Table 2**). Women with obesity or diastolic hypertension tended to mild albuminuria in general (30 ± 29 mg/l or 23 ± 10 mg/l urinary-albumin). The motivating message was that glomerular filtration rates were in the normal range (107 ± 29 ml/min/1.7 m^2).

Next, urinary calcium was in the normal range indicating normal tubular reabsorption of calcium even during obesity or hypertension (1.7 ± 0.9, 1.7 ± 0.9 mmol/l). Mild increase of urinary calcium was found in the first morning urines only of smoking women (2.1 ± 0.8 mmol/g, n = 3) compared to non-smoking women (1.3 ± 1.1 mmol/g urinary creatinine, n = 14, aged 36 ± 7 years). Normal levels of total urinary calcium were found during oral uptake of contraceptives (1.5 ± 0.9 mmol/l; 1.7 ± 1 mmol/l).

Altogether, hematuria was paralleled with alcohol-related dyslipidemia of recently scored women who had high LDL/HDL, low HDL-C, low Alb/Trig and hypertension. Alcohol-related dyslipidemia or alcohol-related obesity triggered proteinuria and/or hematuria. Obese women reacted highly sensitive to critical alcohol consumption showing then macroalbuminuria.

Medical counseling recommended to cede drinking and smoking and to combine low fat dairy products with certified plant oils comprising healthy lecithins. Alcohol-free liquids were recommended comprising healthy albumin, supplements, minerals and constituents to repair alcohol-related dysfunction of renal endothelium barriers during abstinent periods.

4. Discussion

Women with intolerance to glucose reacted here highly sensitive to hypertension compared to controls whereby elevated LDL-C or smoking showed additive effects. LDL-related intolerance to glucose was associated with diastolic hypertension and with critical fasting blood glucose independently of age. The majority of the current participants disowned daily alcohol consumption showing then dependable benefit with lower rates of diastolic hypertension, of critical glucose profiles and more often healthy morning urines. Overall, alcohol-related hypertriglyceridemia decreased as shown with currently scored women attending the Fida-practice at baseline.

Better rates of urine pathology were paralleled with better rates of alcohol use, alcohol-related smoking, alcohol-related hyperlipidemia (LDL/HDL ≥ 3) or alcohol-related hypertriglyceridemia of current participants who often disowned daily alcohol consumption. The motivating message was that alcohol consumption was reduced of currently scored women and healthy biomarkers were found at baseline.

Intolerance to glucose was compared to controls and dependable variants characterized here primairily non-diabetic women who tended to mild hypertension, critical fasting blood glucose and/or elevated LDL-C. Unhealthy combinations of indicated risk factors were found with currently scored women having LDL-related intolerance to glucose, LDL-related smoking, alcohol-related smoking, alcohol-related obesity and/or triglyceride-related hypertension. Better rates of alcohol problems were found but self-reported smoking was still relevant.

High LDL-C or smoking were additive risk factors placing here women into a higher risk class for sustainable hypertension during intolerance to glucose, smoking, alcohol problems and/or obesity. The present study evaluated opposite plasma compartments (LDL/HDL, Alb/Trig) to better distinguish adverse risk profiles. Alcohol use specifically mediated urine pathology with and without second risk factors here and before [1]-[6].

Evidence has been provided before that combined alcohol-related hyperlipidemia triggered hypertension, critical fasting blood glucose and urine pathology [1]-[6]. Hyperlipidemic versus normolipidemic women show significant rise of diastolic blood pressure ($p = 0.004$), alcohol use or smoking ($p = 0.0001$, $p = 0.0019$), urine pathology ($p = 0.005$) and lower HDL-cholesterol ($p = 0.01$) with higher LDL/HDL ($p = 0.001$) [1]. Hypertriglyceridemia is correlated with hypertension ($p = 0.05$) and with LDL-related intolerance to glucose ($p = 0.021$) whereby urine pathology ($p = 0.07$) overlapped with critical fasting blood glucose ($p = 0.07$) of primairily non-diabetic women who reported alcohol consumption. Urine pathology is associated with critical alcohol consumption ($p = 0.04$) and smoking aggravates alcohol-related urine pathology ($p = 0.001$) [1]. Overlapping risk factors were distinguished here to overcome high variances of isolated risk factors such as fasting blood glucose, of postprandial blood glucose, of high LDL-C, of serum albumin or of triglycerides. In short, alcohol-related hypertriglyceridemia decreased and better risk profiles were currently found.

Medical counseling has motivated middle aged women in good time to overcome mild risk profiles as additive effects were explained of independent risk factors and dependable variants showing here additive effects. Individual counseling informed about personal risk profiles initiating home testing of body weight, blood pressure and morning urines in good time to improve the quality of food and lifestyle (www.fidabus.com, www.fida-aha.com). Healthy exercising was recommended, for example to walk at least 30 minutes per day.

Rather unselected women currently showed here better self assessment at baseline indicating that current participates were initially motivated to cede adverse alcohol consumption. Self assessment was the condition in which combined monitoring was initiated in the Fida-practice. The selection of the current study group was correct and without bias as men currently failed any benefit and did not reduce adverse alcohol consumption [2] [3]. The combination of personal monitoring with telemedical informations increased the value of medical counseling and informed women who aimed to overcome healthcare problems at baseline. Mortality studies can scare and overestimated isolated risk factors can confuse keeping in mind that pooled study groups consisting of elderly ill persons can easily undervalue progress of younger persons [62]. Personal problems were more carefully debated here and informed middle class women translated medical recommendations into the practical life and often asked for combined monitoring at baseline.

The present study confirmed that obesity was an independent risk factor for mild hypertension indicating that obesity impaired dilatory adaptation of small vessels. Pharmacotherapy had to be considered in cases of sustainable, nocturnal hypertension [6] [52]. Unexpected cases of diabetes were found with obese woman to be treated and not evaluated here. Known diabetes and/or nocturnal, sustainable hypertension were initially treated and treated persons were not followed here.

Skilled persons know that adipocytes store lipophilic ether-linked phosphocholines [63]. HDL-particles incorporate triglycerides during hypertriglycridemia and LDL particles express phospholipases on outer endothelial cells so that lipidated HDL-particles were degraded by endothelial lipases and/or by phospholipases in accordance with underlying biomedical pathways [10] [63]-[66]. The motivating message was that hematuria and/or albuminuria can heal as shown before with abstinent former alcohol abusers during antihypertensive pharmacotherapy [52]. Elderly hypercholesterolemic women had to cede smoking to overcome mild diabetes and hematuria and age-related rise of cholesterol needed then pharmacotherapy to reduce LDL-cholesterol in the presence of several risk factors. Regeneration of healthy endothelium barriers was supported with low fat dairy products, certified plant oils comprising lecithins and Ginkgoloides [52]-[54]. The combination of dairy products and certified plant oils formed micelles to increase intestinal absorption of pure albumin with uptake of prehomones and constituents to supplement mild increase of urinary calcium as shown here with smoking women at baseline [17] [67].

Obese women reacted highly sensitive to alcohol-related macroalbuminuria indicating disturbed filtration of renal endothelium barriers and/or declined defense potency of plasma albumin. Hematuria indicated thin basement membranes during alcohol-related dyslipidemia so that long cessation periods were needed without alcohol consumption, without sugar alcohol, saturated fat and transformed phospholipids. Women with albuminuria had to perceive that about 40% of excreted albumin is degraded during glomerular transcytosis and cannot be detected [60] [68] [69]. Urinary albumin cannot be reabsorbed and can trigger tubular fibrosis with disturbed tubular re-adsorption [60]. Other reports suggest that increase of urinary calcium predicts tubular problems as shown here with smoking women and elsewhere with offspring animals after gestational diabetes [68]-[70]. Women with hematuria had to give up drinking and smoking to prevent progression of glomerular filtration problems, of tubular fibroses and/or thin renal basement membranes [60] [71]. Thin basement nephropathy can indicate vulnerable DNA regions of rare cases with critical family history [72].

Dyslipidemia was found here and before with persons who reported drinking and/or smoking during high LDL/HDL, low Alb/Trig and hypertension. Submaximal ratio of serum albumin to triglycerides indicated here overloaded albumin in the presence of obesity or declined potency of albumin during hypertriglyceridema. Steroids or insulin trigger accelerated synthesis and expression of phospholipases/lipases on outer endothelial cells [1]-[6] [10] [12]. Submaximal Alb/Trig triggered hypertension and alcohol-related dyslipidemia impaired the balance of renal endothelium barriers. Women at risk had to give up drinking and smoking to repair defects of renal endothelium barriers in good time.

Rating of risky/critical alcohol problems corresponded here with Official rates (A: 12% of 248: 30 ± 5 g ethanol/day). Middle aged men report higher alcohol consumption and react more sensitive to tobacco-related urine pathology [2] [3] [59]. Consenting women currently reached here a reliable progress as shown with normal plasma compartments, healthy morning urines and normal blood pressure. It is noted that healthy plasma albumin can endogenously strengthen the glycoprotein matrix covering then the entire luminal surface of human endothelium to modulate filtration of plasma compartments [73].

Healthy alcohol free drinks were adapted comprising pure albumin and healthy lecithins to enhance intestinal absorption of pure serum albumin [17]. Low fat goat milk products are recommended comprising healthy phospholipases/acetylhydrolase to increase intestinal excretion of adverse lipid mediators [17] [50]. Ginkgoloides can protect renal endothelium during settled cessation of drinking and smoking composing alcohol-free drinks therewith to overcome urine pathology and healing was shown with abstinent former alcohol abusers and elderly women who had to cede smoking to overcome hematuria and mild diabetes at baseline [6] [52]-[54]. Obese or hyperlipidemic persons had to give up drinking and/or smoking and had to reduce uptake of sodium, cholesterol, saturated fat and adverse carbohydrates during abstinent periods [6] [52]-[54].

Long time incubation of cells with hormones such as insulin or steroids differentiate human endothelial cells and express adhesion molecules [9] [10]. More recent reports confirm that hormones such as insulin and steroids trigger proliferative effects based on signal transduction pathways of cells [74]. Pleiotropic phenotypes indicate vulnerable DNA regions of insulin response elements as those are highly sensitive to hypertriglyceridemia and insulin promotor genes can modulate lipases and/or phospholipases [75]. Families can have favourable gene variants of apoproteins as healthy variants of apoB or of apoC3 reacting then about 39% lowering of postprandial triglycerides and 22% increase of HDL-cholesterol with 11% lowering of LDL-cholesterol compared to controls and these persons show 40% reduced prevalence of cardiovascular disorders [76] [77]. Other DNA regions encode variants of lipases/phospholipases and these regions are sensitive to triglyceride-related metabolic problems [78]. Asian persons with mutations of phospholipases/acetylhydrolases are at risk for hypertension and stroke [79]. Mutants of phospholipases A2 (PNPLA3) of obese persons trigger non-alcoholic fatty liver disease or non-alcoholic hypertriglyceridemia as variable phenotype expression [80]. Vulnerable genotypes of alcohol dehydrogenases are related with alcohol liver cirrhosis and pancreatitis of Caucasians persons at younger age [81].

The rates of LDL-C did not change here over the course of time while hypercholesterolemic women with diastolic hypertension were currently about ten years older and needed phramcotherapy in the presence of additive risk factors in respect to the medical guidelines [82]. Statins can then inhibit cholesterol synthesis (e.g. to 70 - 100 mg/dl) and also accelerated synthesis of phospholipases as shown with benefit during diabetes [82] [83]. Ezetimibe or plant-derived oxysterols can inhibit intestinal adsorption of cholesterol [84] [85]. Combinations with fibrates can further protect persons against small vessel disease showing additive beneficial effects of statins and fibrates [82]. Fibrates inhibit peroxisome proliferator-activated receptors in cells interacting with long-chain fatty acids esterified of triglycerides and/or phospholipids such as alkyl-acyl-long-chain-glycerophosphocholines (LA-paf) [86] [87].

Self-reported smoking was a problem at baseline here and abroad [88]. Smoking aggravated here diastolic hypertension and formed additive risk combinations during critical alcohol consumption. Smoking women with high LDL-C reacted here highly sensitive to diastolic hypertension during prodiabetic glucose profiles. Relatively young women needed more pertinent informations to cede smoking as these women were indifferent to known mortality studies. These non-pregnant women who reported smoking had to perceive that smoking agravated alcohol-related small vessel disease and LDL-related hypertension. Smoking and drinking of hyperlipidemic persons triggered prodiabetic risk profiles independently of age. Heavy smoking directly impaired here cholesterol loading of HDL-particles in the presence of normal lipid profiles, normal blood pressure and normal morning urines for the first time. Other clinical reports confirm with Chinese men who smoke more than 20 cigarettes per day having then coronary heart disease showing then dysfunctional monocytes with disturbed expression of ATP-binding cassette transporters [89]. Women were currently motivated to cede drinking and smoking as shown with pregnant women who did not smoke and who overcome mild intolerance to glucose without hypertension (www.fidabus.com).

Background art discloses that smoking triggers enzymatic beta-oxidation in mitochondrial compartments and degradation of the cellular defense system is shown with alveolar epithelial carcinoma cells [90]. Individual history of depression and/or dosage of psychopharmaca had to be carefully considered to guide persons at risk during long cessation periods [91]. Healthy alcohol free liquids were adapted with xanthines, healthy albumin, calcium, prehormones and constituents to replace smoking and drinking, to repair the female defense system, to equilibrate the mind and to supplement urinary calcium excretion as well as required constituents [17].

The major limitation of the study was that modified phospholipids were not measured in indicated compartments and that pre- or postprandial insulin values were not tested. It is noteworthy that the testing was reimbursed by assurances so that medical standard procedures had to be used in accordance with medical guidelines. Coded medical raw data provided here pertinent testing without undue experiments so that physicians can better find and neutralize mild diastolic hypertension at baseline.

The underlying biomedical pathways of ether-linked phosphocholines are included by citation [1]-[17]. Dehydrated alcohol, so-called aldehydes form ether groups in position 1 and aldehydes further conjugate esterified fatty acids in position 2 of glycerophospholipids [7]. Tobacco-related metabolites enhance betaoxidation of AAGPC leading then to biologically active alkyl-acyl-(short-chain)-glycerophosphocholines [7]. Endogenous transcytosis of albumin-bound lysopaf across endothelium is clinically shown with elevated albumin in cerebrospinal fluids during leakage of endothelial blood brain barriers (CSF: $0.245 \pm 0.05 > 0.15$ mg albumin in 500 µl with 68 ± 7 ng lyso paf per mg albumin n = 3) compared to healthy blood brain barriers of persons without psychiatric symptoms ($0.1 \pm 0.05 < 0.15$ mg albumin in 500 µl CSF with 26 ± 7 ng lyso paf per mg albumin, n = 3) [14]. Plasmatic albumin of healthy volunteers bind lysopaf (116 ± 22 ng lysopaf/mg serum albumin). Urinary albumin carries then at least 26 ng lysopaf per mg urinary albumin.

Imbalance of plasma compartments have been shown before with two mixed study groups, two male study groups and three female study groups [1]-[6]. The currently scored study group showed better rates of critical alcohol consumption, more often healthy morning urines and the majority widely eliminated adverse lipid mediators in good time. The current participants showed better rates of LDL-related smoking because women with high LDL-C less often smoked. The relevant proportion of self-reported smoking was the current problem of relatively young women.

5. Conclusion

Alcohol consumption currently decreased in a reliable manner and hematuria decreased of women who currently attended the practice of General Medicine. Hyperlipidemia and/or obesity were related with high LDL-C, low Alb/Trig and hypertension and these risky women reacted highly sensitive to critical alcohol consumption showing then albuminuria. The majority of current participants disowned daily alcohol consumption showing then healthy morning urines. Relatively young women often reported smoking and tended to mild decrease of HDL-C without reaching significancy. Smoking showed additive effects during intolerance to glucose, high LDL-C and/or alcohol-related urine pathology. Obese or hyperlipidemic women reacted highly sensitive to urine pathology and had to give up adverse alcohol consumption. Healthy alcohol-free liquids were adapted to repair dysfunction of endothelium barriers and the defense potency of healthy serum albumin.

Acknowledgements

The study was presented during the NAVBO meeting in Boston, 2015.

Conflict of Interests

The author has no conflict of interests.

References

[1]   Korth, R.M. (2014) Women with Overweight, Mixed Hyperlipidemia, Intolerance to Glucose and Diastolic Hypertension. *Health*, **6**, 454-467. http://dx.doi.org/10.4236/health.2014.65064

[2]   Korth, R.M. (2006) Gender, Obesity, Alcohol Use, Hyperlipidemia, Hypertension and Decline of Renal Endothelial Barriers. *Journal Men's Health & Gender*, **3**, 279-289. http://dx.doi.org/10.1016/j.jmhg.2005.08.006

[3]   Korth, R.M. (2012) Two Male Study Groups with Adiposity and Hypertriglyceridemia Were at Risk for Hypertension. *Health*, **4**, 1390-1395. http://dx.doi.org/10.4236/health.2012.412A201

[4]   Korth, R.M. (2007) Obesity Mediated Hypertension While Alcohol Use Declined Renal Endothelial Barriers of Women. *The FASEB Journal*, **21**, A1361.

[5]   Korth, R.M. (2002) AHA-Syndromes. *Chemistry and Physics of Lipids*, **118**, 96-97.

[6]   Korth, R.M. (2009) Gender Dyslipidemia and Ether Phospholipids. *The FASEB Journal*, **19**, 109.

[7]   Korth, R., Zimmermann, K. and Richter, W. (1994) Lipoprotein-Associated paf (LA-paf) Was Found in Washed Human Platelets and Monocyte/Macrophage-Like U 937 Cells. *Chemistry and Physics of Lipids*, **70**, 109-119. http://dx.doi.org/10.1016/0009-3084(94)90079-5

[8]   Korth, R.M. (1997) VLDL and PAF Binding to Human Endothelial Cells. *Chemistry and Physics of Lipids*, **88**, 134.

[9]   Korth, R. (1999) Treatment and Prevention of Disorders Mediated by LA-paf or Endothelial Cells. United States Patent Publication No. 5895785.

[10]   Korth, R.M., Hirafuji, M., Benveniste, J. and Russo-Marie, F. (1995) Human Umbilical Vein Endothelial Cells: Specific Binding of Platelet-Activating Factor and Cytosolic Calcium Flux. *Biochem Pharmacol*, **49**, 1793-1799. http://dx.doi.org/10.1016/0006-2952(95)00025-U

[11]   Korth, R.M. (1997) Specific Binding Sites for 1-O-Alkyl-sn-Glyceryl-3-Phosphorylcholine on Intact Human Blood

Neutrophils. *International Archives of Allergy and Immunology*, **113**, 460-464. http://dx.doi.org/10.1159/000237623

[12] Korth, R. and Middeke, M. (1991) Long Time Incubation of Monocytic U 937 Cells with LDL Increase Specific PAF-Acether Binding and the Cellular Acetylhydrolase Activity. *Chemistry and Physics of Lipids*, **59**, 207-213. http://dx.doi.org/10.1016/0009-3084(91)90020-C

[13] Korth, R., Bidault, J., Palmantier, R., Benveniste, J. and Ninio, E. (1993) Human Platelets Release a Paf-Acether: Acetylhydrolase Similar to That in Plasma. *Lipids*, **28**, 193-199. http://dx.doi.org/10.1007/BF02536639

[14] Korth, R.M. (2000) Comparison of Phosphocholines in Plasma and Cerebrospinal Fluids (CSF). *The FASEB Journal*, **14**, A72.

[15] Korth, R. and Benveniste, J. (1987) BN 52021 Displaces [^{3}H]paf-Acether from and Inhibits Its Binding to Intact Human Platelets. *European Journal of Pharmacology*, **142**, 331-341. http://dx.doi.org/10.1016/0014-2999(87)90071-9

[16] Korth, R., Nunez, D., Bidault, J. and Benveniste, J. (1988) Comparison of Three paf-Acether Receptor Antagonists Ginkgolides. *European Journal of Pharmacology*, **152**, 101-110. http://dx.doi.org/10.1016/0014-2999(88)90840-0

[17] Korth, R.M. (2014) Novel compositions against alkyl-acyl-GPC, the derivatives and products thereof. European Patent Publication No. 1965791B1.

[18] Meade, C.J., Heuer, H. and Kempe, R. (1991) Commentary: Biochemical Pharmacology of Platelet-Activating Factor (and paf Antagonists) in Relation to Clinical and Experimental Thrombocytopenia. *Biochemical Pharmacology*, **41**, 657-668.

[19] Ihida, K., Predescu, D., Czekay, R.P. and Palade, G.E. (1999) Platelet Activating Factor Receptor (PAF-R) Is Found in a Large Endosomal Compartment in Human Umbilical Vein Endothelial Cells. *Journal of Cell Science*, **112**, 285-295.

[20] Nistor, A. and Simionescu, M. (1986) Uptake of Low Density Lipoproteins by the Hamster Lung. Interactions with Capillary Endothelium. *The American Review of Respiratory Disease*, **134**, 1266-1272.

[21] Wu, R., Lemne, C., De Faire, U. and Frostegard, J. (1997) Antibodies to Platelet-Activating Factor Are Associated with Borderline Hypertension, Early Atherosclerosis and the Metabolic Syndrome. *Journal of Internal Medicine*, **246**, 389-397. http://dx.doi.org/10.1046/j.1365-2796.1999.00570.x

[22] Me.G., Richard, G. and White, T.W. (2007) Gap Junctions: Basic Structure and Function. *Journal of Investigative Dermatology*, **127**, 2516-2524. http://dx.doi.org/10.1038/sj.jid.5700770

[23] Louis, S.F. and Zaharadka, P. (2010) Vascular Smooth Muscle Cell Motility: From Migration to Invasion. *Experimental & Clinical Cardiology*, **15**, e75-e85.

[24] Pizzimenti, S., Ciamporcero, E., Daga, M., Pettazzoni, P., Arcaro, A. Cetrangolo, G., Minelli, R., Dianzani, C., Lepore, A., Gentile, F. and Barrera, G. (2013) Interaction of Aldehydes Derived from Lipid Peroxidation and Membrane Proteins. *Frontiers in Physiology*, **4**, 242.

[25] van der Vusse, G.J. (2009) Albumin as Fatty Acid Transporter. *Drug Metabolism and Pharmacokinetics*, **24**, 300-307. http://dx.doi.org/10.2133/dmpk.24.300

[26] Ambrosio, G., Oriente, A., Napoli, C., Palumbo, G., Chiarello, P., Marone, G., Conorelli, M., Chiariello, M. and Trigginai, M. (1994) Oxygen Radicals Inhibit Plasma Acetylhydrolase, the Enzyme That Catabolized Platelet Activting Factor. *Journal of Clinical Investigation*, **93**, 2408-2416. http://dx.doi.org/10.1172/JCI117248

[27] Silva, I.T., Mello, A.P.Q. and Damasceno, N.R.T. (2011) Antioxidant and Inflammatory Aspects of Lipoproteins-Associated Phospholipases A2 (LP-PLA2): A Review. *Lipids in Health and Disease*, **10**, 170-175. http://dx.doi.org/10.1186/1476-511X-10-170

[28] Gregson, J., Stirnadel-Farrant, H.A., Doobaree, I. and Koro, C. (2012) Variation of Lipoprotein Associated Phospholipases A2 across Demographic Characteristics and Cardiovascular Risk Factors: A Systematic Review of Literature. *Atherosclerosis*, **225**, 11-21. http://dx.doi.org/10.1016/j.atherosclerosis.2012.06.020

[29] Patja, K., Jousilahti, P., Hu, G., Valle, T., Quiao, Q. and Tuomilehto, J. (2005) Effects of Smoking, Obesity and Physical Activity on the Risk of Type 2 Diabetes in Middle-Aged Finnish Men and Women. *Journal of Internal Medicine*, **258**, 356-362. http://dx.doi.org/10.1111/j.1365-2796.2005.01545.x

[30] Saito, T., Urushihara, M., Kotani, Y., Kagami, S. and Kobori, H. (2009) Increased Urinary Angiotensinogen Is Precedent to Increased Urinary Albumin in Patients with Type 1 Diabetes. *The American Journal of the Medical Sciences*, **338**, 478-480. http://dx.doi.org/10.1097/MAJ.0b013e3181b90c25

[31] Dell'Omo, G., Penno, G., Pucci, L., Mariani, M., Del Prato, S. and Pedrinelli, R. (2014) Abnormal Capillary Permeability and Endothelial Dysfunction in Hypertension with Comorbid Metabolic Syndrome. *Atherosclerosis*, **172**, 383-389. http://dx.doi.org/10.1016/j.atherosclerosis.2003.11.013

[32] Barzilay, J.J., Peterson, D., Cushman, M., Heckbert, S.R., Cao, J.J., Blaum, C., Tracy, R.P., Klein, R. and Herrington, D.M. (2004) The Relationship of Cardiovascular Risk Factors to Microalbuminuria in Older Adults with or without Diabetes Mellitus or Hypertension: The Cardiovascular Health Study. *American Journal of Kidney Diseases*, **44**, 25-34.

http://dx.doi.org/10.1053/j.ajkd.2004.03.022

[33] Kristjansson, K., Ljungmann, S., Bengtsson, C., Björkel, C. and Sigurdsson, J.A. (2001) Microproteinuria and Long-Term Prognosis with Respect to Renal Function and Survival in Normotensive and Hypertensive Women. *Scandinavian Journal of Urology and Nephrology*, **35**, 63-70. http://dx.doi.org/10.1080/00365590151030868

[34] Uribarri, J., Woodruff, S., Goodman, S., Cai, W., Chen, X., Pyzik, R., Yong, A., Striker, G.E. and Vlassara, H. (2010) Advanced Glycation End Products in Foods and a Practical Guide to Their Reduction in the Diet. *Journal of the Academy of Nutrition and Dietetics*, **110**, 911-916. http://dx.doi.org/10.1016/j.jada.2010.03.018

[35] Faure, P., Troncy, L., Lecomte, M., Wiernsperger, N., Lagarde, M., Ruggerio, D. and Halimi, S. (2005) Albumin Antioxidant Capacity Is Modified by Methylglyoxal. *Diabetes & Metabolism*, **31**, 169-177. http://dx.doi.org/10.1016/S1262-3636(07)70183-0

[36] Muoio, D.M. (2010) Intramuscular Triacylglycerol and Insulin Resistance: Guilty as Charged or Wrongly Used. *Biochimica et Biophysica Acta* (*BBA*)-*Molecular and Cell Biology of Lipids*, **180**, 281-288. http://dx.doi.org/10.1016/j.bbalip.2009.11.007

[37] Berenson, G.S., Srinivasan, S.R., Bao, W., Newmann, W.P., Tracy, R.E. and Wattigney, W.A. (1998) Association between Multiple Cardiovascular Risk Factors and Atherosclerosis in Children and Young Adults. *The New England Journal of Medicine*, **338**, 1650-1656. http://dx.doi.org/10.1056/NEJM199806043382302

[38] Woo Baidal, J.A. and Taveras, E.M. (2014) Protecting Progress against Childhood Obesity—The National School Lunch Program. *The New England Journal of Medicine*, **371**, 1862-1865. http://dx.doi.org/10.1056/nejmp1409353

[39] Volek, J.S., Fernandez, M.L., Feinman, R.D. and Phinney, S.D. (2008) Dietary Carbohydrate Restricition Induces a Unique Metablic State Positively Affecting Atherogenic Dyslipidemia, Fatty Acid Partioning, and Metabolic Syndrome. *Progress in Lipid Research*, **47**, 307-318. http://dx.doi.org/10.1016/j.plipres.2008.02.003

[40] Shufelt, C.J. and Merz, N.B. (2009) Contraceptive Hormone Use and Cardiovascular Disease. State-of-the-Art-Paper. *Journal of the American College of Cardiology*, **53**, 221-231. http://dx.doi.org/10.1016/j.jacc.2008.09.042

[41] Georgieva, A.M., Cate, H.T., Keulen, E.T.P., van Oerle, R., Govers-Riemslag, J.W.G., Hamulyak, K., van der Kallen, C.J.H., van Greevenbrock, M.M.J. and de Bruin, T.W.A. (2004) Prothrombotic Markers of Familial Combined Hyperlipidemia. Evidence of Endothelial Cell Activation and Relation to Metabolic Syndrome. *Atherosclerosis*, **175**, 345-351. http://dx.doi.org/10.1016/j.atherosclerosis.2004.04.006

[42] Heydarkhan-Hagvall, S., Helenius, G., Johansson, B.R., Li, J.Y., Mattson, E. and Risberg, B. (2003) Co-Culture of Endothelial Cells and Smooth Muscle Cells Affects Gene Expression of Angioneic Factors. *Journal of Cellular Biochemistry*, **89**, 1250-1259. http://dx.doi.org/10.1002/jcb.10583

[43] Canaud, G., Bienaime, F., Tabarin, F., Bataillon, G., Seilhean, D., Noel, L.H, Dragon-Durey, M.L., Snanoudi, R., Friedländer, G., Halbwacgs-Mecarelli, L., Legendre, C. and Terzi, F. (2014) Inhibition of the mTORC Pathway in the Antiphospholipid Syndrome. *The New England Journal of Medicine*, **371**, 303-312. http://dx.doi.org/10.1056/NEJMoa1312890

[44] Sacks, F.M., Svetkey, L.P., Vollmer, W.M., Appel, L.J., Bray, G.A., Harsha, D., Obarzanek, E., Conlin, P.R., Miller, E.R., Simons-Morton, D.G., Karanja, N., Lin, P.-H., *et al.*, DASH-Sodium Collaboration Research Group (2001) Effects on Blood Pressure of Reduced Dietary Sodium and the Dietary Approaches to Stop Hypertension (DASH) Diet. *The New England Journal of Medicine*, **344**, 3-10. http://dx.doi.org/10.1056/NEJM200101043440101

[45] Salmon, A.H.J., Ferguson, J.K., Burford, J.L., Gevorgyan, H., Nakiano, D., Harper, S.J., Bates, D.O. and Peti-Peterdi, J. (2012) Loss of the Endothelial Glycocalyx Links Albuminuria and Vascular Dysfunction. *Journal of the Amercian Society of Nephrology*, **23**, 1339-1350. http://jasn.asnjournals.org

[46] Man, R.Y.K. (1988) Lysophosphatidylcholine-Induced Arrhythmias and Its Accumulation in the Rat Perfused Heart. *British Journal of Pharmacology*, **93**, 412-416. http://dx.doi.org/10.1111/j.1476-5381.1988.tb11448.x

[47] Chen, Y., Zhang, H., Zhang, Y., Lu, N., Zhang, L. and Shi, L. (2015) Exercise Intensity-Dependent Reverse and Adverse Remodeling of Voltage-Gated Ca^{2+} Channels in Mesenteric Arteries from Spontaneously Hypertensive Rats. *Hypertension Research*, **38**, 656-665. http://dx.doi.org/10.1038/hr.2015.56

[48] Dominiczak, A.F., Negrim, D.C., Clark, J.S., Brosnan, J., McBride, M.W. and Alexander, M.Y. (2000) State-of-the-Art Lectures: Genes and Hypertension. *Hypertension*, **35**, 164-172. http://dx.doi.org/10.1161/01.HYP.35.1.164

[49] Nebte, A., O'Donnell, M.J., Rangarajan, S., McQueen, M.J., Poirier, P., *et al.* (2014) Association of Urinary Sodium and Potassium Excretion with Blood Pressure. *The New England Journal of Medicine*, **371**, 601-611. http://dx.doi.org/10.1056/NEJMoa1311989

[50] Furukawa, M., Narahara, H., Yasuda, K. and Johnston, J. (1993) Presence of Platelet-Activating Factor-Acetylhydrolase in Milk. *The Journal of Lipid Research*, **34**, 1603-1609.

[51] Fruhwirth, B. and Hermetter, A. (2007) Seeds and Oil of the Syrian Oil Pumpkin: Components and Biological

Activities. *European Journal of Lipid Science and Technology*, **109**, 1128-1140.
http://dx.doi.org/10.1002/ejlt.200700105

[52] Korth, R.M. (2003) Alcohol, Obesity, Hypertension and Endothelial Irritation. *The FASEB Journal*, **17**, 4-5.

[53] Korth, R.M. (2006) Association of Intolerance to Glucose with Rising Blood Pressure or Proteinuria/Hematuria. *Journal of Vascular Research*, **43**, S90.

[54] Korth, R.M. (2007) PO3-59 Smoking, Borderline LDL Levels and Renal Small Vessel Disease of Women with Overweight. *Atherosclerosis Supplements*, **8**, 32-33. http://dx.doi.org/10.1016/S1567-5688(07)71069-3

[55] Korth, R.M. (2008) Aging Women with LDL-Related Borderline Syndromes. *Chemistry and Physics of Lipids*, **154**, S47-S48. http://dx.doi.org/10.1016/j.chemphyslip.2008.05.129

[56] Chopra, S., Cherian, D. and Jacob, J.J. (2011) The Thyroid Hormone, Parathyroid Hormone and Vitamin D Associated Hypertension. *Indian Journal of Endocrinology and Metabolism*, **15**, S354-S360.

[57] Evans, R. (1988) The Steroid and Thyroid Hormone Receptor Superfamily. *Science*, **240**, 889-895. http://dx.doi.org/10.1126/science.3283939

[58] Visser, M., Bouter, L.M., McQuillan, G.M., Wener, M.H. and Harris, T.B. (1990) Elevated C-Reactive Protein Level in Overweight and Obese Adults. *JAMA*, **282**, 2131-2135.

[59] Kraus, A.R. (2008) Alkoholkonsum, alkoholbezogene Probleme und Trends. Ergebnisse des epidemiologischen Suchtsurvy 2003. Robert Koch Institut, Gesundheitsberichterstattung des Bundes 2008, Heft 40.

[60] Go, A.S., Chertow, G.M., Fan, D., McCulloch, C.E. and Hsu, C.Y. (2004) Chronic Kidney Disease and the Risks of Death, Cardiovascular Events and Hospitalization. *The New England Journal of Medicine*, **351**, 1296-1305. http://dx.doi.org/10.1056/NEJMoa041031

[61] Sava, L., Pillai, S., More, U. and Sontakke, A. (2005) Serum Calcium Measurement: Total versus Free (Ionized) Calcium. *Indian Journal of Clinical Biochemistry*, **20**, 158-161. http://dx.doi.org/10.1007/BF02867418

[62] Cook, N.R. and Ridker, P.M. (2014) Further Insight into Cardiovascular Risk Calculator: The Roles of Statins, Revascularizations and Underascertainment in the Women's Health Study. *JAMA Internal Medicine*, **174**, 1964-1971. http://dx.doi.org/10.1001/jamainternmed.2014.5336

[63] Chapman, M.J., Ginsberg, H.N., Amareno, P., *et al.* (2011) Triglyceride-Rich Lipoproteins and High-Density Lipoprotein Cholesterol in Patients at High Risk of Cardiovascular Disease: Evidence and Guidance for Management. *European Heart Journal*, **32**, 1345-1361. http://dx.doi.org/10.1093/eurheartj/ehr112

[64] Bartz, R., Li, W.H., Venable, B., Zehmer, J.K., Welti, M.R., Aderson, R.G.W., Liu, P. and Chapman, K.D. (2007) Lipidomics Reveal That Adiposome Store Ether Lipids and Mediate Phospholipid Traffic. *The Journal of Lipid Research*, **48**, 837-847. http://dx.doi.org/10.1194/jlr.M600413-JLR200

[65] Vergeer, M., Holleboom, A.G., Kastelein, J.J.P. and Kuivenhoven, J.A. (2010) The HDL Hypothesis: Does High-Density Lipoprotein Protect from Atherosclerosis. *The Journal of Lipid Research*, **51**, 2058-2073. http://dx.doi.org/10.1194/jlr.R001610

[66] Lamarche, B. and Paradi, M.E. (2007) Endothelial Lipase and the Metabolic Syndrome. *Current Opinion in Lipidology*, **18**, 298-303. http://dx.doi.org/10.1097/MOL.0b013e328133857f

[67] Slattery, C., Zhang, L.A., Kelly, D.J., Thorn, P., Nikolic-Paterson, D.J., Tesch, G.H. and Poronnik, P. (2008) *In Vivo* Visualization of Albumin Degradation in the Proximal Tubule. *Kidney International*, **74**, 1480-1486. http://dx.doi.org/10.1038/ki.2008.463

[68] Osicka, T.M., Panagiotopoulos, S., Jerums, G. and Comper, W.D. (1997) Fractional Clearance of Albumin Is Influenced by Its Degradation during Renal Passage. *Clinical Science*, **93**, 557-564. http://dx.doi.org/10.1042/cs0930557

[69] Bond, H., Sibley, C.P., Balment, R.J. and Ashton, N. (2005) Increased Renal Tubular Reabsorbation of Calcium and Magnesium by the Offspring of Diabetic Rat Pregnancy. *Pediatric Research*, **57**, 890-895. http://dx.doi.org/10.1203/01.PDR.0000157720.50808.97

[70] Savige, J., Rana, K., Tonna, S., Buzza, M., Daghar, H. and Wang, Y.Y. (2003) Thin Basement Membrane Nephropathy. *Kidney Inernational*, **64**, 1169-1178. http://dx.doi.org/10.1046/j.1523-1755.2003.00234.x

[71] Collar, J.R., Ladva, S., Cairns, T.D. and Cattell, V. (2001) Red Cell Traverse through Thin Glomerular Basement Membranes. *Kidney International*, **59**, 2069-2072.

[72] Jacob, M., Bruegger, D., Rehm, M., Stoeckelhuber, M., Welsch, U., Conzen, P. and Becker, B.F. (2007) The Endothelial Glycocalyx Affords Compatibility of Starling's Principle and High Cardiac Interstitial Albumin Levels. *Cardiovascular Research*, **73**, 575-586. http://dx.doi.org/10.1016/j.cardiores.2006.11.021

[73] Shukla, A., Grisouard, J., Ehemann, V., Hermani, A., Enzmann, H. and Mayer, D. (2009) Analysis of Signaling Pathways Related to Cell Proliferation Stimulated by Insulin Analogs in Human Mammary Epithelial Cell Lines. *Endocrine-Related Cancer*, **16**, 429-441. http://dx.doi.org/10.1677/ERC-08-0240

[74] Waterworth, D.M., Talmud, P.J., Luan, J., Flavell, D.M., Byrne, C.E., Humphries, S.E. and Wareham, N.J. (2003)

Variants in the *APOC*3 Promoter Insulin Responsive Element Modualte Secretion and Lipids in Middle-Aged Men. *Biochimica et Biophysica Acta* (*BBA*)-*Molecular Basis of Disease*, **1637**, 200-206. http://dx.doi.org/10.1016/S0925-4439(03)00021-8

[75] The TG and HDL Working Group of the Exome Sequencing Project, National-Heart, Lung and Blood Institute (2014) Loss-of-Function Mutations in *APOC*3, Triglycerides, and Coronary Disease. *The New England Journal of Medicine*, **371**, 22-31. http://dx.doi.org/10.1056/NEJMoa1307095

[76] Fouchier, S.W., Sankatsing, J., Peter, J., Castillo, S., Pocovi, M., Alonos, R., Kastelein, J.J.P. and Defesche, J.C. (2005) High Frequency of APOB Gene Mutations Causing Familial Hypobetalipoproteinaemia in Patients of Dutch and Spanish Descent. *Journal of Medical Genetics*, **42**, e23.

[77] Chen, P., Jou, Y.-S., Fann, C.S., Chen, J.-W., Chung, C.-M., Lin, C.-Y., Wu, S.-Y., Kang, M.-J., Chen, Y.-C., Jong, Y.-S., Lo, H.-M., Kang, C.-S., Chen, C.-C., Chang, H.-C., Huangk, N.-K., Wu, Y.-L. and Pan, W.-H. (2009) Lipo-protein Lipase Variants Associated with an Endophenotype of Hypertension: Hypertension Combined with Elevated Triglycerides. *Human Mutation*, **30**, 49-55. http://dx.doi.org/10.1002/humu.20812

[78] Hiramoto, M., Yoshida, H., Imaizumi, T., Yoshimizu, N. and Satoh, K. (1997) A Mutation in Plasma Platelet Activat-ing Factor Acetylhydrolase (Val^{279}-Phe) Is a Genetic Risk Factor for Stroke. *Stroke*, **28**, 2417-2420. http://dx.doi.org/10.1161/01.STR.28.12.2417

[79] Romeo, S., Kozlitina, J., Xing, C., Pertsemlidis, A., Cox, D., Pennachio, L.A., Boerwinkle, E., Cohen, J. and Hobbs, H. (2008) Genetic Variation in *PNPLA*3 Confers Susceptibility to Nonalcoholic Fatty Liver Disease. *Nature Genetics*, **40**, 1461-1465. http://dx.doi.org/10.1038/ng.257

[80] Cichoz-Lach, H., Partyck, J., Nesina, I., Celinski, K., Slomka, M. and Wojcierowsli, J. (2007) Alcohol Dehydrogenase and Aldehyde Dehydrogenase Gene Polymorphism in Alcohol Liver Cirrhosis and Alcohol Chronic Pancreatitis among Polish Individuals. *Scandinavian Journal of Gastroenterology*, **42**, 493-498. http://dx.doi.org/10.1080/00365520600965723

[81] The ACCORD Study Groupand ACCORD Eye Study Group (2010) Effects of Medical Therapies on Retinopathy Progression in Type 2 Diabetes. *The New England Journal of Medicine*, **363**, 233-244. http://dx.doi.org/10.1056/NEJMoa1001288

[82] Winkler, K., Abletshauser, C., Friedrich, I., Hoffmann, M.M., Wieland, H. and Marz, W. (2004) Fluvastatin Slow-Release Lowers Platelet-Activating Factor Acetylhydrolase Activity: A Placebo-Controlled Trial in Patients with Type 2 Diabetes. *The Journal of Clinical Endocrinology & Metabolism*, **89**, 1153-1159. http://dx.doi.org/10.1210/jc.2003-031494

[83] Cole, P. and Rabassada, X. (2005) Enhanced Hypercholesterolemia Therapy: The Ezetimibe/Simvastatin Tablet. *Drugs Today*, **41**, 317-327. http://dx.doi.org/10.1358/dot.2005.41.5.893614

[84] Weingärtner, O., Böhm, M. and Lauf, U. (2009) Controversial Role of Plant Sterols Esters in the Management of Hypercholestrolemia. *European Heart Journal*, **40**, 404-409.

[85] Brand-Herrmann, S.M., Kuznetsova, T., Wiechert, A., Stolarz, K., Tikhonoff, V., Schmidt-Peterson, K., Telgmann, R., Casiglia, E., Wang, J.G., Thijs, L., Staessen, J.A. and Brand, E. (2005) Alcohol Intake Modulates the Genetic Association between HDL Cholesterol and the PPARγ2 Pro12Ala Polymorphism. *The Journal of Lipid Research*, **46**, 913-919. http://dx.doi.org/10.1194/jlr.M400405-JLR200

[86] Davies, S.S., Pontsler, A.V., Marathe, G.K., Harrison, K.A., Murphy, R.C., Hinshaw, J.C., Prestwich, G.D., Hilaire, A.S.T., Prescott, S.M., Zimmerman, G.A. and McIntyre, T.M. (2001) Oxidized Alkyl Phospholipids Are Specific High Affinity Peroxisome Proliferator-Activated Receptor γ Ligands and Agonists. *The Journal of Biological Chemistry*, **276**, 16015-16023. http://dx.doi.org/10.1074/jbc.M100878200

[87] Cepeda-Benito, A., Reynoso, J.T. and Erath, S. (2004) Meta-Analysis of the Efficacy of Nicotine Replacement Therapy for Smoking Cessation: Differences between Men and Women. *Journal of Consulting and Clinical Psycho-logy*, **72**, 712-722. http://dx.doi.org/10.1037/0022-006X.72.4.712

[88] Song, W., Wang, L., Dou, L.-Y., Wang, Y., Xu, Y., Chen, L.F. and Yan, X.W. (2015) The Implication of Cigarette Smoking and Cessation on Macrophage Cholesterol Efflux in Coronary Artery Disease Patients. *The Journal of Lipid Research*, **56**, 682-691. http://dx.doi.org/10.1194/jlr.P055491

[89] Bundeszentrale für gesundheitliche Aufklärung. Internet Presentation 2015. www.rauchfrei-info.de

[90] Vulimir, S.V., Misa, M., Hamm, J.T., Mitchell, M. and Berger, A. (2009) Effects of Mainstream Cigarette Smoke on the Global Metabolome of Human Lung Epithelial Cells. *Chemical Research in Toxicology*, **22**, 492-503. http://dx.doi.org/10.1021/tx8003246

[91] Fragerström, K. and Aubin, H.J. (2009) Management of Smoking Cessation in Patients with Psychiatric Disorders. *Current Medical Research and Opinion*, **25**, 511-518. http://dx.doi.org/10.1185/03007990802707568

13

The Role of Health Inequality in the Maternal Health Services Provided by Public Institutions in Mexico

Graciela Freyermuth-Enciso[1], Mónica Carrasco-Gómez[2], Martín Romero-Martínez[3]

[1]Centro de Investigaciones y Estudios Superiores en Antropología Social (CIESAS) sede SURESTE, San Cristóbal de las Casas, México
[2]Cátedras CONACYT/Centro de Investigaciones y Estudios Superiores en Antropología Social sede SURESTE, San Cristóbal de las Casas, México
[3]National Public Health Institute's Research Center in Evaluations and Surveys, Cuernavaca, México
Email: gracielafreyermuth54@hotmail.com, lazulblues@yahoo.com.mx, martin.romero@insp.mx

Abstract

This work aims to determine the role of inequality in the provision of maternal health services among five regions in Mexico (northwest, northeast, central, the Mexico City-State of Mexico region and the south). We consider the most important service providers corresponding to the main health institutions in Mexico (IMSS, ISSSTE, SESAS, IMSS-Oportunidades). Therefore, a cross-sectional prospective study was conducted to analyze eight intervention packages (Prenatal Care, Syphilis, Influenza, Obstetric Urgent Care, HIV in pregnancy, delivery care, neonatal care and accessibility) offered by the Maternal and Perinatal Health (MPH) program. A quantitative analysis demonstrates low to marginal performance of the MPH program in three regions (South, Mexico City-State of Mexico and the Northwest) and marginal in two other regions (Central and Northeast). Furthermore, four of the intervention packages presented the lowest performance in the South (Prenatal Care, Syphilis, Influenza and Obstetric Urgent Care), as did the average of the total of the MPH packages. The performance of HIV in Pregnancy package was marginal in the Southern and Mexico City-State of Mexico regions and Neonatal Care was low in the Northwest. The assessment of the MPH intervention packages allows us to identify their strengths and weaknesses. This information allows us to identify similarities and differences among the geographical regions in order to describe and analyze the strengths, weaknesses, opportunities and threats in the current system and hence to improve the decision making regarding the Maternal and Perinatal Health Programs in Mexico. The results suggest that a homogenization has taken place in terms of the low quality of the services.

Keywords

Health Inequality, Evaluation of Health Services, Maternal and Perinatal Health, Quality of Care

---

1. Introduction

The public health system in Mexico has been segmented through institutions that provide social security to different users (*i.e.*, patients) according to their work assignment and also to those who lacked affiliation to a social security institution. Therefore, until the beginning of XXI century the health care services for the Mexicans were differential for population with social security (attended by IMSS and ISSSTE) and without social security who were attended by the Health Secretary and the IMSS-Oportunidades. López Acuña (1986) pointed out the inequalities in the health spending and the resources available for health care in Mexico [1].

In recent decades, we have witnessed structural changes in the organization of the Mexican health system, which have been influenced by international organizations and multilateral agencies of cooperation. The latter has been reflected in public policies and programs in order to strengthen local systems of health and to reduce the gaps among different geographical regions.

The aim of this article is to assess if public health policy focused on maternal and perinatal health in the 1980-2010 period has contributed to reducing inequality of care within different geographical regions in Mexico. An overview of the political context and the changes that have been promoted through the decentralization of health services since the eighties is presented in Section 2. Then, the methodology employed in this work is described (Section 3). An assessment on the performance of services in the five geographical regions of the country through the analysis of intervention packages in the four major public institutions is presented in Section 4. Finally, discussion and conclusions are presented in Sections 5 and 6, respectively.

2. Background of the Decentralization of Health Services in Mexico

Public policies have been created in Mexico to strengthen the governance of the health system as well as decrease inequalities among regions and institutions since the 1980s. The purpose of Mexico's health system, its governance, financing, and provision of services has been changing over the past three decades. These changes have been made based on studies that propose more efficient ways to administer resources in order to provide health care coverage to the Mexican population. These include deconcentration (1984), decentralization (1996), universal coverage (1994), universal insurance "Seguro Popular" (2003), and more recently the functional integration of the health system (2011) [2]-[4].

In 1981, President López Portillo implemented a series of health measures that established the basis for this new reform, which was aimed at providing coverage for the entire population [5]. For instance, the Department of Health Services (Coordinación para los Servicios de Salud) was created in order to develop normative, administrative, financial and technical guidelines which soon thereafter made it possible to integrate public health services under the National Health System. Decrees issued in 1983 and 1984 aimed to establish the basis for the decentralization of the Secretary of Public Education, Secretary of Agrarian Reform and the Secretary of Health and Welfare (SSA, Spanish acronym) [6] [7]. This first decentralization phase was supported not only by the Presidency of the Republic but also by the World Health Organization (WHO) [5]. By 1986, the states were expected to have consolidated their own health systems by establishing their health laws and decentralizing services for the general population without social security.

One problem that arose from the decentralization process was the heterogeneity of the conditions in the health sectors in each state, as well as the need to strengthen services before decentralizing them. Cardozo Brum and González Block *et al.* (cited by Homedes, 2008) [8] found that the states that decentralized services were wealthier, had a greater capacity to provide services to the uninsured population and had the support of the governor at that time; although they also had little infrastructure from the IMSS-Coplamar [9] [10]. During this stage decentralization was implemented in 14 states from 32.

Nevertheless, the process was interrupted due to lack of experience of decentralized states and/or the economic crisis in the country that took place the second half of the 1980s. The latter was accompanied by cuts in the health budget from 2.5% to 1.3% in the percentage of the gross domestic product allocated to health care and social security between 1980 and 1988 [11]. By the end of the 1980s, a process to modernize health services was initiated during President Salinas' administration (1988-1994), which was said to be a continuation of the plan presented by the previous government. The first agreement with the World Bank was also reached during this government's term, which was aimed at expanding the coverage of services in those states with problems in health care services. This established the foundation to strengthen the infrastructure in states with the greatest deficiencies in health services and infrastructure. Moreover, the institutional capacities of the states were promoted by decentralizing the acquisition of basic supplies and improving capacities to manage information systems.

During 1995-2000 period, the National Development Plan called for a new federalism to emerge out of the recognition of autonomous spaces in political communities and the respect for the various powers ascribed to each level of government. The aim was to harmoniously and effectively bring together the sovereignty of states and municipalities with the constitutional powers of the federal government. This was also intended to promote social participation and to define a new framework for relationships between the State and its citizens and organizations [12]. It was the 1996 National Accord[1] that gave a new impetus to the decentralization process [13] and agreements between the federation and the states were signed, the last of which was by Chihuahua in February of 1999 [8].

Previous studies [14]-[16] pointed out that the majority of Latin American countries were pressured to reform health services, and one of the components of this reform was decentralization. The promoters of these initiatives were the World Bank, the Inter-American Development Bank and certain bilateral and multilateral development agencies. They proposed decentralization as part of a structural adjustment that would make it possible to free up federal resources to pay external debts. Decentralization would also facilitate the privatization of the health system, which is considered by neoliberal theory to be more efficient than public services (Collins 1989; Griffin, 1999; Ugalde and Homedes N. 2002).

It was believed that decentralization would facilitate a more reasonable and equitable distribution of the federal expenditures on health by taking into account mortality and marginalization indicators. It was also considered as a way to help balance per capita expenditures on health, thereby increasing both efficiency and equity. The decentralization process included the state governments' creation of legislative initiatives, or creation decrees, the formation of a government entity and the administration of federal resources through the SSA and the state governments. In turn, the SSA would decentralize the operations of health services from the federal to the state level and stipulate the priorities to be followed by the decentralized agencies. The SSA would also grant programming and budgeting functions to the states according to established federal guidelines [17].

Decentralization made it possible to allocate funds to the states in a more equitable manner. Thus, income improved for state governments with fewer resources. In terms of programming, the most important policies continued to be generated by the federal government but without the control mechanisms needed for them to be carried out in the states.

In 2003 during Vicente Fox's term (2000-2006) the Social Health Protection System (Sistema de Protección Social en Salud; SPSS, Spanish acronym) and Seguro Popular de Salud (its operational arm) were approved in order to create medical insurance for the population without social security, through the reform of the General Health Law (Ley General de Salud; LGS Spanish acronym). Similar to enrollees in the IMSS and the ISSSTE, the SPSS is a financial instrument aimed at providing a *per capita* amount to Seguro Popular enrollees. This would standardize the financial structure of these three insurance systems.

The purpose of these reforms were to provide universal coverage for Mexicans through medical insurance with a financial structure similar to that of social security, in order to advance the functional integration of the health system.

The Health Sector Program (Programa Sectorial de Salud; PROSESA) was established in the 1980s to maintain the regulatory role of the Secretary of Health, consolidate the National Health System (SNS, Spanish acronym) and guarantee mechanisms to implement the right to health protection. PROSESA has 13 substantive programs and 3 support programs, including maternal and child health. This program was consolidate in accordance with Mexican Official Norm NOM-007-SSA2-1993 which was established by the federal government and

---

[1]National Agreement for the decentralization of health services, Journal of the Federation (DOF, Spanish acronym), September 25, 1996.

stipulates the criteria for treating and monitoring women's health during pregnancy, delivery and the postnatal period, as well as for newborn care.

This program was created through the implementation of Seguro Popular, which has treated the population without social security since 2004, and at that time provided access to 20 interventions for maternal and child health. Additional initiatives were developed in 2008 and 2009 to decrease economic barriers and thereby improve access: 1) Healthy Pregnancy (Embarazo Saludable) which enabled pregnant women and their families to affiliate and 2) General Agreement on Inter-institutional Collaboration for Obstetric Emergency Care which established treatment for all women experiencing obstetric complications regardless of their affiliation in any of the health institutes (IMSS, ISSSTE or State Health Services [SESA]).

Nevertheless, at both the IMSS and the ISSSTE (institutions coordinated at the federal level, that is, they are not decentralized) maternal health care is based on prenatal health services at the primary level and delivery care at the secondary level, while obstetric emergencies are treated only at the secondary level where the timely treatment of obstetric emergencies and the public health perspective of the The Maternal and Perinatal Health Program (MPH) are not included in their guidelines. However, some of the components of the IMSS-O program are similar to the MPH, such as the organization of social community networks to transport the women and even community promoters to identify risks among pregnant women [18].

This article is focused on describing the availability of the interventions established by the regulations. It includes the four largest public and social security institutions in the country (IMSS, ISSSTE, SESAS, IMSS-Oportunidades) and encompasses five regions in Mexico (northwest, northeast, central, the Mexico City-State of Mexico region and the south) (See **Table 1**). This will allow us to identify similarities and differences among the regions in order to describe and analyze the strengths, weaknesses, opportunities and threats in the system and thereby suggest improvements that will ensure that the goods and services established by the regulations are provided in the various regions and health care subsystems.

3. Methodology

A cross-sectional prospective study was conducted using quantitative research methods. The Maternal and Perinatal Health Program was analyzed based on guidelines by the maternal and perinatal program, the Official Mexican Norms (Normas Oficiales Mexicanas; NOM, Spanish acronym), and clinical practice guidelines (CPG). Intervention packages were defined which were composed of a set of the marginal essential interventions needed for the adequate provision of services [19].

3.1. Instruments

Four instruments were designed to collect the information: 1) checklists, 2) questionnaires, 3) observation guides, and 4) interview guides to obtain information from the various actors. Nineteen areas were also defined to collect information, with specific informants at each establishment and according to level of care. The instruments were adapted and validated based on consensus with those responsible for the programs at each institution.

Eight health care packages covering a total of 134 primary level and 164 hospital level interventions were defined for the maternal and perinatal program[2]: 1) Accessibility: knowledge of the health care staff and population about the Healthy Pregnancy strategy (Embarazo Saludable) and the General Agreement on Inter-institutional Collaboration for Obstetric Emergency Care (Convenio General de Colaboración Interinstitucional para la Atención de Emergencias Obstétricas) as well as no physical, economic and cultural barriers to accessing health facilities; 2) Prenatal care: interventions aimed at identifying the skills and competencies needed to treat urinary infections and to determine risk factors for preeclampsia and hemorrhage. Other packages that represent some of the new challenges in prenatal care were included separately, such as the next three; 3) HIV-STI in Pregnancy: universal access to antiretroviral medication, adequate prevention campaigns and prevention of vertical transmission; 4) Syphilis: resources needed to perform the VDRL blood test for syphilis as well as early treatment; 5) Influenza in Pregnancy: early detection of cases, detection of complications and case referrals, adequate treatment, sufficient and adequate information aimed at the general public; 6) Delivery Care: a) the availability of supplies and instruments, b) the basic knowledge needed to provide medical attention as indicated by norms and

---

[2]These can be consulted in-depth in the technical report.

Table 1. Evaluation of the performance of intervention packages, by region.

Intervention Package	Significance Tests by Region					
	Northwest	Northeast	Central	MexCty-St of Mex	South	Overall Significance
Mean for prenatal Care:	**0.6834**	**0.7236**	**0.6959**	**0.7127**	**0.5979**	
Northwest		0.277	0.662	0.512	0.003***	
Northeast			0.247	0.776	0.000***	
Central				0.572	0.000***	0.000***
MexCty-St of Mex					0.000***	
South						
Mean for HIV in Pregnancy:	**0.5223**	**0.7197**	**0.6447**	**0.5052**	**0.5304**	
Northwest		0.005***	0.053*	0.814	0.858	
Northeast			0.235	0.003***	0.000***	
Central				0.041**	0.007***	0.001***
MexCty-St of Mex					0.563	
South						
Mean for Syphilis:	**0.5782**	**0.6426**	**0.3966**	**0.5019**	**0.3744**	
Northwest		0.136	0.000***	0.100*	0.000***	
Northeast			0.000***	0.004***	0.000***	
Central				0.005***	0.439	0.000***
MexCty-St of Mex					0.002***	
South						
Mean for influenza:	**0.5221**	**0.684**	**0.5508**	**0.4499**	**0.4068**	
Northwest		0.007***	0.601	0.331	0.038**	
Northeast			0.001***	0.000***	0.000***	
Central				0.051*	0.001***	0.000***
MexCty-St of Mex					0.442	
South						
Mean for delivery care:	**0.6911**	**0.7887**	**0.7415**	**0.747**	**0.7012**	
Northwest		0.365	0.496	0.496	0.783	
Northeast			0.646	0.721	0.094*	
Central				0.948	0.3	0.582
MexCty-St of Mex					0.284	
South						
Mean for neonatal care:	**0.4853**	**0.6645**	**0.7742**	**0.7819**	**0.6074**	
Northwest		0.41	0.072*	0.046**	0.28	
Northeast			0.434	0.454	0.697	
Central				0.943	0.13	0.099
MexCty-St of Mex					0.068*	
South						

Continued

Mean for Obstetric Emergency:	**0.4167**	**0.5202**	**0.4933**	**0.5217**	**0.3982**	
Northwest		0.003***	0.035**	0.039**	0.616	
Northeast			0.419	0.975	0.001***	
Central				0.544	0.006***	0.001***
MexCty-St of Mex					0.012**	
South						
Mean for accessibility:	**0.4672**	**0.4839**	**0.4983**	**0.4299**	**0.5149**	
Northwest		0.64	0.147	0.284	0.092*	
Northeast			0.653	0.279	0.394	
Central				0.031**	0.506	0.123
MexCty-St of Mex					0.029**	
South						
Mean for all SMP packages:	**0.5572**	**0.6308**	**0.5923**	**0.5492**	**0.5058**	
Northwest		0.009***	0.178	0.815	0.040*	
Northeast			0.15	0.021*	0.000***	
Central				0.191	0.000***	0.000***
MexCty-St of Mex					0.169	
South						

Significance ***p value ≤0.01, **p ≤ 0.05, *p ≤ 0.10.

to ensure adequate care and the privacy and comfort of the mothers, c) the availability of checkups and monitoring procedures to ensure the early detection of complications); 7) Neonatal Care: interventions that help to identify the neonate's availability to receive checkups (those born with and without complications) and the availability of supplies and strategies for the screening and early detection of hypothyroidism; and 8) Obstetric Emergency Care: the availability of the instruments, supplies and knowledge that enable the physician to make decisions related to the most common obstetric emergencies and the availability of medications to treat those problems.

3.2. Sampling Methods

The sampling framework was dictated by the health sector national directory of health care facilities (http://clues.salud.gob.mx/). Stratified and clustered sampling methods were used. Five regions were defined (as described in **Figure 1**) and 10 municipalities were chosen from each region. The facilities were selected with probability proportional to the population of the municipality. In each municipality, one medical establishment was selected for each one of eight strata defined by institution criteria (IMSS, IMSS-Prospera, ISSSTE, SESA) and type of establishment (primary care and hospitalization).

The medical establishments were selected with probability proportional to their size, defined as the inverse square root of the frequency of their typology, as presented by the SSA webpage (http://clues.salud.gob.mx/).

Each unit in the sample was then assigned a weight (w) based on the selection probability. The directory of national medical establishments in the health sector provided by the SSA webpage (http://clues.salud.gob.mx/) was used as the sampling framework.

The sample was composed of 205 medical units, 50 municipalities and 23 states and Mexico City. Responses were obtained from 201 medical units (2% non-response). The sample size was defined based on a study of the performance of maternal services and was nationally representative of institutions providing these services and the types of populations they treat.

The fieldwork was conducted from September to December 2010. The CSPro Census and Survey Processing System (www.census.gov/population/international/software/cspro/) was used for the data entry.

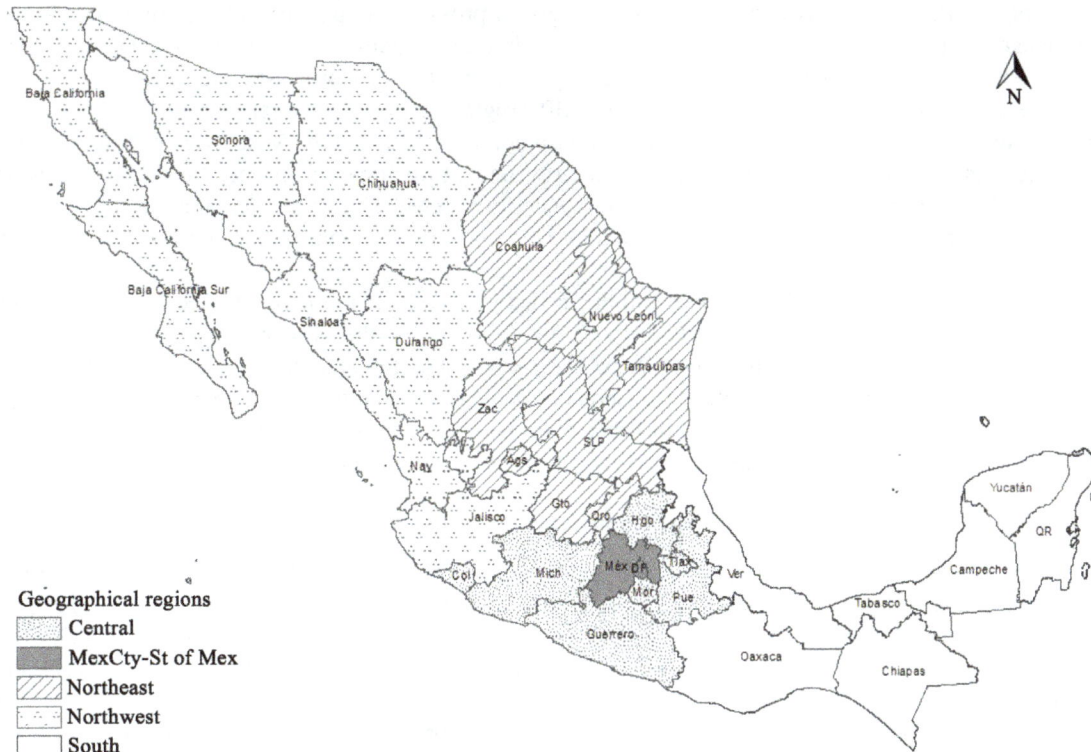

Figure 1. Regional distribution of the states.

3.3. Data Analysis

The scores for each region were estimated for each of the intervention packages (Prenatal Care, Syphilis, Influenza, Obstetric Urgent Care, HIV in pregnancy, delivery care, neonatal care and accessibility). The intervention packages were evaluated using indices that represented a relative score with respect to the total items evaluated, according to the services provided by each unit. This was obtained by calculating the quotient of the sum of points accumulated by a medical unit divided by the number of items evaluated in that unit (minimum value = 0 and maximum value = 1). A detailed description of this analysis can be found in Freyermuth *et al.* (2011) [18].

Two levels of analyses were performed. The first consists on a statistical, significance test for a regional comparison of the indices through the obtainment of the T-Student[3] test considering the design effect, since the primary units in the sample were the municipalities and not the medical units. All of the T-Student test were run but only tests that were significant for a level of .01 were discussed. The second level of analysis was qualitative, through the traffic light system described above, which explored the deficiencies in the contents of the intervention packages in order to drive public policies. The performance scale proposed by the National Council for the Evaluation of Social Policy (Consejo Nacional de Evaluación de la Política de Desarrollo Social; CONEVAL, Spanish acronym) was used to create a traffic light system based on the indices. A score equal to or more than 0.85 was an indicator of good performance, 0.70 to 0.84 adequate performance, 0.50 to 0.69 marginal performance and low performance is indicated by values under 0.50.

This research was approved by the ISSSTE Research Ethics Committee and written consent to conduct the evaluation was obtained from each institution. The confidentiality of the participants was maintained.

4. Results

4.1. Performance of the MPH Program

The mean index for the program was 0.56 (95%CI; 0.48, 0.64), which can be interpreted as the middle value.

---

[3]The T-student is computed as $t = (x - y)/\mathrm{sqrt}(\mathrm{Var}(x - y))$ where x and y are mean scores of different programs and Var() is estimated taking into account the sampling design.

This is noteworthy since it is one of the oldest programs provided by public health institutions. According to confidence levels, its performance was low to marginal in three regions (South (with a mean of .50), MexCty-St of Mex and the Northwest) and marginal in two regions (Central and Northeast). Significant differences in the performance of the entire set of packages in the SMP program were found when comparing the South to three other regions (Northeast, Northwest and Central). Also noteworthy is that the MexCty-St of Mex region was not one of the regions with better performance in the provision of this type of service. No differences were found between this region and the South and the performance in both MexCty-St of Mex and the Northwest was significantly lower than in the Northeast. The order of how well this program performed was: Northeast, Central, Northwest, MexCty-St of Mex and South.

Furthermore, four of the eight packages had the lowest performance in the South (Prenatal Care, Syphilis, Influenza and Obstetric Urgent Care), as did the average of the total of the MPH packages. HIV in Pregnancy had marginal performance in the South and the MexCty-St of Mex region and Neonatal Care had low performance in the Northwest. Although no significant differences were found among regions for three packages (delivery care, newborn care and accessibility), we describe them based on the second level of analysis which is aimed at establishing a performance range for the intervention packages and monitoring the components of the program.

4.2. Overall Performance of the Intervention Packages in the MPH Program

In the provision of services related to delivery care, which can be considered to be a traditional maternal-infant care service, adequate performance was found with no significant differences among regions. Furthermore, other traditional intervention packages exist, such as prenatal care which resulted in indices of 0.68, 0.72, 0.70, 0.71 and 0.60 in the Northwest, Northeast, Central, MexCty-St of Mex and Southern regions, respectively, indicating marginal and adequate performance. In the case of neonatal services, the average indices were 0.49, 0.66, 0.77, 0.78 and 0.60 in the above regions, respectively. Thus the extremes were the Northwest with very low performance and the Central and MexCty-St of Mex regions with adequate performance. Nevertheless, it is worth mentioning that the South was notable for having the lowest prenatal care performance index of all the regions.

Obstetric Emergency Care is one of the intervention packages recently implemented in the health sector, which was established in 2006. This package resulted in low performance in the Northwest (0.47), Central (0.49) and especially the South (0.39) and marginal performance in the Northeast and the MexCty-St of Mex regions (0.52).

In terms of **prenatal care**, the interventions that determined its marginal performance in three of the regions were knowledge about high-risk factors for preeclampsia and about medications indicated for urinary infections during pregnancy. At the hospital level, interventions classified as low performance were also related to a lack of knowledge about detecting risk factors for preeclampsia and treating urinary infections, as well as a failure to indicate to women at their first prenatal checkup (at 24 weeks gestation) the laboratory tests to be performed. Nevertheless, the other interventions presented adequate performance, as mentioned previously, indicating that the prevention of neural tube problems and the availability of supplies for their prevention were adequate for interventions related to the health of the baby.

As mentioned previously, **delivery care** was the package which presented adequate performance in four of the five regions, with no differences among the regions. This demonstrates the availability of supplies and equipment, having basic knowledge about the medical care indicated in the NOM-007, and the availability of checkups and monitoring procedures to ensure the early detection of complications. Nevertheless, some of the individual interventions resulted in low performance in all of the regions, including insufficient walking space in delivery rooms for women in labor and a lack of partograms (except in MexCty-St of Mex and the Northwest). In the CE[4], there was a lack of oxytocin in the Northwest and Central regions and both oxytocin and ergonovine in MexCty-St of Mex, which compromises women's comfort and puts their lives in risk because of hemorrhage.

For **neonatal care**, adequate performance was found in the Central and MexCty-St of Mex regions, marginal in the South and Northeast and low in the Northwest. This indicates the need to improve the immediate care of neonates by providing interventions that guarantee the treatment of complications, the provision of supplies and strategies for the screening and early detection of hypothyroidism. The interventions with the lowest indices in all the regions were the lack of medical certificates, neonatal resuscitation equipment and Silverman Anderson and Apgar evaluation tables.

---

[4]CE refers to the Rural Medical Units run by the IMSS-*Oportunidades* program and Health Centers that provide hospitalization for primary care delivery.

Regarding of **Obstetric Emergency** care, marginal performance was found only in the Northeast and MexCty-St of Mex regions. Performance was low in the other regions and the South had the lowest average index (0.39), where medical staff did not have the competencies needed to make decisions about the most common obstetric emergencies, such as what to do in case of hemorrhaging and toxemia and risk factors for postpartum hemorrhaging. Medications to treat these problems were lacking as well as manuals and algorithms related to obstetric hemorrhage, sepsis and miscarriage. In terms of supplies, plasma expanders, cephalexin and gentamicina were not available or free substitutes were not provided. There was also an inability to perform blood cultures, urine cultures and antibiograms, as well as to identify serum lactate. In addition, ultrasounds were not available 24 hours per day 7 days per week for emergencies.

Intervention packages for prenatal care that have been recently and systematically more implemented include the detection and treatment of HIV-AIDS and syphilis and the prevention of influenza in pregnant women. In the case of HIV detection, interventions related to checkups and early treatment for women who test positive as well as measures to prevent vertical transmission performed adequately in the Northeast and had marginal performance in the other four regions. The main weaknesses in this package were: not offering the rapid HIV test to all pregnant women; deficiency in availability of rapid tests for HIV; lack of informed consent forms for HIV diagnoses; lack of a guide for the use of rapid tests; laboratories without the capacity to perform viral load tests, TCD4 and TCD8 counts and western blot tests; and the unavailability of antiretroviral drugs, including HIV STI/zidovudine (AZT)+lamivudine (3tc)+lopinavir (saquinavir, ritonavir).

A similar situation was found for the **influenza** packages, which had marginal performance in the Northwest (0.52), Northeast (0.68) and Central (0.55) regions and low performance in MexCty-St of Mex (0.45) and the South (0.40). These differences in performance were primarily associated with the availability of treatment and the timely referral in the event of complications. The main deficiencies were: insufficient information related to recognizing and preventing the transmission of influenza; the absence of oseltamivir, zanamivir and the vaccine; and a lack of clinical guides for treatment and referrals as well as visible algorithms that facilitate diagnosis and treatment.

Even though it has been mandatory for decades, the intervention package to detect and treat **syphilis** was found to have low performance in the Central (0.39) and South (0.37) and marginal in the Northeast (0.68), Northwest (0.52) and MexCty-St of Mex (0.55) regions. The interventions identified as being most deficient were not performing VDRL syphilis detection tests and not having diagnostic and treatment guides or adequate dosages of medications such as penicillin G benzathine, ceftriaxone (500 mg) and azithromycin (500 mg).

Lastly, the performance of the **accessibility** package was low in four of the five regions and marginal only in the South, although the difference was not significant. This is important given that difficulties with access have been one of the main problems in the early treatment of obstetric emergencies. In 2010 when the information was collected, two strategies were implemented to improve universal coverage of the service and its functional integration Healthy Pregnancy (Embarazo Saludable) and the Inter-Institutional Agreement for Obstetric Emergency Care (Convenio Interinstitucional para la Atención de la Urgencia Obstétrica). Therefore, in addition to monitoring whether or not physical, economic and cultural barriers to the facilities existed, health care staff and the populations were also evaluated as to whether or not they knew about these strategies (free, support from health staff, ambulance service, telephone, etc.).

The low performance by the **accessibility** package was primarily due to not visibly displaying hours, lack of staff who spoke the local indigenous language, poor dissemination of information about the Healthy Pregnancy program and insufficient information about the signs and symptoms of obstetric emergencies. It is also worth mentioning that health care staff were not aware of the IMSS-ISSSTE-SESA agreement regarding obstetric emergency care and information was lacking about where to go for delivery care as well as about Seguro Popular and enrollment and complaint procedures.

5. Discussion

The proposed methodology contributes to rapidly identify interventions considered by the health sector to be essential to the performance of services. The methodology can be used to make synthetic comparisons, in this case among regions, as well as institutional comparisons among health care services and among medical units.

While in some ways decentralization tried to homogenize the regions' institutional capacities to produce services, in the case of maternal and perinatal services significant differences were found when comparing the

Northwest, Northeast and Central regions with the South and the Northeast and MexCty-St of Mex regions, in which the MPH program performed lowest in the South. What is notable is a homogenization in the performance of regions with marginal to low indices. None of the intervention packages showed good performance and, at best, three of the eight packages studied had adequate performance in the Northeast and the MexCty-St of Mex region.

Although the differences among regions would be expected to range from good and adequate to marginal and low, the quality of maternal-infant services was found to be heterogeneous even within the same region. In addition, all regions had some intervention packages with low performance while most of the services were classified as marginal.

Homedes and Ugalde (2008) concluded that, 25 years after implementing decentralization in Mexico, inequalities in the health system have increased due to an unclear process and ineffective strategies to compensate for inequalities among the decentralized states. We suggest that while these inequalities have continued, the present study shows that the services generally tend to have marginal and low performance in all regions. Thus, not only has there been a failure to homogenize quality and decrease gaps, we consider these results to be more indicative of a homogenization in terms of the low quality of the service than of a deepening of inequalities.

While it is the case that low performance was found in the South for four of the eight intervention packages (Prenatal Care, Syphilis, Influenza, Obstetric Emergencies), the other four were found to have low performance in other regions. The performance of accessibility was low even in the Northeast, which had the highest quality ranking.

The "Evaluation of Women's Health Care Programs" presented results by level of care (primary and secondary) and by the type of population receiving the services (insured and uninsured). This evaluation found significant differences between the secondary level and insured population (IMSS/ISSSTE) as compared to the primary care level and uninsured population, in which the former had better performance. Nevertheless, a worrisome trend was found similar to that presented by the regional findings, in which there was low performance in the capacity to offer Obstetric Emergency Care, especially by institutions aimed at the uninsured population. Furthermore, although the performance of the IMSS/ISSSTE was classified as marginal, this also cannot be considered satisfactory [20].

Performance in the accessibility to the health system continues to be low, especially in terms of what the National Aboriginal Health Organization refers to as cultural security, which is understood as the capacity of service providers to communicate with patients according to their political, economic, social, spiritual and linguistic perspectives [21]. This has even been associated with resistance towards adhering to portions of the NOM-007, including adopting the position desired by the woman in labor [18], weaknesses in the infrastructure and placing furniture in such a way that makes it difficult for women to walk during labor. These infrastructure and supply problems have been recognized by the Mexican Collegiate Federation of Obstetrics and Gynecology (Federación Mexicana de Colegios de Obstetricia y Ginecología, A.C.; FEMECOG, Spanish acronym)[5].

It is also important to mention that communication within institutions and among their own members was found to be insufficient and it was evident that primary- and secondary-level health care staff in MexCty-St of Mex and the Southern regions lacked knowledge about policy agreements to improve performance and access (such as the Inter-Institutional Agreement for Obstetric Emergency Care). This has also been reported in the states of Guerrero, Oaxaca and Veracruz [22].

The low performance evident in primary-level obstetric emergency care demonstrated little knowledge on the part of health care staff about protocols used to treat the most common causes of obstetric emergencies and a lack of guides to manage these emergencies and the supplies needed to treat them. In an evaluation of participatory actions related to the MPH program, the measures used to support obstetric emergencies had an influence on the availability of transportation and housing for pregnant women, which helped to obtain international certification of Arranque Parejo en la Vida actions [23]. This information could be compared to our findings, nevertheless while both studies refer to obstetric emergency care they do not evaluate the same actions.

At the hospital level, the low performance by the HIV package indicated deficiencies in the capacity to perform tests and in the availability of antiretroviral drugs, even though a strategy existed and resources were allocated [24]. Deficiencies were also identified in the influenza package, in spite of the severity of the epidemic

---

[5]We are referring to the announcement issued on June 10, 2015 about obstetric violence and legislative initiatives in some states, available in http://www.femecog.org.mx/docs/FEMECOG%20pronunciamiento.pdf

and its political visibility in 2009 [25]. Therefore, further research, monitoring by citizens and social accountability continue to be necessary not only to see whether the public resources allocated to the programs are being adequately distributed and used but also in order to design and create processes and indicators that evaluate their impacts [26].

In the South, specifically in the case of Chiapas, Freyermuth identified particular social and political situations as having contributed to a substantial increase in the health budget through the Ramo 33 Health Services Fund (Fondo de Aportaciones para los Servicios de Salud; FASSA, Spanish acronym) [6] such as the Zapatista uprising in 1994 and the decentralization of state services in 1998. While this could have signified an improvement in the performance of the services provided, it is important to note that deficiencies were found in the South, especially at the primary care level of the new programs (syphilis, influenza and obstetric emergency care programs).

In addition, even though the national SPSS budget increased over 600%[6] between 2004 and 2010, the IMSS and ISSSTE were the institutions that continued to show better performance.

Therefore, differences in performance among regions could be identified in spite of several attempts to improve the health system. These regional differences persisted even after performing interventions, increasing budgets and implementing programs to attempt to address the lack of coverage by decentralizing the National Health System and implementing Seguro Popular. And even after attempts to improve maternal-infant care by integrating the system through a variety of strategies, such as the Agreement, the 2006 Medical Insurance for a New Generation in 2006 and Healthy Pregnancy in 2009, it can be identified that there are different performances between regions. In this regard, it is important to mention that the region which presented the poorest performance was the South. This can be interpreted as a failure of the concentration of resources to bring about the short-term results expected and the need to ensure a more effective allocation of the budget and to target resources towards the most vulnerable populations.

This inequality has also been identified by recent studies focused on particular programs aimed at combating inequalities in municipalities with a lower human development index, which found that inequality increased [27]. Gwatkin and Ergo (2011) called this phenomenon "regressive universalization," in which programs aimed at universal coverage largely end up benefiting less disadvantaged populations to a greater degree than more vulnerable populations [28].

6. Conclusions

In this work, an assessment of the interventions in the SMP program allows us to identify their strengths and weaknesses. This analysis provided useful information for policy-makers and health program decision-makers in order to improve the provision of health services of pregnant women and neonates. Surprisingly, regions with the more important health care facilities (i.e., MexCty-St of Mex) presented low to marginal performance in the MPH program with similar scores to the poorest region (South). Four of the eight packages had the lowest performance in the South (Prenatal Care, Syphilis, Influenza and Obstetric Urgent Care), as did the average of the total of the SMP packages.

Despite preeclampsia being the second leading cause of maternal death in Mexico, the evaluation in the prenatal care package showed shortcomings in the knowledge about high-risk factors for preeclampsia and indicated medications for urinary infections during pregnancy. On the other hand, in delivery care, which can be considered to be a traditional maternal-infant care service, adequate performance was found with no significant differences among regions.

We suggest that while these inequalities have continued, the present study shows that the services generally tend to have marginal and low performance in all regions. These results suggest that a homogenization has taken place in terms of the low quality of the service than of a deepening of inequalities.

These monitoring exercises need to be continued at the academic level in order to evaluate the performance of maternal and neonatal programs, so as to identify progress and setbacks and suggest control measures. Lastly, the national health system needs to be strengthened so it can function as a single system operated with public financing.

---

[6]Comparison in constant pesos from the year 2004 to 2009 of the total budget allocated to the SPSS, with data from the SHCP from the years 2004 to 2008. From the federal treasury department account, 2009, PEF APROBADO (approved federal expense budget). Source: Diaz, D., Pérez, M. A. C., & Navarro, S. M. (2010) p. 39.

Acknowledgements

The authors want to acknowledge to the authorities of the Federal Ministry of Health, IMSS-Oportunidades IMSS, ISSSTE and state health services for the facilities provided in the implementation of this evaluation work. And, for their financial support, to the Women's National Institute (INMUJERES), CIESAS and Catedras program of CONACYT.

References

[1]   López Acuña, D. (1986) La salud desigual en México. Siglo Veintiuno Editores, México.

[2]   Londoño, J.L. and Frenk, J. (1997) Structured Pluralism: Towards an Innovative Model for Health System Reform in Latin America. *Health Policy*, **41**,1-36. http://dx.doi.org/10.1016/S0168-8510(97)00010-9

[3]   Soberón, G. and Valdéz, C. (2007) Evidencias y salud, ¿Hacia dónde va el sistema de salud en México? *Salud Pública de México*, **49**, 5-27. http://dx.doi.org/10.1590/S0036-36342007000700002

[4]   Secretary of Health (2011) Hacia la integración funcional del Sistema Nacional de Salud. Secretaría de Salud, México.

[5]   Soberón-Acevedo, G. and Martínez-Narváez, G. (1996) La descentralización de los servicios de salud en México en la década de los ochenta. *Salud Pública de México*, **38**, 371-378.

[6]   Freyermuth Enciso, M.G., Sánchez Pérez, H. and Argüello Avendaño, H. (2015) Transparencia y rendición de cuentas en salud materna: El caso del AFASPE en Chiapas. *Revista Pueblos y Fronteras*, **9**, 79-93. http://www.pueblosyfronteras.unam.mx/v09n17/05art.html

[7]   Diario Oficial de la Federación (DOM) (1983) Decreto por el que el Ejecutivo Federal establece bases para el programa de descentralización de los Servicios de salud de la SECRETARÍA DE SALUBRIDAD Y ASISTENCIA. México. http://www.dof.gob.mx/nota_to_imagen_fs.php?cod_diario=207621&pagina=11&seccion=0

[8]   Homedes Beguer, N. and Ugalde, A. (2008) 25 años de descentralizacion del sistema de salud mexicano: Una experiencia para analizar. *Revista Gerencia y Políticas de Salud*, **7**, 26-43.

[9]   Cardozo, M. (1993) Análisis de la política descentralizadora del sector salud: Centro de Investigación y Docencia Económicas. México, D.F.

[10] González Block, M.A., Leyva, R., Zapata, O., Loewe, R. and Alagón, J. (1989) Health Services Decentralization in México: Formulation, Implementation and Results of Policy. *Health Policy and Planning*, **4**, 301-315. http://dx.doi.org/10.1093/heapol/4.4.301

[11] López Arellano, O. and Blanco Gil, J. (1993) La modernización neoliberal en salud: México en los ochenta. México Universidad Autónoma Metropolitana, México.

[12] Diario Oficial de la Federación (DOM) (1995) Plan Nacional de Desarrollo 1995-2000 (Separata), México. http://www.dof.gob.mx/nota_detalle.php?codigo=4874791&fecha=31/05/1995

[13] Sales Heredia, F.J. (2012) A 30 años de la descentralización de los servicios de salud. Centro de Estudios Sociales y de opinión Pública de la Cámara de Diputados, LX Legislatura. Documento de trabajo núm. 140.

[14] Collins, C.D. (1989) Decentralization and the Need for Political and Critical Analysis. *Health Policy and Planning*, **4**, 168-171. http://dx.doi.org/10.1093/heapol/4.2.168

[15] Griffin, C. (1999) Empowering Mayors, Hospital Directors, or Patients? The Decentralization of Health Care. In: Burki, S.J., Perry, G. and Dillinger, W., Eds., *Beyond the Center: Decentralizing the State*, World Bank, Washington DC.

[16] Ugalde, A. and Homedes, N. (2002) Descentralización del sector salud en América Latina. *Gaceta Sanitaria*, **16**, 18-29. http://dx.doi.org/10.1016/S0213-9111(02)71629-4

[17] Escalante, E. (2000) El Ramo 33 Aportaciones Federales para Entidades Federativas y Municipios y Avances en el Federalismo. Crónica Legislativa. Cámara de Diputados LVIII Legislatura No. 12, México, 77-81. http://www.diputados.gob.mx/cronica57/contenido/cont12/leer8.html

[18] Freyermuth, G., *et al.* (2011) Monitoreo de la atención a las mujeres en servicios públicos del sector salud. Cuadernos de Trabajo 29, Instituto Nacional de las Mujeres—Centro de Investigaciones y Estudios Superiores en Antropología Social, México. http://www.inmujeres.gob.mx/images/stories/cuadernos/c29_o.pdf

[19] Oohna, C. and Graham, W. (2006) Strategies for Reducing Maternal Mortality: Getting on with What Works. *The Lancet*, **368**, 1284-1299. http://dx.doi.org/10.1016/S0140-6736(06)69381-1

[20] Freyermuth Enciso, G., Meneses Navarro, S. and Romero Martínez, M. (2015) Evaluation of Women's Health Care Programs in the Main Institutions of the Mexican Health System. *Cadernos de Saúde Pública*, **31**, 71-81.

[21] National Aboriginal Health Organization (2008) Cultural Competency and Safety: A Guide for Health Care Administrators Providers and Educator. National Aboriginal Health Organization, Otawa.

[22] Rodríguez Soriano, D., Freyermuth Enciso, M.G. and Argüello Avendaño, H. (2013) Monitoreos al acuerdo para el fortalecimiento de las acciones de salud pública en los estados y al convenio general de colaboración interinstitucional para la atención de la emergencia obstétrica. Un ejercicio de contraloría social. Observatorio de Mortalidad Materna en México.
http://www.omm.org.mx/images/stories/Documentos%20grandes/ANA%20Informe%20integrado%20AFASPE%20C ONVENIO%20AEO%20VERSI%C3%93N%20FINAL%20mayo%2016,%202013-2.pdf

[23] Orozco-Nuñez, E., González-Block, M.A., Kageyama-Escobar, L.M. and Hernández-Prado, B. (2009) Participación social en salud: La experiencia del programa de salud materna Arranque Parejo en la Vida. *Salud Pública de México*, **51**, 104-113. http://dx.doi.org/10.1590/S0036-36342009000200005

[24] Secretary of Health (2008) Programa de acción específico Arranque Parejo en la Vida, SSA, México.

[25] Torres Ramírez, A. (2010) La influenza pandémica A (H1N1) en mujeres embarazadas. *Ginecología y Obstetricia de México*, **78**, 121-127.

[26] Freyermuth, G. and Sesia, P., Eds. (2013) Monitoreos, diagnósticos y evaluaciones en salud maternal y reproductiva: Nuevas experiencias de contraloría. Centro de Investigaciones y Estudios Superiores en Antropología Social/Comité Promotor por una Maternidad Segura-México, Observatorio de Muerte Materna-México.

[27] Meneses Navarro, S., González Block, M.A., Quezada Sánchez, A.D. and Freyermuth Enciso, G. (2014) Evolución de la equidad en el acceso a servicios hospitalarios según composición indígena municipal en Chiapas, México: 2001 a 2009. In: Page Pliego, J.T., Ed., *Enfermedades del rezago y emergentes desde las ciencias sociales y la salud pública*, Programa de Investigaciones Interdisciplinarias sobre Mesoamérica y el Sureste, Instituto de Investigaciones Antropológicas, Universidad Nacional Autónoma de México, México, 17-35.

[28] Gwatkin, D. and Ergo, A. (2011) Universal Health Coverage: Friend or Foe of Health Equity? *The Lancet*, **377**, 2160-2161. http://dx.doi.org/10.1016/S0140-6736(10)62058-2

14

Prevalence of Menstrual Pain among Saudi Nursing Students and Its Effect on Sickness Absenteeism

Samantha Ismaile*, Seham Al-Enezi, Wajdan Otaif, Albandari Al-Mahadi, Nada Bingorban, Nourah Barayaan

The College of Nursing, Princess Nourah Bint Abdulrahman University, Riyadh, Saudi Arabia
Email: *SQIsmail@pnu.edu.sa, *samantha.ismaile@ymail.com

Abstract

Background: Primary menstrual pain is a well-known gynecological disorder among adult females including nursing undergraduate students. Nursing students tend not to seek medical treatment. As a result, this affects their quality of academic life and also absenteeism rate is increased. Objectives: To evaluate the prevalence of menstrual pain and its effect on sickness absenteeism on nursing student. Methods: This is a descriptive survey research design study by means of using a validated and modified questionnaire. Questionnaire information regarding menstrual pain severity, history and absenteeism were included. The research took place in the collage of nursing at the largest University in the world, Princess Nourah Bint Abdelrahman University, Riyadh, Saudi Arabia. A total of 100 single, female, unmarried undergraduate nursing students (Year 1, 2, 3, 4) were recruited by personal invitation during lectures. Result: The prevalence of menstrual pain was 92%. Most of the nursing students 27% had menstrual pain of moderate grade 5 - 6 and 38% of nursing students did not take pain medication for it. Lecture and collage absenteeism due to menstrual pain was present in 9% and 30% respectively. Finally, there was no significant correlation between menstrual pain and age of menarche, age and height. Conclusion: Menstrual pain is widely common prevalent among nursing undergraduates. As a result, it affects the quality of students' day-to-day life routine. The majority of nursing students' rarely seeks medical treatment. Providing health and patient education to improve awareness on managing menstrual period might help in avoiding students' absence from classes.

Keywords

Nursing Students, Primary Menstrual Pain, Sickness Absenteeism

---

*Corresponding author.

1. Introduction

Menstrual pain and also referred to as dysmenorrhea is a well-known gynecological disorder among adult females. There are two types of menstrual pain namely: primary and secondary menstrual pain. The primary menstrual pain is related to normal ovulatory cycles without pelvic pathology whereas secondary menstrual pain is "associated with pelvic pathology" [1]. The most common type of menstrual pain among undergraduate university students is the primary menstrual pain. According to French in 2008, there are many risk factors associated with primary menstrual pain such as heavy bleeding and pain during menses [2]. Moreover, mental stress was also reported as one of the main risk factors as a consequence of menstrual pain [3].

According to the literature, there are many published articles in regards to the effect of menstrual pain on student attendance grades and achievement [1] [4] [5]. Menstrual pain is common among adult undergraduate students [1] [2] [5] [6]. This deserves careful consideration as un-dealt menstrual pain may negatively affect the day to day routine and thus the quality of life. Hence, there are many researchers who report that the most common effect of menstrual pain is on the adverse effect on daily routine, which is experienced as "prolonged resting hours" and inability to cope with lectures, assignments and sometimes collage attendance [5].

In nursing undergraduate students, the most common gynecological problem was on menstrual pain. It is reported by [1] [5] that menstrual period is "highly prevalent" among female nursing students. Moreover, both researchers highlight that nursing undergraduate students do not usually seek medical treatment and as a consequence it affects their quality of academic life [1] [5]. They also, stated that, as a result of menstrual pain, absenteeism rate is increased among adult undergraduate students and this can be prevented and thus improve the quality of life [1] [5] [7].

A list of recommendation solutions to manage menstrual pain is listed by Gangwar *et al.* in 2014. This includes "mental preparation and by appropriate change in life style like de-stressing the person through relaxation exercise, yoga and breathing exercises" [1].

The choice of investigating undergraduate nursing students' is made because these students' are normally under huge psychological pressure without sufficient support. Menstrual pain affects student achievement, attendance and grades. However, the researches were unable to find any studies in Saudi Arabia regarding the menstrual pain and the effect of it among undergraduate students. Therefore, this research study is unique to conduct.

2. Aim and Objectives

The purpose of this study was to assess the prevalence of menstrual pain and to determine the sickness absenteeism as a result of menstrual pain among undergraduate nursing students.

3. Methods

This is a quantitative research study by using descriptive survey research.

3.1. Sample

The number of participants' in this research study were 100 female undergraduate nursing students' form Princess Nourah University (PNU) in Saudi Arabia. The inclusion criteria for this study were; female and single undergraduate nursing students, age range from 18 - 25 years old and without any history of pelvic pathology. While, the exclusion criteria were; participants who are less than 18 or more than 25 years old, married or those who were reported to have pelvic pathology. The nursing program at PNU is divided into 8 levels. Each academic year consist of 2 levels. In this research study, students were in their 4th year, level7. The overall grade at PNU is a GPA value of maximum 5.

3.2. Protocol

Questionnaires were distributed by face-to-face personal invitation during lectures in all different nursing students' years. Data took place at the middle weeks of the first academic in 2015. Sample rate depended on attendance rate of the lectures. All participants were given consent form and information sheet before taking part in the research study. In case participants felt any discomfort during completing the questionnaires; participants were allowed to withdraw freely without any pressure. Hence, no cases were reported. All participants took part in this study voluntary and were advised in case they have ethical concerns about this study that they can contact the nursing ethics committee. Ethical approval was obtained through the nursing collage ethics committees at Princess Nourah University.

3.3. Questionnaire

A validated questionnaire and Basic Information (BI) was used after gaining permission from the original authors [1]. The validated questionnaire and BI was then modified to the research aim. Face expert validity [8] for BI and the modified questionnaire was sought out before conducting the research.

The BI included demographic data in regards to weight, height and history of menstrual cycle. It also included any use of medication for menstrual pain and family history of menstrual pain. The BI total scores ranges from 0 - 44. The highest score for student level is 8. Students' grade (4 - 5) maximum score is 3. Height (180 - 190 cm) maximum score is 3 and weigh (80 - 100 kg) maximum score is 3. Maximum age score is 25. Finally, first monarch age (14 years old) highest score is 2.

The questionnaire questions related to the length of menstrual cycle, period of bleeding, history of menstrual pain and absenteeism from lectures or classes as a result of menstrual pain. The maximum score for the regularity of menstrual cycle is 1 and for the frequency of the presence of menstrual pain is also 1. The highest score for grades of menstrual pain (9 - 10 pain scale) is 4 and for experiencing strong pelvic cramping with sharp pains maximum score is1. The highest score for using of any of self-medication experiencing period pain that is soothed by warmth and pressure is 1, using medication maximum score is 1, and sickness absenteeism maximum score is 2. The total questionnaire scoring including the BI section is from 0 - 55.

Data analysis was done by the using of Statistical Package for the Social Sciences (SPSS), version 2015. This is most widely used program for statistical analysis to social study. An expert Advice from a scientific research statistician was sought out when needed.

4. Results

4.1. The Results of the Frequency, Mean, Median and Standard Deviation

The results of this research study was as the following; the mean of student's level is 6.06, the overall grade is 1.27, the age of the students is 21.81, the weight is 50 and height is 150 summarized in **Table 1**. There was no significant correlation of menstrual pain with height, weight, menstrual regularity.

4.2. The Results of Sample Distribution

A summary of the nursing students distribution according to student's level, student's overall grade, age, height, weight and age when first period are presented in **Table 2**. As shown, the highest sample has respond to the questionnaires were from the seventh level, where as many as 53 students by 61% and were the least of the second level and the number was 2 with average of 2.3%. As it can be seen that the highest sample has respond to the questionnaires were aged 22 years by 39%, and least of the 19-year by 1%. It also is clear that the higher sample has respond to the questionnaires were weight ranging from 40 - 60 kg by up to 50%, and less sample was weighing between 20 - 40 number 1 and 1%. Moreover, higher sample has respond to the questionnaires

Table 1. Statistics of the study frequency, mean, median and standard deviation.

		Student Level	Overall Grade	Age	Weight	Height	Age when first period
N	Valid	87	99	94	100	100	100
	Missing	13	1	6	0	0	0
Mean		6.06	1.27	21.81	1.51	1.31	0.95
Median		7.00	1.00	22.00	1.00	1.00	1.00
Std. Deviation		1.306	0.586	1.212	0.577	0.563	0.730

Table 2. Statistics of the study frequency, mean, median and standard deviation.

Factors	Average	Frequency
	2.3	2
	3.4	3
Student's Level	2.3	2
	31.0	27
	60.9	53
	7.1	7
Student's Overall Grade	58.6	58
	34.3	34
	1.1	1
	12.8	12
	24.5	23
Age	39.4	37
	13.8	13
	5.3	5
	3.2	3
	1.0	1
	71.0	71
Height	24.0	24
	4.0	4
	1.0	1
	50.0	50
Weight	46.0	46
	3.0	3
	29.0	29
Age when first period	47.0	47
	24.0	24

was the first menstrual period at age of 13 - 14 where as many as 47 students by 47%.

4.3. Results of the Means and Standard Deviation of Sentences Mentioned in the Questioners and Ranked by Their Means (N = 100)

The means and standard deviation of sentences mentioned in the questioners and ranked by their means (N = 100) are summarized in **Table 3**. Accordingly, the overall average for all paragraphs amounted is 0.55 and a standard deviation of 0.589. The highest paragraph received the highest average arithmetic was "Grades of menstrual pain" a mean of 1.83 and a standard deviation of 1.248, less paragraph was "Presence of menstrual pain". With an average standard of 0.08, and a standard deviation of 0.273. Moreover, there was no significant correlation of the absenteeism with the grades of menstrual pain among undergraduate nursing students'.

Table 3. Means and Standard deviation of sentences mentioned in the questioners and ranked by their means (N = 100).

Number	Sentences	Mean	Standard Deviation	Rank
1	Menstrual cycle regulating	0.20	0.404	6
2	Presence of menstrual pain.	0.08	0.273	7
3	Grades of menstrual pain.	1.83	1.248	1
4	Do experience strong pelvic cramping with sharp pains and/or nausea during your period?	0.32	0.467	4
5	Do you use any of self-medication for menstrual pain?	0.38	0.489	3
6	Do you experience period pain that is soothed by warmth and pressure, such as hugging a hot water bottle?	0.30	0.461	5
7	Sickness absenteeism (absence from the class) due to menstrual pain.	0.72	0.781	2

4.4. The Results of Regularity of Menstruation, Frequency of the Presence of Menstrual Pain and Grades of Menstrual Pain among Nursing Students

According to **Table 4**, it is obvious that 79% of the sample has respond to questionnaires and mentioned that the menstrual cycle is a regular with 80%. Interestingly, the majority of the sample 92% of those who responded to the questionnaire mentioned that the menstrual pain is preset **Table 5**. The highest sample chose 5 - 6 as a grade of menstrual pain were they reached number of 27 with an average of 27% **Table 6**.

4.5. The Results of Experiencing Menstrual Pain Signs & Symptoms, Self-Medication and Sickness Absenteeism Results among Nursing Students

The majority of nursing students 67% of participant has experienced strong pelvic cramping with sharp pains and/or nausea during their period **Table 7**. Moreover, the majority of participants with an average of 61% use self-medication for menstrual pain **Table 8**. An exact number of, 70 participants with average of 70 soothed menstrual pain by warmth and pressure, such as hugging a hot water bottle **Table 9**. Finally, 46% of the participants live normal day to day life routine even with the menstrual pain, and don't need to get absent of college or classes (**Table 10**).

5. Discussion

Menstrual pain is the most common gynecological problem in adult females. There are many side effects of menstrual pain and the most common one is on causing mental stress among nursing undergraduate students' and thus effecting the quality of life and day to day routine. Interestingly, a prevalence of a total of 92% of those who responded to the questionnaire mentioned that the menstrual pain is present. Nursing students in our study reported experiencing menstrual pain. While, other studies on the prevalence of menstrual pain among students reported 85.1% [1], 67.5% [6] and 62.02% [9].

The mean age of menarche was 13.50 years while other study was 13.88 years [1]. Menstrual pain grades are categorized as the following 3 - 4 as mild 5 - 6 as moderate and 7 - 10 as severe. In this study, the highest grade among nursing students had menstrual pain selected 5 - 6 as a grade of menstrual pain was they reached number of 27 with an average of 27% **Table 6**. Therefore, this indicates that nursing students in our research suffers moderates grade of menstrual pain. In the other hand, this result was not similar to the study by [1] as the majority of the students' experienced moderate grade of menstrual pain.

There was no significant correlation between the first age of menstrual period and menstrual pain. Similarly, a recent study reported the same results [1]. In the other hand, other studies [6], and [9] reported the opposite.

This research reports that 46% of menstrual pain nursing students have a normal day to day routine life, and only 19% reported class and 30% lecture and college absenteeism.

A recent study done in India [1] reported that over than 76% of undergraduate medical students seek medical treatment. In our research, nursing undergraduate students around 61% administrate medication self-prescription to relive menstrual pain. Interestingly, the majority of 70 participants with average of 70% of the undergraduate nursing students took no medication for pain and menstrual pain was soothed by the application of warmth

Table 4. Frequency of the regularity of menstrual cycle among nursing students'.

		Frequency	Percent	Valid Percent	Cumulative Percent
	Regular	79	79.0	79.8	79.8
Valid	Irregular	20	20.0	20.2	100.0
	Total	99	99.0	100.0	
Missing	9	1	1.0		
Total		100	100.0		

Table 5. Frequency of the presence of menstrual pain among nursing students.

		Frequency	Percent	Valid Percent	Cumulative Percent
	Present	92	92.0	92.0	92.0
Valid	Absent	8	8.0	8.0	100.0
	Total	100	100.0	100.0	

Table 6. Grades of menstrual pain among nursing students.

		Frequency	Percent	Valid Percent	Cumulative Percent
	0 - 2	18	18.0	18.0	18.0
	3 - 4	23	23.0	23.0	41.0
	5 - 6	27	27.0	27.0	68.0
Valid	7 - 8	22	22.0	22.0	90.0
	9 - 10	10	10.0	10.0	100.0
	Total	100	100.0	100.0	

Table 7. Percentage of experiencing strong pelvic cramping with sharp pains and/or nausea during your period among nursing students'.

		Frequency	Percent	Valid Percent	Cumulative Percent
	Yes	67	67.0	68.4	68.4
Valid	No	31	31.0	31.6	100.0
	Total	98	98.0	100.0	
Missing	9	2	2.0		
Total		100	100.0		

Table 8. Percentage of using of any of self-medication for menstrual pain among nursing students'.

		Frequency	Percent	Valid Percent	Cumulative Percent
	Yes	61	61.0	61.6	61.6
Valid	No	38	38.0	38.4	100.0
	Total	99	99.0	100.0	
Missing	9	1	1.0		
Total		100	100.0		

Table 9. Percentage of experiencing period pain that is soothed by warmth and pressure, such as hugging a hot water bottle nursing students.

		Frequency	Percent	Valid Percent	Cumulative Percent
	Yes	70	70.0	70.0	70.0
Valid	No	30	30.0	30.0	100.0
	Total	100	100.0	100.0	

Table 10. Percentage of Sickness absenteeism (absence from the class) due to menstrual pain among nursing students'.

		Frequency	Percent	Valid Percent	Cumulative Percent
	Normal daily life	46	46.0	48.4	48.4
	College absenteeism	30	30.0	31.6	80.0
Valid	Class absenteeism	19	19.0	20.0	100.0
	Total	95	95.0	100.0	
Missing	9	5	5.0		
Total		100	100.0		

and pressure, such as hugging a hot water bottle. Less than half of the sample 46% of the participants live normal day to day life routine even with the menstrual pain, and didn't need to get absent of college or classes. A study done by [10] reported that, over half of the participants in their study reported absenteeism from collage. Improving students nursing knowledge and awareness can lead to changing attitudes and behaviors' [11]. This can be done through improving the knowledge and awareness on menstrual pain management.

There was no significant correlation of menstrual pain with height, weight, menstrual regularity. Other studies reported similar findings [1] [6].

6. Conclusions and Implication

Menstrual pain is a common problem among female nursing undergraduate students and it is the main cause for students to be absents from college and attending classes. Therefore, students might miss attending classes and thus effect their overall achievements and grades.

Female adult health education and health promotion on managing menstrual pain might help in avoiding students absents from classes. It would also be beneficial to conduct the health education on the natural sources for managing menstrual pain among undergraduate students.

Health education on menstrual problem by health care providers can help prevent absenteeism.

To enhance the reliability and the validity of this research findings, adding a qualitative research arm with one-to-one and focus groups interviews' might enhance this research study.

Conflicts of Interest

There is no conflict of interest.

Acknowledgements

The authors would like to thank the Collage of Nursing represented by the Dean Dr. Hana Al-Sobayel and the Vice Dean of Academic Affairs Dr. Sana Hawamdeh, Princess Nourah University, for motivating both their students and staff to engage in a world class academic research.

References

[1] Gangwar, V., Kumar, D., Gangwar, R., Arya, M. and Banoo, H. (2014) Prevalence of Primary Dysmenorrhea among

the Undergraduate Medical Students and Its Impact on Their Performance in Study. *International Journal of Physiology*, **2**, 14-18. http://dx.doi.org/10.5958/j.2320-608X.2.1.004

[2]   French, L. (2001) Dysmenorrhea in Adolescents: Diagnosis & Treatment. *Paediatric Drugs*, **810**, 1-7.

[3]   Alonso, C. and Coe, C. (2001) Disruptions of Social Relationships Accentuates the Association between Emotional Distress and Menstrual Pain in Young Women. *Health Pscychology*, **42**, 871-881. http://dx.doi.org/10.1037/0278-6133.20.6.411

[4]   Balbi, C., Musone, R., Menditto, A. and Prisco, L.D. (2000) Cassese E. Influence of Menstrual Factors and Dietary Habits on Menstrual Pain in Adolescence Age. *European Journal of Obstetrics &Gynecology and Reproductive Biolog*, **91**, 143-148. http://dx.doi.org/10.1016/S0301-2115(99)00277-8

[5]   Sharma, A., Taneja, A., Sharma, P. and Saha, R. (2008) Problems Related to Menstruation and Their Effect on Daily Routine of Students of a Medical College in Delhi, India. *Asia-Pacific Journal of Public Health*, **20**, 1-8. http://dx.doi.org/10.1177/1010539508316939

[6]   Shrotriya, C., Ray, A. and George, A. (2012) Menstrual Characteristic' and "Prevalence and Effects of Dysmenorrhea" on Quality of Life of Medical Students. *International Journal of Collaborative Research on Internal Medicine & Public Health*, **4**, 276-286.

[7]   Agarwal, A. and Agarwal, A. (2010) A Study of Dysmenorrhea during Menstruation in Adolescent Girls. *Indian Journal of Community Medicine*, **35**, 159-164. http://dx.doi.org/10.4103/0970-0218.62586

[8]   Neuman, W. (1997) Social Research Methods: Qualitative and Quantitative Approaches. Allyn and Bacon, Boston.

[9]   Kumbhar, S., Redd, M., Sujana, B., Reddy, K. and Balkrishna, C. (2011) Prevalence of Dysmenorrhea among Adolescent Girls (14-19 Years) of Kapada District and Its Impact on Quality of Life: A Cross Sectional Study. *National Journal of Community Medicine*, **2**, 265-268.

[10]   Banikarim, C., Chacko, M. and Kelder, S. (2000) Achieves of Prevalence and Impact of Dysmenorrhea on Hispanic Female Adolescents. *Pediatrics & Adolescent Medicine*, **154**, 1226-1229. http://dx.doi.org/10.1001/archpedi.154.12.1226

[11]   Ismaile, S. (2015) Nursing Studies: Factors Promoting and Inhibiting Adherence to Clinical Practice Guidelines among the Nursing Profession. Ph.D. Dissertation, Medicine, Pharmacy and Health School, Durham University, UK.

15

Change in Preoperative Nervousness: A Randomized Controlled Trial in Gynecological Cancer Patients

Marianne K. Thygesen[1,2]*, René De Pont Christensen[3], Lone Hedemand[1], Ole Mogensen[1,2]

[1]Institute of Clinical Research, Faculty of Health Sciences, University of Southern Denmark, Odense, Denmark
[2]Department of Obstetrics and Gynaecology, Odense University Hospital, Odense, Denmark
[3]Research Unit of General Practice, University of Southern Denmark, Odense, Denmark
Email: *marianne.thygesen@rsyd.dk

Abstract

Patients are often nervous prior to surgery and females might suffer the most. Increased nervousness needs attention as it can negatively affect postoperative recovery. Support from nurses, *i.e.* being present, attentive, empowering and helpful to the patient, and talking about what is on the patient's mind, might help to reduce nervousness. However, there is a lack of evidence as to the ideal level of attention and resources to reduce preoperative nervousness. The objective of the current study was to compare a range of care combinations with standard care to female patients prior to sedation and cancer surgery primarily on difference in change in nervousness from admission until sedation before cancer surgery, measured on a Visual Analouge Scale. Using simple randomization and numbers in sealed envelopes, adult gynaecological patients scheduled for open cancer surgery were allocated to care provided by a nurse anaesthetist and: A) a surgical nurse, B) no additional care, C) a known nurse , and D) a relative. Only the statistician was blinded. The trial stopped when the calculated numbers were included. In the full analysis set, compared to standard care A) (n = 61), we observed the following mean changes and [95% confidence intervals]: B) (n = 65) 1.05 [CI: 0.298 to 1.794] with $p = 0.006$, C) (n = 61): −0.38 [−1.140 to 0.385] with $p = 0.330$, D) (n = 71): 0.23 [−0.498 to 0.967] with $p = 0.528$. Female cancer patients will benefit from supportive care by a surgical nurse from the time of arrival on the operating ward plus supportive care from a nurse anesthetist from 5 - 10 minutes after entering the operating ward. It is not recommended at any time to rely fully on the support of relatives. The effect on adults of preoperative painful procedures and patients' time alone on the operating ward should be further investigated.

Keywords

Anxiety, Cancer, Perioperative Care, Randomized Controlled Trial, Women's Health

*Corresponding author.

1. Introduction

Preoperative nervousness and anxiety are common [1]-[8]. Anxiety is "a feeling of worry, nervousness, or unease about something with an uncertain outcome" [9] and nervousness is found to express essential elements of anxiety [3] [10]. Increased preoperative anxiety or nervousness can lead to deterioration in the patient's postoperative situation, e.g. increased pain, decreased mood, or negatively affected patient satisfaction [11]-[14]. However, we do not know the ideal level of attention and resources that should be made available to alleviate this situation. In meeting the challenges involved in sedation and surgery, patients will ideally be provided with suitable techniques aimed at helping them to manage, or decrease, their anxiety or nervousness. Many such techniques exist [4] [5] [12] [15]-[19]. One technique is the provision of support, *i.e.* for a nurse to be present, attentive, empowering and otherwise helpful towards the patient and to talk about what is on the patient's mind. Such support could be of a therapeutic nature, and gives the patient the opportunity to initiate a close bond with the healthcare professional [1] [15] [20] [21]. However, the time spent on the operating ward might be too short for patients to create a close psychological bond and obtain the optimum benefit from it [5]. Multiple studies have tested interventions to reduce preoperative anxiety or nervousness. A literature review of anxiety-reducing techniques primarily found tests of premedication and distraction and concluded that anxiety management was "dominated more by the desire for clinical efficiency than by effective individual requirements" [4]. A more active and less helpless attitude on the part of patients might be of the most benefit to them [4] [22]. Recent systematic reviews of patient education find information techniques to be promising but not convincing [17] [23] and, again, the authors emphasize the importance of meeting individual support needs. Others found the supportive element and the patient-nurse relationship to be important [1] [24], as this might allow healthcare professionals to choose appropriate techniques. Close relatives might also be a valuable support for patients before anesthesia, as they already know each other and often have affectional bonds, and relatives might intuitively support the patient in the way best suited to the patient [20] [25]. Moreover, from the patients point of view, there might be differences between sex in preoperative anxiety and preferences for support, and women might suffer the most [7] [18] [26]-[28]. Therefore, the objective of this research was to investigate the effectiveness of different care combinations delivered by nurses and relatives to adult females awaiting cancer surgery, and we had chosen the gynecological field. Standard care comprised situational support delivered by a nurse anesthetist in combination with a surgery nurse and we aimed to test the hypothesis: Situational support before sedation and surgery by a nurse anesthetist alone or in combination with a relative or a nurse known to the patient will prove superior to standard care, primarily with regard to a reduction of patient nervousness before anesthesia and, secondarily, with regard to global patient satisfaction before discharge.

2. Methods

2.1. Trial Design and Participants

A study with simple randomization was conducted in a large university hospital in Denmark that serves 1.2 million people. Patients were included in this study if they were offered open surgery for gynecological cancer, could communicate in Danish, and accepted the ward standard of anesthesia without anxiolytic premedication. Moreover, participants should have an adult close relative who agreed to accompany the patient to the operating ward on the day of surgery, if necessary. Exclusion criteria were permanent mental disability and those under the age of 18. No changes were made after commencement.

2.2. Interventions and Standard Care

All the participating nurses were educated in Denmark and had a bachelor in nursing minus three months. No special training was performed in regard to this study. They all worked with gynecological cancer care and had the intention to support patients in the best possible way during the perioperative period. They used their resources and competences in interaction with individual patients; *i.e.* they were present, attentive and helpful, and chatted at the patient's convenience. Moreover, they used additional anxiety-reducing strategies appropriate to the immediate situation: informed (provided factual information), predicted (predicted a better outcome than what the patient expected), empowered (gave information about a matter of course before explaining options available for action, and eventually encouraged to take action), and/or distracted (talked about something other than the threatening situation).

Prior to accept of participation all patients were informed about the different support combinations and how these potentially could benefit the patients.

In all groups: a hospital porter transferred the patient in bed from the ward to the operating ward. Five to ten minutes later, a nurse anesthetist came and stayed with the patient throughout the patient's remaining period on the ward an in theatre. The nurse anesthetist had a list of questions to put to the patient, inserted a drip and assisted the anesthesiologist in inserting, if appropriate, an epidural catheter. The operating nurse and the surgeon would stop by to ask some questions, which is required by law, and would leave. In the operating theatre, the operating nurse and the nurse anesthetist would help the patient to be warm and to lie in a way that would avoid pressure sores. All those involved stayed with the patient until she was heavily sedated.

The differences between groups:

1. *Standard care*: a surgical nurse met the patient on arrival on the operating ward, and stayed with the patient until she was sedated at the operating theatre. As standard, we have long had an idea of this care as optimal.

2. *The Ward Model*: a nurse known to the patient accompanied her to the operating ward. A project nurse with several years of experience in gynecological cancer care met the patient at the outpatient clinic prior to scheduled surgery in order to establish a connection and to answer questions. On the day of surgery, approximately 15 minutes before transfer from the gynecology ward, the same project nurse visited the patient again and accompanied her to the operating ward, and into the operating theatre. This care combination might be superior, as a known nurse might be beneficial for patients.

3. *The Caregiver Model*: a relative accompanied the patient to the operating ward.

On the day of surgery, a close relative of the patient's choosing was prepared to follow the patient. (S)he was shown a photo of the operating theatre, was asked to put on protective clothing, and was informed to leave the operating theatre quietly once the patient was heavily sedated. The close relative accompanied the patient to the operating ward and into the operating theatre, and acted according to the patient's wishes and as appropriate to the situation. As a close relative know the patient and *visa versa*, it might be beneficial to patients to have a close relative by their side at the theatre.

4. *The Anaesthesia Model*: only the nurse anesthetist attended to the patient 5 - 10 minutes after arrival on the operating ward. The nurse anesthetist and the operating nurse accompanied the patient from the operating ward into the operating theatre. In this care combination the nurse anesthetist and the patient had undisturbed time to establish a relationship, which might be beneficial to patients, as the nurse anesthetist would be the one keeping a special eye on the patient when she would become sedated.

2.3. Outcomes

Patient measures and data collection

The primary outcome was a change in nervousness from admission to immediately prior to anesthesia and cancer surgery. Patients expressed their nervousness intensity as a VAS (Visual Analog Scale) score, ranging from zero to ten, where zero meant not at all nervous and ten meant the most nervous the patient thought she could ever be. This measure was collected with one decimal upon admission (primarily noted by the same secretary for all patients) and immediately before being anaesthetized (noted by the nurse anesthetist who was present). The VAS score was tested in the study population before study start (n = 20), and a clinically meaningful difference was stated to be 0.9 - 1.0. The secondary outcome was global satisfaction at discharge, measured by use of a questionnaire filled in by the patients immediately before discharge and handed to a nurse in a sealed envelope. The questionnaire had a four-point Likert scale, including the possibility to choose "don't know" and included the five items: global questions regarding information received practical help, support, surgery and medicine, as well as the overall impression of the hospital visit. It was qualitatively validated in the study population (n = 12) before study start using a think-aloud test with silent observations, retrospective interviewing, and a small correction to one question after testing on the first four patients [29].

Patient characteristics and time spent

Specific patient characteristics were given by the patients before randomization and collected later from the electronic patient journal. The nurses involved measured time spent on support that was in addition to that provided by the nurse anesthetist in each group.

2.4. Sample Size

Based on a prior study [10], we assumed a mean change of three on the VAS scale in the standard care group, and a common standard deviation of two. With these assumptions, we calculated that, with 64 patients in each group, we would have 80% power at the two-sided 5% level to detect a difference of at least one in mean change of nervousness.

2.5. Randomization and Masking

Participants were assigned to one of the four groups using simple randomization via a computer-generated random number list that was printed out and placed in numbered sealed envelopes by the first author. Nurses at the outpatient clinic collected written informed consent, and telephoned the study nurse who allocated patients to a group using the next numbered sealed envelopes. Patients became participants as soon as the envelope was opened. The nature of the interventions made it impossible to mask either patients or healthcare professionals. The statistician was masked until the analyses and interpretations were completed.

2.6. Control of Complex Intervention

All the nurses were regularly verbally incited to keep the interventions as described and to report immediately, if any deviations were observed. Moreover, first author made three to five minutes semi-structured interviews with random participants in all groups with the prompt: Please describe for me, the care you received before anesthesia.

2.7. Statistical Analyses

Specific patient characteristics were summarized by descriptive statistics number and percentage for categorical parameters and mean, range of scores, and standard deviation for continuous parameters. VAS score at admission and immediately prior to surgery were summarized, together with the corresponding change. The primary analysis was by linear regression of the difference in VAS score adjusted for group and baseline score, with the standard care group as reference. The difference in change in VAS score between the groups is given by the mean, together with the 95% CI. The normality assumption of the difference was checked by visual inspection of the quantile-quantile plot. The primary analysis was on the full analysis set, *i.e.* only those with two VAS score measurements. Additionally, we assumed that missing scores were "Missing At Random" *i.e.* the missing values did not depend on unobserved data. Under this assumption, the missing values were imputed using multiple-imputation with a model containing group and baseline value. Linear regression was performed, including the imputed values of the difference adjusted for group and baseline value. Furthermore, we repeated the primary analysis with the Minimal Model as reference. The questionnaire scores were summed and both a Kruskal-Wallis equality-of-populations rank test and pairwise Wilcoxon rank sum tests were performed. Stata 13.1 StataCorp LP, College Station TX USA was used for all statistical analyses.

2.8. Ethical Issues

Before randomization, patients were informed of the standard care to non-participants, including the possibility to be accompanied by a relative up to (but not into) the operating theatre. The study number at the Biomedical Research Committee System Act at the Scientific Committee for Southern Region in Denmark is S-20082000-41, and the study adheres to the Declaration of Helsinki [30] and the Ethical Guidelines for Nursing Research in the Nordic Countries [31]. It was ethical acceptable to ask patients about their nervousness right before anesthesia as this theme had been addressed to the patients earlier, the question was asked friendly by the nurse anesthetist, and it is not necessarily desirable to remove nervousness entirely before sedation [11] [22].

3. Results

In total, 1116 patients were assessed for eligibility from December 2008. In May 2012, the desired sample size was reached and inclusion ceased. In total, 350 patients provided written informed consent and were randomized (**Figure 1**). Among the non-participants, many were offered minimal invasive surgery, some stated that they did not have relatives, several declined to participate without giving a reason, and some did not want to rely on help from relatives. Of those randomized, 13 did not want to participate in the end (due to overwhelming developments in their disease or unspecified situations), and 42 experienced changes in treatment plan (to minimal inva-

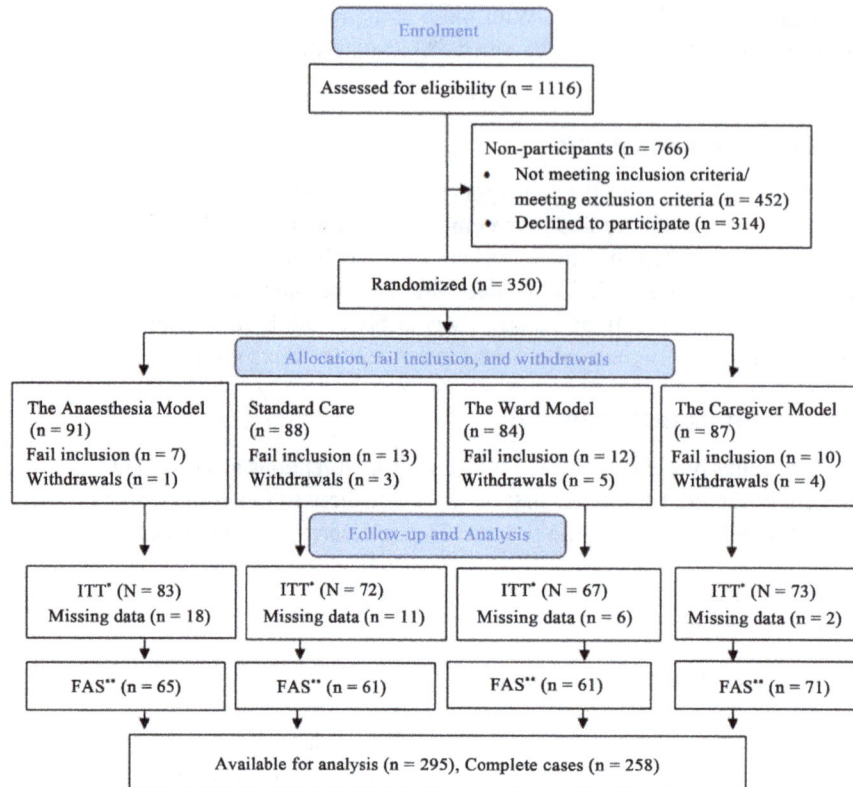

Figure 1. Flow chart. *ITT: Intention to treat, **FAS: Full Analysis set.

sive surgery or surgery at another hospital). A total of 295 patients provided specific characteristics and these were well balanced across the randomization groups (**Table 1**). All 295 patients provided a VAS score on admission, and approximately 1.5 days passed between this and the next VAS measures. A total of 37 patients were lost to follow-up, primarily due to business on the ward and premedication given before the VAS evaluation, leaving 258 as complete cases. Patients were in 73 cases follow by a relative of their choice, which were mainly a husband or a daughter. Only few had chosen a friend to follow them. The interventions were delivered consistently apart from four cases where other nurses reported the care to be not as attentive as it could be (one in the ward model and one in standard care) or the care could not be delivered by the same nurse at the outpatient clinic and in the ward (two in the ward model). All interviewed patients (n = 30) described the right care according to their allocation, and a few of those receiving the caregiver model commented, that they were surprised about their relatives reaction which could be both positive and negative.

Descriptive statistics for VAS of nervousness reveals no apparent clinically relevant difference on admission (**Table 2**). We observed a mean increase in nervousness in all four groups. The largest increase related to the Anesthesia Model, where only a nurse anesthetist was present. This is depicted, for illustration purposes only, by the regression lines in **Figure 2**. Patients who received supportive care in the form of the Ward Model exhibited the greatest benefit, with a mean difference in change in nervousness of −0.38 [CI: −1.140 to 0.385] $p = 0.330$, but no experimental model proved to be superior to standard care with statistical significance or clinical relevance. The Caregiver Model achieved a mean difference of 0.23 [CI: −0.498 to 0.967] $p = 0.528$, and the Anesthesia Model achieved a mean difference of 1.05 [CI: 0.298 to 1.794] $p = 0.006$. In the additional analysis, the Anesthesia Model was found to be significantly inferior to all the other care combinations. However, in those receiving support from the Caregiver Model, the difference was not clinically relevant: −0.81 [CI: −1.532 to −0.011] $p = 0.027$. The Ward Model achieved a mean difference of 1.42 [CI: −2.174 to −0.674] $p < 0.001$. When we performed an analysis for robustness by multiple imputations, no substantial changes were found (data not shown). With regard to patient satisfaction, we found a similar picture. No experimental models proved superior to standard care (**Table 3**), but in the additional analysis, the Anesthesia Model proved significantly inferior to both standard care ($p = 0.013$), the Ward Model ($p \leq 0.001$), and the Caregiver Model ($p = 0.004$). The

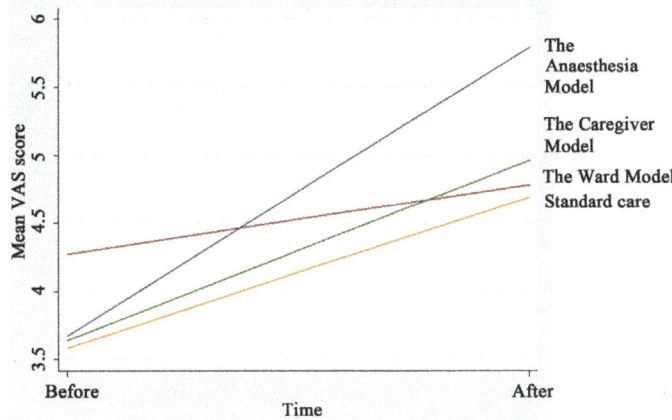

Figure 2. Regression lines for differences in Visual Analogue Score (VAS) in the four groups at the time before and after intervention.

Table 1. Patient characteristics at admission and at discharge, and the staging.

Characteristics at admission in groups	The Anaesthesia Model N = 83, n (%)	Standard care N = 72, n (%)	The Ward Model N = 67, n (%)	The Caregiver Model N = 73, n (%)
Live alone	14 (16.9)	12 (16.7)	12 (17.9)	15 (20.6)
Under 60 years of age	40 (48.2)	38 (52.8)	31 (46.3)	41 (56.2)
Previous surgery	53 (63.9)	51 (70.8)	51 (76.1)	53 (72.6)
Diagnosed cancer before surgery	37 (44.6)	31 (43.1)	24 (35.8)	25 (34.3)
Characteristics at discharge				
Benign diagnosis before discharge	13 (15.7)	6 (8.3)	13 (19.4)	15 (20.6)
Postoperative infection or reoperation	8 (9.6)	8 (11.1)	7 (10.5)	10 (13.7)
Diagnosis				
Tumour delimited to the affected organ	8 (9.6)	5 (6.9)	6 (9.0)	5 (6.9)
Tumour is spread outside the affected organ	59 (51.8)	47 (48.6)	38 (47.8)	48 (49.3)

Table 2. Distribution of the Visual Analogue Score (VAS[a]) of nervousness and the differences between them within the original assigned groups.

	The Anesthesia Model N (range) Mean, SD	Standard care N (range) Mean, SD	The Ward Model N (range) Mean, SD	The Caregiver Model N (range) Mean, SD
Hospitalization				
FAS[b]	65 (0 to 10) 3.7, 2.5	61 (0 to 10) 3.6, 2.8	61 (0 to 10) 4.3, 3.1	71 (0 to 10) 3.6, 2.8
ITT[c]	83 (0 to 10) 3.8, 2.5	72 (0 to 10) 3.5, 2.7	67 (0 to 10) 4.2, 3.1	73 (0 to 10) 3.6, 2.8
Preoperative				
FAS[b]	65 (0 to 8.2) 5.8, 2.9	61 (0 to 10) 4.7, 2.7	61 (0 to 10) 4.8, 3.0	71 (0.5 to 10) 5.0, 2.8
ITT[c]	65 (0 to 10) 5.8, 2.9	61 (0 to 10) 4.7, 2.7	61 (0 to 10) 4.8, 3.0	71 (0.5 to 10) 5.0, 2.8
Difference				
FAS[b]	65 (−2 to 8.2) 2.1, 2.5	61 (−4.9 to 8.2) 1.1, 2.3	61 (−4.4 to 6) 0.5, 2.0	71 (−5.2 to 6.4) 1.3, 2.4
ITT[c]	65 (−2 to 8.2) 2.1, 2.5	61 (−4.9 to 8.2) 1.1, 2.3	61 (−4.4 to 6) 0.5, 2.0	71 (−5.2 to 6.4) 1.3, 2.4

[a]VAS score of nervousness is from 0 to 10, with 0 as no nervousness at all and 10 as the most extreme nervousness patients could ever think of, [b]FAS: Full Analysis Set, [c]ITT: Intention to Treat.

Table 3. Distribution of patient satisfaction score in the four original assigned groups and differences between groups.

Group	N	Mean[a]	SD	Median	p-value	
					Compared to the Anaesthesia Model	Compared to standard care
The Anaesthesia Model	83	11.4	5.5	14		0.013
Standard care	72	13.1	4.1	15	0.013	
The Ward Model	67	13.9	2.7	15	<0.001	0.351
The Caregiver Model	73	13.8	2.7	15	0.004	0.850

[a]Score min = 0, max = 15.

Anesthesia Model was the most economically efficient, as it involved no additional time to that spent by the nurse anesthetist, while, for standard care, the Ward Model and the Caregiver Model, respectively, 35, 57, and 6 additional minutes per patient were spent by staff.

4. Discussion

We investigated the effect of different healthcare combinations and the involvement of a relative on the nervousness of cancer patients before anesthesia and cancer surgery and we were not able to show that any of the tested interventions were better than standard care. In our additional analyses, standard care, the Ward Model and the Caregiver Model proved significantly better than the Anesthesia Model on both measures: global satisfaction at discharge and VAS of nervousness before sedation and surgery. However, a clinically relevant improvement was reached only by standard care and the Ward Model. Patients' nervousness was not eradicated, but an increase in nervousness was to some degree counteracted. Preoperative anxiety and recovery have been in focus in research for more than fifty years. Within the last two decades, reviews acknowledge that, a reduction of preoperative anxiety to zero would not necessarily be of benefit to patients [11] [22]. Preoperative anxiety is, nevertheless, a good predictor of recovery [11] [13] [14] [32] [33], and a recent systematic review recommends a reduction in higher levels of anxiety before sedation for surgery for a life-threatening disease [34]. Because anxiety level is influenced by personality characteristics [35], a recommended preoperative anxiety level would be misleading. Our study adds more scientifically tested care combinations to support patients in counteracting an increase in preoperative anxiety. The procedures carried out by the nurse anesthetist could be painful. Moreover, in our study, the anesthetist came to the patient five to ten minutes after the patient arrived on the operating ward. Pain inflicted by healthcare professionals might provoke anxiety, and in our unconscious mind, pain might be linked to threat and danger [36]. Research on patients' experiences of dialogues prior to, during and after surgery with the same nurse, however, revealed that patients considered the talks they had and the continuity to be anxiety-reducing [37] [38] and even that they "prevented and alleviated suffering in surgical procedures" [37]. This idea is supported in a study about children's healthcare. It is less the case that the patient suffers pain from the actual procedures conducted, but from the environment in which they take place [39]. The inherent waiting time at the operating ward before the anesthetist nurse showed up may have contributed to patients' perception of the situation. This is supported by research performed by Cobley et al., who interviewed 124 patients by means of a 16-item questionnaire within 36 hours of surgery and found that arrival at the operating ward was a distressing time for patients, and for some it was even unbearable [40]. Having someone to talk to during the perioperative period is preferred by females [27], and females might indeed benefit by not being left alone at the final preoperative stage. However, we lack research on adult patients' experiences in general, the effects of unpleasant or painful preoperative procedures, and being left alone on the operating ward.

We found no statistical or clinically relevant difference between standard care and the Ward Model or the Caregiver Model. These interventions both offered ongoing attention and care from the time before leaving the ward and until the patient was anaesthetized. In this way, support was provided throughout the period that Coleby et al. identified as specifically distressing before surgery: waiting on the ward and being transferred to, and arriving at, the operating ward [40]. Moreover, the patients who received these support interventions had the opportunity to make a connection with their respective supporters, which might also be beneficial for patients [20] [25]. However, compared to standard care, the benefit for patients was not statistically significant or clinically relevant in counteracting an increase in nervousness and did not show an increase in global satisfaction with the healthcare. It is notable that compared to the Anesthesia Model in the additional analyses; the Caregiver Model did not result in clinically relevant changes in patients' experienced nervousness. Relatives might have more personal strength than patients, but new research has found a link between the level of anxiety in cancer patients and their relatives [41]. Moreover, a new systematic review did not find a convincing effect of family caregivers' supportive care in cancer [42]. Therefore, it is not recommended to rely fully on supportive care from relatives in the preoperative period.

Strengths and Limitations

We planned the sample size assuming a standard deviation of two. Evidently, this was optimistic for some groups (**Table 2**). Thus, the study is slightly under-powered. However, apart from the Minimal Group, none of the experimental groups show clinically relevant differences compared to the standard care group. Hence, higher power would not be likely to alter the clinical conclusions.

The satisfaction questionnaire used was only qualitatively validated. However, the few questions were validated in the study population ahead of study start. Both of the patient measures were based solely on self-report and therefore influenced by personality. Given the size of the study, we can be fairly confident that any unobserved characteristics were well-balanced across the groups. However, we acknowledge that there is some potential for bias because our randomization was not blinded to the patients, the healthcare professionals or the relatives. Patients might have been more nervous by knowing they were allocated to the model with only one supporting nurse. Patients were, however, informed about the possible benefits of *all* the care combinations, and one good care relation is expected to be enough [20] [21]. Moreover, following this logic, patients who knew they were to receive care from an additional person and even be followed from the ward might have been even less nervous, but we did not observe this. The healthcare professionals could have promoted their own intervention and disturbed others', but this was not reported. On the contrary, others performance was reported if it was not as attentive as possible judged by their healthcare professional co-workers. At the study site, each nurse's primary aim was to strive to help the individual patients as well as possible, and the study's aim was secondary to this, which is reflected in the missing VAS scores from the operating room. The fact that these are missing, of course, constitutes a limitation in its own right, but the number of complete cases is still convincing, and the robustness analysis did not hint at any problems with reliability. Our interventions ran over more years. The intervention did not change, but the context changed slightly with a few changes in staff, and increased offers of minimal invasive surgery which excluded such patients and left those with larger tumors as participants in our study. However, all changes would have affected even in the four arms, due to the study design. The interventions were complex and it was not possible to control whether the best possible anxiety reduction strategy was used in the specific interactions. However, we expected that the healthcare professionals would need to be free to use their knowledge and skills to adapt care to suit individual patients' needs [27] [43]. Our approach was to stay as close as possible to usual clinical practice and this enhanced the ecological validity of the study, and, consequently, its external validity [44]. Of females acceptable for inclusion, 47% declined to participate. As is inherent in almost all such research, we may therefore have included only the strongest.

Previous studies report that females have a greater tendency to have preoperative anxiety, a tendency to higher anxiety, and more females than males prefer to have a partner by their side in the preoperative period [26]-[28]. Eventually generalizability to male patient populations should therefore be done with great caution.

5. Conclusion

Supportive care by a surgery nurse, from the time of arrival at the operating ward, and by a nurse anesthetist, from 5 - 10 minutes after the arrival and until the patient has been anesthetized, will help female cancer patients to counteract an increase in preoperative nervousness and feel satisfied at discharge. The support and company of a ward nurse from ten minutes before leaving the ward and until the patient is anesthetized provide a similar level of benefit. However, support from a surgery nurse and a nurse anesthetist might be attractive to offer as standard, because this is the most time efficient of the four care combinations. Relatives might, to some degree, be helpful in alleviating female patients' preoperative suffering due to nervousness, but it is not recommended at any time to rely fully on their support. Furthermore, the sole support of a nurse anesthetist from 5 - 10 minutes after arrival at the operating ward is not recommended. How nurse anesthetists' procedures and patients' time alone on the operating ward affect adult patients in general should be the focus of further research.

Acknowledgements

We thank the patients and the relatives who participated in this study. Moreover, we thanks Jette Johansen, Annette Henriksen, Inger Juhl and Kristian Kidholm who contributed to the study's conception and we acknowledge the important collaboration in randomization and data collection with nurse anesthetists, surgery nurses, ward nurses, and the secretary where the study took place. Lorna Campbell copy-edited this article. The study was financially supported by non-partisan funds: The Tryg Foundation and Sister Marie Dalgaard's Foundation.

References

[1]   Carr, E., Brockbank, K., Allen, S. and Strike P. (2006) Patterns and Frequency of Anxiety in Women Undergoing Gynaecological Surgery. *Journal of Clinical Nursing*, **15**, 341-352. http://dx.doi.org/10.1111/j.1365-2702.2006.01285.x

[2]   Thygesen, M.K., Pedersen, B.D., Kragstrup, J., Wagner, L. and Mogensen, O. (2011) Utilizing a New Graphical Elicitation Technique to Collect Emotional Narratives Describing Disease Trajectories. *The Qualitative Report*, **16**, 596-608. http://nsuworks.nova.edu/cgi/viewcontent.cgi?article=1076&context=tqr

[3]   Mackenzie, J.W. (1989) Daycase Anaesthesia and Anxiety. A Study of Anxiety Profiles amongst Patients Attending a Day Bed Unit. *Anaesthesia*, **44**, 437-440.

[4]   Mitchell, M. (2003) Patient Anxiety and Modern Elective Surgery: A Literature Review. *Journal of Clinical Nursing*, **12**, 806-815. http://dx.doi.org/10.1046/j.1365-2702.2003.00812.x

[5]   Grieve, R.J. (2002) Day Surgery Preoperative Anxiety Reduction and Coping Strategies. *British Journal of Nursing*, **11**, 670-678. http://dx.doi.org/10.12968/bjon.2002.11.10.670

[6]   Mertz, B.G., Bistrup, P.E., Johansen, C., Dalton, S.O., Deltour, I. and Kehlet, H. (2012) Psychological Distress among Women with Newly Diagnosed Breast Cancer. European *Journal of Oncology Nursing*: *The Official Journal of European Oncology Nursing Society*, **16**, 439-443. http://dx.doi.org/10.1016/j.ejon.2011.10.001

[7]   Rosen, S., Svensson, M. and Nilsson, U. (2008) Calm or Not Calm: The Question of Anxiety in the Perianesthesia Patient. *Journal of Perianesthesia Nursing*: *Official Journal of the American Society of PeriAnesthesia Nurses/American Society of PeriAnesthesia Nurses*, **23**, 237-246. http://dx.doi.org/10.1016/j.jopan.2008.05.002

[8]   Haugen, A.S., Eide, G.E., Olsen, M.V., Haukeland, B., Remme, A.R. and Wahl, A.K. (2009) Anxiety in the Operating Theatre: A Study of Frequency and Environmental Impact in Patients Having Local, Plexus or Regional Anaesthesia. *Journal of Clinical Nursing*, **18**, 2301-2310. http://dx.doi.org/10.1111/j.1365-2702.2009.02792.x

[9]   Oxford Dictionaries (2015) Oxford University Press. http://www.oxforddictionaries.com

[10] Videbech, M., Carlsson, P.S., Jensen, N.C. and Videbech, P. (2003) [Measuring of Preoperative Anxiety by Three Self-Reporting Scales: State Trait Anxiety Inventory, Symptoms CheckList 92 and Visual Analogue Scale]. *Ugeskrift for Laeger*, **165**, 569-574.

[11] Munafo, M.R. and Stevenson, J. (2001) Anxiety and Surgical Recovery. Reinterpreting the Literature. *Journal of Psychosomatic Research*, **51**, 589-596. http://dx.doi.org/10.1016/S0022-3999(01)00258-6

[12] Markland, D. and Hardy, L. (1993) Anxiety, Relaxation and Anaesthesia for Day-Case Surgery. *British Journal of Clinical Psychology*, **32**, 493-504. http://dx.doi.org/10.1111/j.2044-8260.1993.tb01085.x

[13] Kil, H.K., Kim, W.O., Chung, W.Y., Kim, G.H., Seo, H. and Hong, J.Y. (2012) Preoperative Anxiety and Pain Sensitivity Are Independent Predictors of Propofol and Sevoflurane Requirements in General Anaesthesia. *British Journal of Anaesthesia*, **108**, 119-125. http://dx.doi.org/10.1093/bja/aer305

[14] Li, C., Carli, F., Lee, L., Charlebois, P., Stein, B. and Liberman, A.S. (2013) Impact of a Trimodal Prehabilitation Program on Functional Recovery after Colorectal Cancer Surgery: A Pilot Study. *Surgical Endoscopy*, **27**, 1072-1082. http://dx.doi.org/10.1007/s00464-012-2560-5

[15] Teasdale, K. (1995) Theoretical and Practical Considerations on the Use of Reassurance in the Nursing Management of Anxious Patients. *Journal of Advanced Nursing*, **22**, 79-86. http://dx.doi.org/10.1046/j.1365-2648.1995.22010079.x

[16] Nilsson, U., Rawal, N., Enqvist, B. and Unosson, M. (2003) Analgesia Following Music and Therapeutic Suggestions in the PACU in Ambulatory Surgery: A Randomized Controlled Trial. *Acta Anaesthesiologica Scandinavica*, **47**, 278-283. http://dx.doi.org/10.1034/j.1399-6576.2003.00064.x

[17] Ayyadhah Alanazi, A. (2014) Reducing Anxiety in Preoperative Patients: A Systematic Review. *British Journal of Nursing*, **23**, 387-393. http://www.magonlinelibrary.com/doi/pdf/10.12968/bjon.2014.23.7.387

[18] Jlala, H.A., French, J.L., Foxall, G.L., Hardman, J.G. and Bedforth, N.M. (2010) Effect of Preoperative Multimedia Information on Perioperative Anxiety in Patients Undergoing Procedures under Regional Anaesthesia. *British Journal of Anaesthesia*, **104**, 369-374. http://dx.doi.org/10.1093/bja/aeq002

[19] Lin, S.Y., Huang, H.A., Lin, S.C., Huang, Y.T., Wang, K.Y. and Shi, H.Y. (2016) The Effect of an Anaesthetic Patient

Information Video on Perioperative Anxiety: A Randomised Study. *European Journal of Anaesthesiology*, **33**, 134-139. http://dx.doi.org/10.1097/EJA.0000000000000307

[20] Bowlby, J. (1989) The Making and Breaking of Affectional Bonds. Routledge, London.

[21] Thygesen, M.K., Pedersen, B.D., Kragstrup, J., Wagner, L. and Mogensen, O. (2011) Benefits and Challenges Perceived by Patients with Cancer When Offered a Nurse Navigator. *International Journal of Integrated Care*, **11**, e130. http://www.ncbi.nlm.nih.gov/pmc/articles/PMC3225241/pdf/ijic2011-2011130.pdf

[22] Salmon, P. (1993) The Reduction of Anxiety in Surgical Patients: An Important Nursing Task or the Medicalization of Preparatory Worry? *International Journal of Nursing Studies*, **30**, 323-330. http://dx.doi.org/10.1016/0020-7489(93)90104-3

[23] Guo, P. (2015) Preoperative Education Interventions to Reduce Anxiety and Improve Recovery among Cardiac Surgery Patients: A Review of Randomised Controlled Trials. *Journal of Clinical Nursing*, **24**, 34-46. http://onlinelibrary.wiley.com/doi/10.1111/jocn.12618/epdf http://dx.doi.org/10.1111/jocn.12618

[24] Rudolfsson, G., von Post, I. and Eriksson, K. (2007) The Perioperative Dialogue: Holistic Nursing in Practice. *Holistic Nursing Practice*, **21**, 292-298. http://dx.doi.org/10.1097/01.HNP.0000298613.40469.6c

[25] Lindwall, L. and von Post, I. (2009) Continuity Created by Nurses in the Perioperative Dialogue—A Literature Review. *Scandinavian Journal of Caring Science*, **23**, 395-401. http://dx.doi.org/10.1111/j.1471-6712.2008.00609.x

[26] Karanci, A.N. and Dirik, G. (2003) Predictors of Pre- and Postoperative Anxiety in Emergency Surgery Patients. *Journal of Psychosomatic Research*, **55**, 363-369. http://dx.doi.org/10.1016/S0022-3999(02)00631-1

[27] Mitchell, M. (2013) Anaesthesia Type, Gender and Anxiety. *Journal of Perioperative Practice*, **23**, 41-47.

[28] Blais, M.C., St-Hilaire, A., Fillion, L., De Serres, M. and Tremblay, A. (2014) What to Do with Screening for Distress Scores? Integrating Descriptive Data into Clinical Practice. *Palliative & Supportive Care*, **12**, 25-38. http://dx.doi.org/10.1017/S1478951513000059

[29] Drennan, J. (2003) Cognitive Interviewing: Verbal Data in the Design and Pretesting of Questionnaires. *Journal of Advanced Nursing*, **42**, 57-63. http://dx.doi.org/10.1046/j.1365-2648.2003.02579.x

[30] WMA Declaration of Helsinki (2013) Ethical Principles for Medical Research Involving Human Subjects. http://www.wma.net/en/30publications/10policies/b3/index.html

[31] Northern Nurses' Federation (2003) Ethical Guidelines for Nursing Research in the Nordic Countries. *Nordic Journal of Nursing Research & Clinical Studies/Vaard i Norden*, **23**, 1-5.

[32] Granot, M. and Ferber, S.G. (2005) The Roles of Pain Catastrophizing and Anxiety in the Prediction of Postoperative Pain Intensity: A Prospective Study. *The Clinical Journal of Pain*, **21**, 439-445. http://dx.doi.org/10.1097/01.ajp.0000135236.12705.2d

[33] Pearson, S., Maddern, G.J. and Fitridge, R. (2005) The Role of Pre-Operative State-Anxiety in the Determination of Intra-Operative Neuroendocrine Responses and Recovery. *British Journal of Health Psychology*, **10**, 299-310. http://dx.doi.org/10.1348/135910705X26957

[34] McKenzie, L.H., Simpson, J. and Stewart, M. (2010) A Systematic Review of Pre-Operative Predictors of Post-Operative Depression and Anxiety in Individuals Who Have Undergone Coronary Artery Bypass Graft Surgery. *Psychology, Health & Medicine*, **15**, 74-93. http://dx.doi.org/10.1080/13548500903483486

[35] King, F.J., Heinrich, D.L., Stephenson, R.S. and Spielberger, C.D. (1976) An Investigation of the Causal Influence of Trait and State Anxiety on Academic Achievement. *Journal of Educational Psychology*, **68**, 330-334. http://dx.doi.org/10.1037/0022-0663.68.3.330

[36] Collen, M. (2014) Pain and Treatment from a Human Primate Perspective. *Journal of Pain & Palliative Care Pharmacotherapy*, **28**, 152-157. http://dx.doi.org/10.3109/15360288.2014.911237

[37] Lindwall, L., von Post, I. and Bergbom, I. (2003) Patients' and Nurses' Experiences of Perioperative Dialogues. *Journal of Advanced Nursing*, **43**, 246-253. http://dx.doi.org/10.1046/j.1365-2648.2003.02707.x

[38] Rudolfsson, G., Hallberg, L.R.M., Ringsberg, K.C. and von Post, I. (2003) The Nurse Has Time for Me: The Perioperative Dialogue from the Perspective of Patients. *Journal of Advanced Perioperative Care*, **1**, 77-84.

[39] Rennick, J.E., Johnston, C.C., Dougherty, G., Platt, R. and Ritchie, J.A. (2002) Children's Psychological Responses after Critical Illness and Exposure to Invasive Technology. *Journal of Developmental and Behavioral Pediatrics: JDBP*, **23**, 133-144. http://dx.doi.org/10.1097/00004703-200206000-00002

[40] Cobley, M., Dunne, J.A. and Sanders, L.D. (1991) Stressful Pre-Operative Preparation Procedures. The Routine Removal of Dentures during Pre-Operative Preparation Contributes to Pre-Operative Distress. *Anaesthesia*, **46**, 1019-1022. http://dx.doi.org/10.1111/j.1365-2044.1991.tb09913.x

[41] Cormio, C., Romito, F., Viscanti, G., Turaccio, M., Lorusso, V. and Mattioli, V. (2014) Psychological Well-Being and

Posttraumatic Growth in Caregivers of Cancer Patients. *Frontiers in psychology*, **5**, 1342.
http://dx.doi.org/10.3389/fpsyg.2014.01342
http://www.ncbi.nlm.nih.gov/pmc/articles/PMC4238371/pdf/fpsyg-05-01342.pdf

[42] Griffin, J.M., Meis, L.A., MacDonald, R., Greer, N., Jensen, A. and Rutks, I. (2014) Effectiveness of Family and Care-giver Interventions on Patient Outcomes in Adults with Cancer: A Systematic Review. *Journal of General Internal Medicine*, **29**, 1274-1282. http://dx.doi.org/10.1007/s11606-014-2873-2

[43] Stoddard, J.A., White, K.S., Covino, N.A. and Strauss, L. (2005) Impact of a Brief Intervention on Patient Anxiety Prior to Day Surgery. *Journal of Clinical Psychology in Medical Settings*, **12**, 99-110.
http://link.springer.com/article/10.1007/s10880-005-3269-6#page-1
http://dx.doi.org/10.1007/s10880-005-3269-6

[44] Bowling, A. (2002) Research Methods in Health. Investigating Health and Health Services. 2nd Edition, Open University Press, Maidenhead.

16

Two NGO-Run Youth-Centers in Multicultural, Socially Deprived Suburbs in Sweden—Who Are the Participants?

Susanna Geidne*, Ingela Fredriksson, Koustuv Dalal, Charli Eriksson

School of Health and Medical Sciences, Örebro University, Örebro, Sweden
Email: *susanna.geidne@oru.se, ingela.fredriksson@oru.se, koustuv.dalal@oru.se, charli.eriksson@oru.se

Abstract

Objective: Leisure-time is an important part of young people's lives. One way to reduce social differences in health is to improve adolescents' living conditions, for example by enhancing the quality of after-school activities. Multicultural, socially deprived suburbs have less youth participation in organized leisure-time activities. This study explores who the participants are at two NGO-run youth-centers in multicultural, socially deprived suburbs in Sweden and whether socio-demographic, health-related, and leisure-time factors affect the targeted participation. Methods: The study can be seen as an explanatory mixed-methods study where qualitative data help explain initial quantitative results. The included data are a survey with youth (*n* = 207), seven individual interviews with staff, and six focus-groups interviews with young people at two youth-centers in two different cities. Results and Conclusions: The participants in the youth-centers are Swedish born youths having foreign-born parents who live with both parents, often in crowded apartments with many siblings. Moreover they feel healthy, enjoy school and have good contact with their parents. It seems that strategies for recruiting youths to youth-centers have a large impact on who participates. One way to succeed in having a more equal gender and ethnicity distribution is to offer youth activities that are a natural step forward from children's activities. The youth-centers' proximity is also of importance for participation, in these types of neighborhoods.

Keywords

Youth-Center, Leisure-Time, Participation, Suburbs, NGO

1. Introduction

Leisure-time is important for young people's psychological, cognitive, and physical development [1]. Individuals

---
*Corresponding author.

outside the family become more important to adolescents, and leisure-time can therefore have a greater impact on their beliefs and behavior [2]. Most children and youth can decide how they want to spend this time, which gives the content of leisure activities an important role in youth development [3] [4]. Leisure-time also comprises a large part of young people's lives today and differs in some ways from that of earlier generations [4] [5]. However, there is no guarantee that young people will use their leisure-time beneficially, for example by choosing activities that challenge them [6].

Multicultural, socially deprived suburbs have less youth participation in organized leisure-time activities than other areas, due to both their higher proportion of immigrants and lower socioeconomic status (SES) [7]-[9]. Young people do not choose their leisure activities randomly; social circumstances are one of the determinants that matter [10]. Children's activities are also often chosen by their parents [11]. One way to reduce social differences in health is to improve children's and adolescents' living conditions, for example by enhancing the quality of school and after-school activities [12]. Much of the variation in health among children and adolescents can be explained by social factors (cf. [13] [14]).

Studies of adolescents' participation in leisure-time activities often examine organized sports activities and confirm that participants to a greater extent are male and have high SES background (cf. [15]-[18]). Adolescents who participate in both sports and other organized activities have been found less likely to use alcohol and drugs [19]. Moreover, harmful use of alcohol is less common among adolescents born outside of Sweden than adolescents born in Sweden [20]. Participation in leisure-time activities is associated with better academic achievement [21] [22]. It can be of particular significance for adolescents with lower SES [15].

Participation in structured activities relates to low levels of antisocial behavior [23] and to having a clear idea of what to do after leaving compulsory school [24]. It seems as if it is the psychologically healthy adolescents who tend to be involved in structured activities [25]. On the other hand, participants in low-structured activities were characterized by deviant peer relations and poor relations between parents and children [23]. They also more often lived in two homes and had an unemployed mother [24]. One reason that participation in structured activities relates to good adjustment is self-selection, because well-adjusted youth choose structured activities [26]. A medium level of participation in organized leisure activities is most favorable for adolescents' health and well-being [24]. Youth-centers are often less structured than organized sports and other leisure-time activities. However, they have opportunities to reach youth who are not interested in sports or other leisure activities.

Leisure-time activities for adolescents are constituted differently in different parts of the world. In countries like USA, extracurricular activities and out-of-school time [27] are two concepts. In Sweden, two orientations can be identified as important. On the one hand there is the widespread tradition of non-governmental organizations (NGOs), which run leisure-time activities, for example within sports. On the other hand, there are youth-centers, which are often run by municipalities.

Leisure-time is an important part of adolescents' lives. Leisure-time activities can be beneficial to young people's development. However, young people, especially girls, living in multicultural, socially deprived suburbs participate less in leisure-time activities. There is a need to understand who the participants are to be able to develop youth-centers in these neighborhoods. Youth-centers located in these neighborhoods can be a way to get young people to participate in leisure-time activities. Therefore this study has aimed to explore who participate in two NGO-run youth-centers in multicultural, socially deprived suburbs in Sweden with special focus on socio-demographic factors, health-related factors, or leisure-time factors.

2. Methods

This study is part of a study focusing on "Leisure-time as a setting for alcohol and drug prevention" in a special venture financed by the Swedish government [28]. The research program will answer a series of questions as why do young people participate in this type of activity and what particular strategies do the different youth-centers use in their everyday work. A three year longitudinal study will also try to answer the question what the young people gain from being participants in youth-center activities, The study was approved by the regional ethical committee in Uppsala in January 2012 (reg. No. 2011/475).

This study can be seen as an explanatory mixed-methods study, using Creswell and Plano Clark's approach [29], whereby qualitative data helps to explain initial quantitative results. Data were collected at the two youth-centers using surveys, individual interviews, and focus-groups interviews.

The study has also used a participatory and practice-based approach. This involves cooperating with youth-center staff on survey questions, data collection procedures, and samples (**Figure 1**). It also includes regular feedback to the youth-centers within six months after data collection, as well as extra feedback upon request. This approach was chosen for two reasons: (1) people are experts on their own settings, and (2) it is of great importance that the research results be of practical use for the setting, in this case the youth-centers.

2.1. The Study Context

The two youth-centers in this study are located in suburbs in two of the top-ten cities (by population) in Sweden. Both of these suburbs are characterized by apartment blocks and a high proportion of residents with immigrant backgrounds (60% - 90% compared with 20% for Sweden as a whole). The most frequent countries of origin are Iraq and Somalia [30]. The youth-centers are run by two different NGOs. The first, hereafter called T, is located in the neighborhood's central shopping area. T's activities cater to young people in the area aged 12 - 16 years. The second NGO, hereafter called V, has two different premises, one for youth up to 13, and another for youth between 13 and 18 years. Both youth-centers provide structured activities, such as dance groups, travel groups, tutoring, exhibitions, and leadership training, as well as unstructured activities, such as playing games, watching television, or just hanging out with friends. The youth-centers have both paid and volunteer staff. The paid staffs have educational training and the volunteer staffs are older youth, former participants, with internal leadership training. T primarily has employed leaders. V has few employed leaders, but many volunteer youth leaders.

2.2. Sample

The study used purposive sampling; those who came to the youth-centers during a defined time period were invited to take part, the idea being to reach people in voluntary and partly unstructured activities. Both youth-centers are member-based, and lists of all members in the targeted age group (12 - 16 years) were provided by each youth-center (**Table 1**). Since not all members visited the youth-centers on a regular basis, we chose to use the member lists to broaden the sample as much as possible.

Parents of youth who had not reached 15 years of age (62% of the sample) received information about the study. Due to the high proportion of immigrants, information was sent in five different languages: Swedish, English, Turkish, Arabic, and Somali. The choice of languages was decided in cooperation with the staff at each youth-center. Parent could refuse consent by returning a form stating that they did not want their child to participate (5% did so).

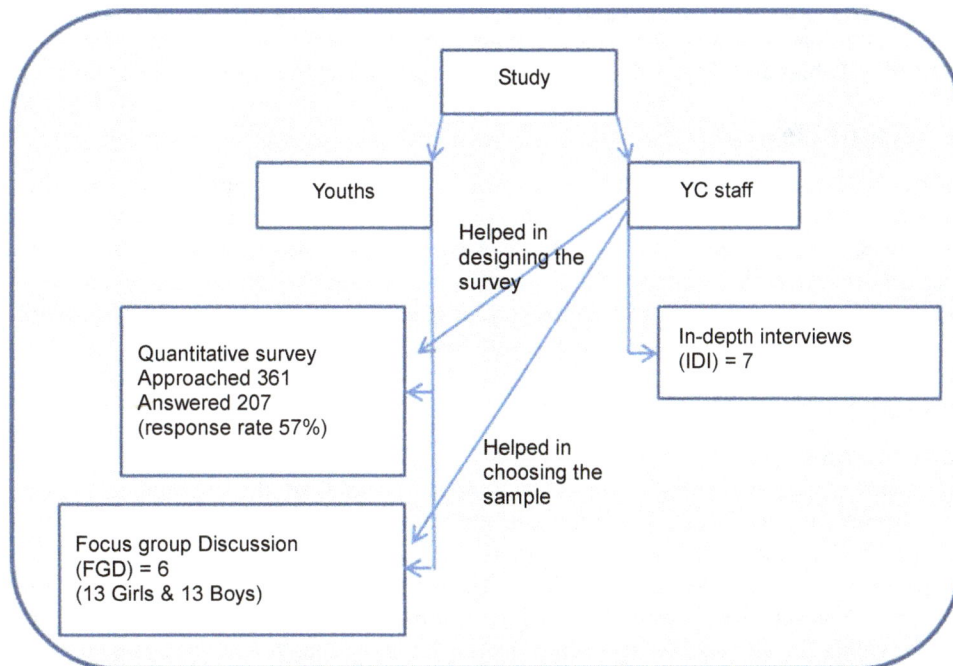

Figure 1. Samples and data collection with a participatory approach.

Table 1. Demographic factors of the respondents.

Youth center	Original sample	Response rate	Girls	Boys	Younger (<15 years)	Older (>15 years)	Total
V	271	144 (53%)	61 (42%)	83 (58%)	86 (60%)	57 (40%)	70%
T	90	63 (70%)	28 (44%)	35 (56%)	28 (44%)	35 (56%)	30%
Total	**361**	**207 (57%)**	**89 (43%)**	**118 (57%)**	**114 (55%)**	**92 (45%)**	**207 (100%)**

Staff members were instructed by the researchers to choose youth of different ages for the youth focus-groups. There was to be one group of girls and one of boys per youth-center location, *i.e.* three groups of girls and three groups of boys in total. (One center had two separate premises.) Center staff recommended that the groups be homogenous with regard to gender instead of age. The focus-groups contained three to five members. The sample for individual interviews was decided jointly by researchers and staff, but was to include both paid and volunteer staff as well as both genders. In total seven staff members, either paid or volunteers, were interviewed.

2.3. Data Collection

Data was collected through a survey in spring 2012. The questionnaires were distributed by the center leaders during a period of six weeks at V and 10 weeks (not open on weekends) at T. The young people who voluntarily visited the centers during this time were requested to fill in the questionnaires on the premises. The length of the data collection was decided upon together with the staff of the youth-centers in order to reach as many participants as possible.

The in-depth interviews of the staff were conducted by SG and IF in all but two cases. Two interviews were conducted by IF alone. Focus-group interviews were conducted by SG or IF at the premises. The interviews were conducted in February 2013, recorded with the permission of the respondents, and then transcribed verbatim. Both in-depth interviews and focus-group interviews lasted for around an hour each.

No individuals were paid for their participation, but the youth-centers received a small sum depending on the young people's level of participation.

2.4. Questionnaire

The questions used in this particular analysis concerned the three categories: the young person's socioeconomic background, health-related factors such as alcohol and tobacco use, and leisure-time interests and habits (thorough described in **Tables 2-6**). Many of the questions have previously been used in earlier studies (cf. [31] [32]).

2.5. Interview Guide

The semi-structured interview guide included questions about who participates and why they participate in youth-center activities. It also focused on what the young people gained, and what particular strategies the different youth-centers use in their everyday work. The questions specifically focusing on who participates concerned age, gender and birth countries. But also questions on other leisure-time interests, frequency of attendance, who stays and who drops out, and if who participates differ from year to year. The same interview guide was used for both in-depth interviews and focus-group interviews.

2.6. Analysis

2.6.1. Statistical Analyses

Descriptive statistics were employed using chi-square tests to find out if there were any differences between gender or frequency of attendance and the independent variables. Logistic regression analyses were conducted with the dependent variable gender. First, unadjusted odds ratios with 95% confidence intervals were estimated for all independent variables. Then three different logistic regression analyses were performed using three categories of independent variables (socio-demographic, health-related, and leisure-time factors). Only individuals with full information for all variables were included in the logistic regression analyses. It was not possible to enter all variables in all categories into the same model due to the low number of participants in relation to the large number of variables.

2.6.2. Qualitative Analysis

The interviews were recorded and transcribed verbatim. An inductive qualitative content analysis was performed to analyze both the in-depth interviews and the focus-group interviews and describe variations by identifying differences and similarities in the interviews [33].

Each interview, in its entirety, was used as a units of analysis. Meaning units were first identified in accordance with the study aim of who participates and then condensed. The condensed meaning units were then abstracted into codes. Interviews were jointly analyzed into codes from whole units of analysis by two authors (SG and IF). In moving from codes to categories, other researchers were involved to validate and discuss the results and together create categories. The codes were color-marked concerning which youth-center the respondents belonged to and whether the respondents were staff, female adolescents or male adolescents to be able to see if any categories were shared by all groups or were unique to a specific group.

3. Results

3.1. Who Are the Participants?

The survey includes 207 youth, 57% boys and 43% girls. Most participants come from youth-center V (70%, **Table 1**). The gender distribution is similar, but there are a higher proportion of younger participants in the sample from youth-center V.

However, the young people from the two youth-centers share many features. The majority was born in Sweden, but have foreign-born parents. Most of them live with both their parents and have fathers who work. They feel healthy, enjoy school, and feel quite safe in their neighborhoods. Almost none of them use tobacco and a small proportion has tried alcohol. Their parents know what they do in their leisure-time.

There are also some differences worth noticing between the adolescents at the two youth-centers. At V there is a higher proportion of youth who were born in Sweden, but a lower proportion whose parents were born in Sweden or Europe. At V there are also more young people who live with both parents and fewer who live in a rented apartment. More of the youth at V also have mothers who work and they enjoy school to a greater extent. Almost everyone at T lives within walking or biking distance of the youth-center; at V more than a third live farther away. The young people's frequency of attendance has significantly different distributions at the two youth-centers (**Figure 2**). At V more than one third of the adolescents participate less than once a week, compared to one tenth at T.

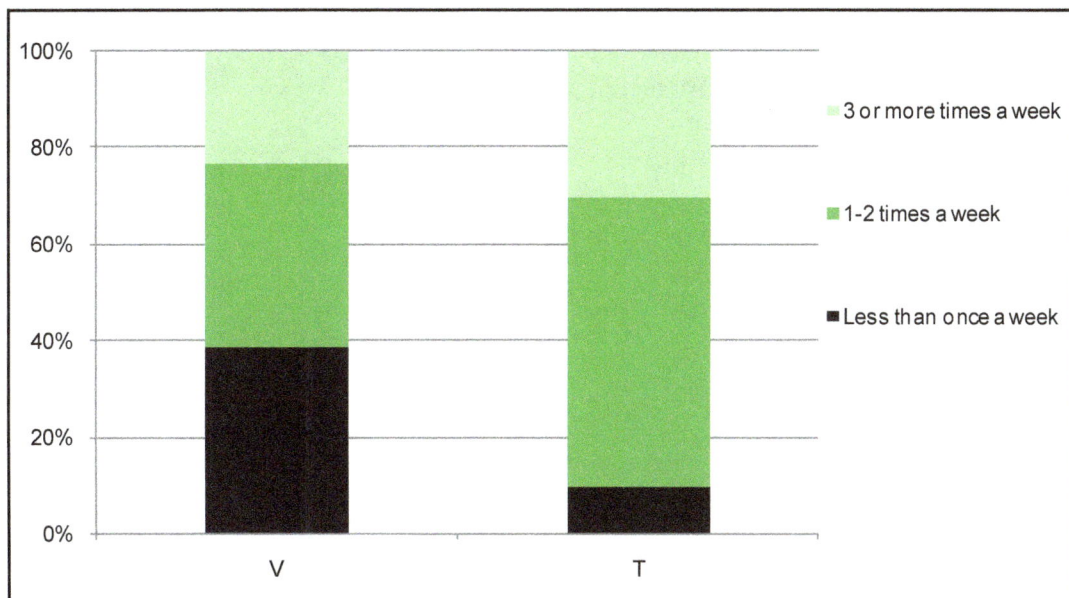

Figure 2. Frequency of attendance at the two youth-centers (in percent) $n = 181$.

3.2. Are There Gender Differences?

Concerning socio-demographic factors, more girls than boys have fathers born in Sweden and live in an owned residence. Regarding health-related factors, the girls agree to a greater extent that they feel safe in their neighborhood during daytime. A higher proportion of the boys exercise more than once a week, and they are also members of a sports club to a greater extent than the girls. Other leisure-time factors that differ are that girls visit friends at home more often in the evenings, and more of them use computers more than four hours a day. The girls state to a greater extent that their parents know what they are doing in their leisure-time (**Table 2**).

The socio-demographic factors that remain significant after controlling for the other socio-demographic factors in a logistic regression (**Table 3**) are that girls are more likely to have a father born in Sweden (OR = 5.1) and to live in an owned residence (OR = 2.5). There were difference between girls and boys with regard to health-rated factors (**Table 4**). Girls were more likely to exercise infrequently (OR = 2.6) and were more likely to feel safe in their neighborhood during daytime (OR = 0.2). The only leisure-time factor that remains significant when controlling for other leisure-time factors is that girls to a lesser extent than boys are members of sports clubs (OR = 14.7, **Table 5**).

Table 2. All independent variables compared between girls and boys (in %) with chi square tests.

Socio-demographic factors		N	Boys	Girls	p-value
Age	Younger (Years 6 - 7)	114	55	56	0.932
	Older (Years 8 - 9 + 1)	92	45	44	
Birth country	Sweden	172	81	85	0.435
	Other country	35	19	15	
Mother's birth country	Sweden	17	5	13	0.053
	Other country	178	95	87	
Father's birth country	Sweden	14	4	12	**0.028**
	Other country	175	96	88	
Lives with both parents all the time	Yes	176	87	84	0.569
	No	29	13	16	
Type of housing	Rented apartment	122	67	51	**0.02**
	Owned residence or both	82	33	49	
Mother's employment	Working	125	62	65	0.69
	Other	73	38	35	
Father's employment	Working	158	84	82	0.69
	Other	32	16	18	
Perceived economic status	Worse/much worse than friends	13	9	3	**0.042**
	About equal to friends	114	49	65	
	Better/much better than friends	77	43	32	
Has a smartphone	Yes	132	67	72	0.466
	No	60	33	28	
Hashis/her own room	Yes	122	39	39	0.974
	No	77	61	61	
Health-related factors					
Feels safe in neighborhood (daytime) in daytime	Strongly agree/Agree	156	83	95	**0.021**
	Disagree/Strongly disagree	21	17	5	
Feels safe in neighborhood in evenings	Strongly agree/Agree	138	77	80	0.602
	Disagree/Strongly disagree	38	23	20	
Self-perceived health	Neither good nor bad, or not good	15	5	11	0.327

Continued

		N	Boys	Girls	p-value
	Feels well	41	20	22	
	Feels very well	140	75	67	
Enjoys school	Very/Pretty much	178	96	89	0.069
	Neither good nor bad or pretty/very bad	13	4	11	
Good in school compared	Among the best/better than most	106	60	54	0.445
to classmates	Equal, worse or among the worst	79	40	46	
Exercise	≤1 time a week	56	22	38	**0.015**
	>1 time a week	139	78	62	
Alcohol consumer	Yes, have drunk at least once	38	18	22	0.457
	No or just tasted	157	82	78	
Tobacco consumer	Yes, party or regular	5	2	4	0.449
	No, tried or stopped	193	98	96	
Leisure-time factors		N	Boys	Girls	p-value
Youth-center	V	144	70	69	0.781
	T	63	30	31	
Frequency of attendance	Less than once a week	57	28	37	0.345
	1 - 2 times a week	79	44	43	
	More than 3 times a week	45	28	21	
Close to youth-center	Yes, walking or biking distance	137	72	67	0.443
	No	60	28	33	
Peers at school mostly friends	Yes	118	58	71	0.062
	No answer	69	42	29	
Peers at center mostly friends	Yes	84	47	42	0.522
	No answer	103	53	58	
Walks/Bikes to school/leisure	Never/few times a year	56	33	26	0.319
	Once a month or more often	130	67	74	
Goes to parties	Never/few times a year	116	58	63	0.463
	Once a month or more often	76	42	37	
Goes to concerts, museum	Never/few times a year	84	44	48	0.603
	Once a month or more often	99	56	52	
At friend's home in evening	Never/few times a year	61	40	24	**0.02**
	Once a month or more often	122	60	76	
Computer use during week	<1 h a day	32	21	11	**0.015**
	1 - 3 h a day	96	54	46	
	>4 h a day	63	25	43	
Sports club	Never been member	22	5	24	**<0.001**
	Have been member	74	40	46	
	Am member	78	55	30	
Reads for pleasure	Never/few times a year	78	46	33	0.07
	At least some times a month	114	54	67	
Same hobby as parent	Yes	95	47	52	0.477
	No	97	53	48	
Parents know about	Never/rarely/varies	16	12	2	**0.011**
leisure-time	Most of the time/always/almost always	187	88	98	

Table 3. Unadjusted odds ratios and all socio-demographic factors entered (CI 95%).

Socio-demographic factors	Unadjusted = 199	Adjusted = 157
Gender		
Age		
Younger	1.0*	
Older	1.0 (0.6 - 1.7)	0.8 (0.4 - 1.7)
Birth country		
Sweden	1.0	
Other country	0.8 (0.4 - 1.6)	0.5 (0.2 - 1.5)
Mother's birth country		
Other country	1.0	Excluded due to strong correlation to
Sweden	2.7 (0.96 - 7.6)	Father's birth country
Father's birth country		
Other country	1.0	
Sweden	**3.6 (1.1 - 11.9)**	**5.1 (1.2 - 21.8)**
Lives with both parents		
Yes	1.0	
No	0.8 (0.4 - 1.7)	0.5 (0.1 - 1.5)
Type of housing		
Rental	1.0	
Other	**2.0 (1.1 - 3.5)**	**2.5 (1.2 - 5.4)**
Mother's employment		
Work	1.0	
Other	0.9 (0.5 - 1.6)	1.0 (0.5 - 2.2)
Father's employment		
Work	1.0	
Other	1.2 (0.5 - 2.5)	2.0 (0.7 - 5.7)
Perceived economic status		
Better	**1.0**	
Equal	**1.8 (1.003 - 3.3)**	1.7 (0.8 - 3.7)
Worse	0.5 (0.1 - 2.1)	0.6 (0.1 - 2.8)
Has a smartphone		
Yes	1.0	
No	0.8 (0.4 - 1.5)	0.6 (0.3 - 1.2)
Has own room		
Yes	1.0	
No	1.0 (0.6 - 1.8)	1.9 (0.9 - 4.2)

*Reference category: Boys.

Table 4. Unadjusted odds ratios and all health-related factors entered (CI 95%).

Health-related factors		
Feel safe daytime	Unadjusted = 199	Adjusted = 154
Feels safe daytime		
Strongly agree/Agree	1.0*	
Disagree/Strongly disagree	**0.3 (0.1 - 0.9)**	**0.2 (0.03 - 0.8)**
Feels safe evening		
Strongly agree/Agree	1.0	
Disagree/Strongly disagree	0.8 (0.4 - 1.7)	1.7 (0.6 - 5.0)
Self-perceived health		
Feels very well	1.0	
Feels well	1.3 (0.6 - 2.5)	0.7 (0.3 - 1.8)
Neither good nor bad/not good	2.2 (0.7 - 6.5)	2.1 (0.5 - 9.4)
Enjoys school		
Very/pretty much	1.0	
Neither good/bad or pretty/very bad	3.0 (0.9 - 9.9)	2.7 (0.7 - 11.0)
Good in school		
Among the best/better than most	1.0	
Equal, worse or among the worst	1.3 (0.7 - 2.3)	1.0 (0.5 - 2.1)
Exercise		
>1 time per week	1.0	
<= 1 time per week	**2.2 (1.15 - 4.1)**	**2.6 (1.2 - 5.6)**
Alcohol consumer		
No	1.0	
Yes	1.3 (0.6 - 2.7)	1.3 (0.5 - 3.1)
Tobacco consumer		
No	1.0	
Yes	2.0 (0.3 - 12.2)	2.6 (0.2 - 32.3)

*Reference category: Boys.

3.3. Are There Differences between Participants' Frequency of Attendance?

Concerning socio-demographic factors, the chi-square test (**Table 6**) shows that a greater proportion of the young people who participate less than once a week live in an owned residence and have a father who works than those who participate more often. The more often the young people attend the youth-center, the better they seem to rate their health. Those who are at the center often have most of their friends there and live nearby to a greater extent.

3.4. Who Participates at the Youth-Centers According to the Interviews?

The content analysis of qualitative data collected at the two youth-centers resulted in three themes (**Figure 3**) which support the results of the survey on some issues and deepen and widen the understanding of some issues.

Table 5. Unadjusted odds ratios and all leisure-time factors entered (CI 95%).

Leisure-time factors	Unadjusted = 199	Unadjusted = 98
Youth-center		
V	1.0*	
T	1.1 (0.6 - 2.0)	1.4 (0.4 - 4.6)
Frequency of attendance		
<1 time a week	1.0	
1 - 2 times a week	0.7 (0.4 - 1.4)	0.6 (0.2 - 2.3)
>3 times a week	0.6 (0.3 - 1.3)	0.3 (0.07 - 1.2)
Lives close to youth-center		
Yes	1.0	
No	1.3 (0.7 - 2.3)	1.1 (0.4 - 3.4)
Peers in school mostly friends		
Yes	1.0	
No answer	0.6 (0.3 - 1.03)	0.9 (0.3 - 2.7)
Peers at youth-center mostly friends		
Yes	1.0	
No answer	1.2 (0.7 - 2.2)	0.9 (0.3 - 2.5)
Walks/Bikes to school/leisure		
Once a month or more often	1.0	
Never/a few times a year	0.7 (0.4 - 1.4)	0.8 (0.3 - 2.5)
Goes to parties		
Never/a few times a year	1.0	
Once a month or more often	0.8 (0.4 - 1.4)	2.2 (0.7 - 6.7)
Goes to concerts, museums		
Never/a few times a year	1.0	
Once a month or more often	0.9 (0.5 - 1.5)	0.4 (0.15 - 1.2)
At friend's home in evening		
Never/a few times a year	1.0	
Once a month or more often	**2.1 (1.1 - 4.0)**	0.9 (0.3 - 3.4)
Computer use during the week		
<1 h a day	**1.0**	
1 - 3 h a day	1.7 (0.7 - 4.0)	0.9 (0.2 - 3.6)
>4 h a day	**3.4 (1.4 - 8.5)**	1.8 (0.4 - 8.2)
Sports club		
Am member	1.0	**1.0**
Have been a member	**2.1 (1.05 - 4.1)**	2.3 (0.8 - 6.4)
Never been member	**9.2(3.0 - 28.2)**	**14.7 (2.1 - 102.5)**
Reads for pleasure		
Never/a few times a year	1.0	
At least a few times a month	1.7 (1.0 - 3.2)	2.1 (0.7 - 5.8)
Same hobby as parent		
Yes	1.0	
No	0.8 (0.5 - 1.4)	0.5 (0.2 - 1.3)
Parents know about leisure-time		
Most of the time/Always/almost always	1.0	Excluded due to insufficient cell size
Never/Rarely	**0.2 (0.04 - 0.8)**	

*Reference category: Boys.

Table 6. All independent variables compared between three levels of frequency of attendance (in%) with chi square tests.

Socio-demographic factors		<1	1 - 2	>3	p-value
Age	Younger (Years 6 - 7)	61	46	66	0.053
	Older (Years 8 - 9 + 1)	39	54	34	
Gender	Boys	53	61	67	0.345
	Girls	47	39	33	
Birth country	Sweden	84	80	82	0.798
	Other country	16	20	18	
Mother's birth country	Sweden	4	9	7	0.534
	Other country	96	91	93	
Father's birth country	Sweden	4	10	2	0.223
	Other country	96	90	98	
Lives with both parents all the time	Yes	93	85	86	0.327
	No	7	15	14	
Type of housing	Rented apartment	34	77	70	**<0.001**
	Owned residence or both	66	23	30	
Mother's employment	Working	72	66	58	0.347
	Other	28	34	42	
Father's employment	Working	96	83	69	**0.003**
	Other	4	17	31	
Perceived economic status	Worse/much worse than friends	2	9	9	0.343
	About equal to friends	58	49	59	
	Better/much better than friends	40	42	32	
Has a smartphone	Yes	75	70	59	0.220
	No	25	30	41	
Hashis/her own room	Yes	64	57	55	0.593
	No	36	43	45	
Health-related factors					
Feels safe in neighborhood (daytime) in daytime	Strongly agree/Agree	88	88	88	0.998
	Disagree/Strongly disagree	12	12	12	
Feels safe in neighborhood in evenings	Strongly agree/Agree	71	82	83	0.307
	Disagree/Strongly disagree	29	18	17	
Self-perceived health	Neither good nor bad, or not good	11	7	2	**0.009**
	Feeling well	34	16	11	
	Feeling very well	55	77	86	
Enjoy school	Very/Pretty good	93	96	95	0.671
	Neither good nor bad or pretty/very bad	7	4	5	

Continued

Good in school compared	Among the best/better than most	54	60	59	0.769
to classmates	Equal, worse or among the worst	46	40	41	
Exercises	≤1 time a week	31	28	34	0.781
	>1 time a week	69	72	66	
Alcohol consumer	Yes, have drank at least once	22	23	7	0.065
	No or just tasted	78	77	93	
Tobacco consumer	Yes, party or regular	2	5	0	0.199
	No, tried or quit	98	95	100	
Leisure-time factors					
Youth-center	V	91	63	69	**0.001**
	T	9	37	31	
Lives close to youth-center	Yes, walking or biking distance	48	72	14	**<0.001**
	No	52	28	86	
Peers in school mostly friends	Yes	74	57	53	0.065
	No answer	26	43	47	
Peers at center mostly friends	Yes	23	53	58	**<0.001**
	No answer	77	47	42	
Walks/Bikes to school/leisure	Never/a few times a year	42	26	28	0.138
	Once a month or more often	58	74	72	
Goes to parties	Never/few times a year	79	45	60	**0.001**
	Once a month or more often	21	55	40	
Goes to concerts, museum	Never/few times a year	60	42	37	**0.044**
	Once a month or more often	40	58	63	
At friend's home in evening	Never/few times a year	45	19	42	**0.005**
	Once a month or more often	55	81	58	
Computer use during week	<1 h a day	24	10	18	0.056
	1 - 3 h a day	40	53	61	
	>4 h a day	36	37	21	
Sports club	Never been member	15	8	13	0.571
	Have been member	36	44	50	
	Am member	49	48	37	
Reads for pleasure	Never/few times a year	44	44	40	0.914
	At least a few times a month	56	56	60	
Same hobby as parent	Yes	43	51	49	0.627
	No	57	49	51	
Parents know about	Never/rarely/varies	2	10	13	0.083
Leisure-time	Most of the time/always/almost always	92	90	87	

Who are the youth-center participants?

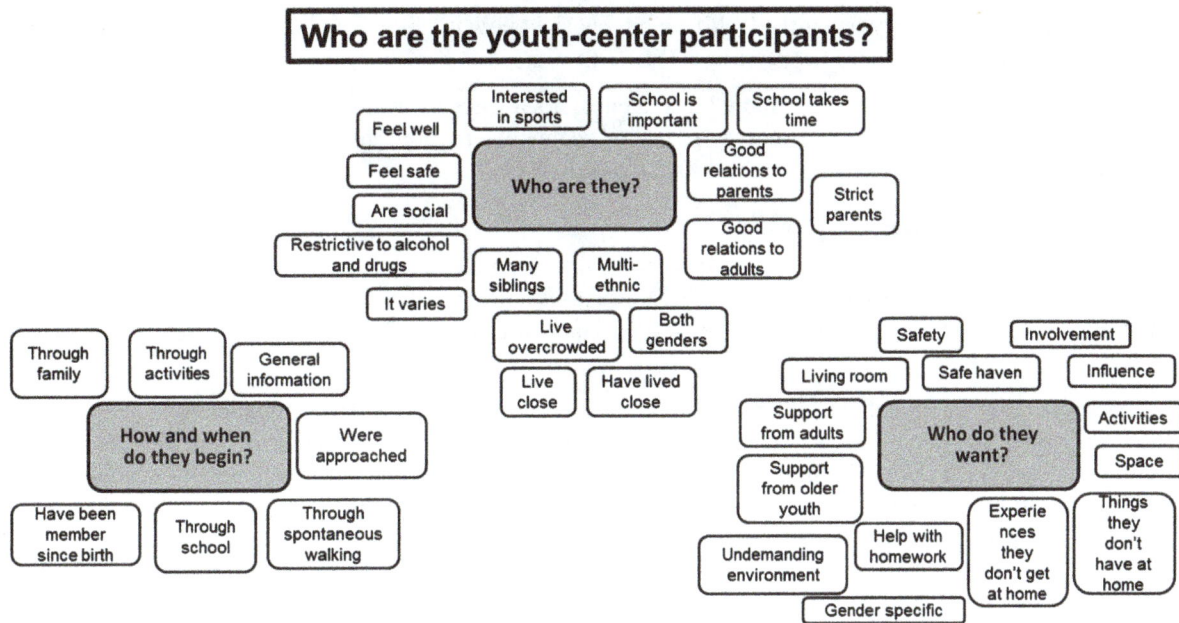

Figure 3. The themes and categories from the qualitative content analysis.

3.4.1. Who Are They?

Many of the youth at both centers come from families with lower SES, and many of them live in crowded apartments with many siblings. They do not attend activities in the city center, where their parents would have to drive them. However most of the young people have good home conditions and enjoy spending time with their families.

> They aren't able to spend time together at home. It's crowded; they have many siblings. (Staff, T)

> They feel comfortable in their homes. They enjoy the company of their parents. Sometimes they think their parents are too strict, but don't almost all young people think that at that age? (Staff, V)

They respect adults and see no problems with adults being present during different activities. Most of the young people are against alcohol, tobacco, and drugs and most abstain completely. Sport is an interest mentioned by many young people at both youth-centers.

> And then you'll skip everything bad, like alcohol, cigarettes, and stuff. Instead of partying on a Friday, you can just come to the center and be with your friends, play FIFA and stuff. (Boy, T)

Especially the boys are members of sport clubs; the girls used to be members, but nowadays they often mention that schoolwork takes a lot of time. Many of the girls find it more difficult to hang out at the center and participate in various activities for reasons related to cultural gender norms.

At both youth-centers many respondents report feeling unsafe in the neighborhood. It is common for the young people accompany each other home from the center in the evenings. The young people feel safe at the centers; the older they are the safer they feel. At V there is no difference between girls' and boys' feeling of safety. But at T boys seem to feel safer than girls.

> Or if some girl from the youth-center is going home, one of us can follow her home. Yes, we usually do. Everyone helps like that. (Boys, V)

At V boys and girls hang out more together. They sit and talk, relax, and watch television or films together, although at T it is more common that girls attend structured activities such as dance, while boys play indoor-football, FIFA (PlayStation), or hang out. At both T and V boys are at the center on weekdays more often than girls. At V they think that all the young people are nice and social, consider everyone friends, and hang out with each other even outside V. At T they think that friends are important and they often come together with friends.

Right now there are very few girls. It shifts a bit, but right now it's like that. And the girls come for directed activities more than perhaps ten years ago. (Staff, T)

They have more boys' activities, more boys' games; it's always FIFA and PlayStation and such, which are not girls' activities; that's a reason why girls don't come; we're more interested in beauty, nails, and such, but it's only on girls' evenings that they do that. (Girls, T)

3.4.2. How and When Do They Begin?

How and when the youth start coming to the centers differs quite a lot. Most of the young people at V have been members and have come to the center's different premises since childhood. They start coming because they had family members and friends there. At T they start to come in grades 6 - 7, and most have been members for 2 - 4 years.

Many have grown up with this; many are members since birth. It's like a second home. (Staff, V)
…the youth who come here now are not…it's different now than 10 - 15 years ago when everyone went to the same school and were in the same classes. Everyone knew everyone, even before they came to us. Now they might know each other, because they live in the same area, but they're not so closely knit and they don't bump into each other every day, because they go to different schools and are in different classes. (Staff, T)

Visiting nearby schools is used as a way of recruiting members to both V and T. At V another active strategy is to take spontaneous walks in the neighborhood.

We usually walk around, spontaneous walks, three or four of us. We may meet some people we know; they have hardly anything to do. We talk to them about V. Tell them it's a place where you can spend time, especially in the winter when it's cold outside. That's one way to spread the message. (Staff, V)

3.4.3. What Do They Want?

The young people want things they don't have at home or experiences they don't get at home.

…if it weren't for V I wouldn't, I'd never go to Dalarna and, like, be there for a week and stay in a cabin. There are such things, experiences; this activity has given me experiences that I otherwise would never get to do (Girls, V)

Not everyone has the resources. For example TV-games, Ping-Pong tables, and so on. You don't have room for that in an apartment. (Staff, T)

Young people at both V and T talk about having a living room. A place where there is space for friends and where the environment is safe and undemanding. They also want adults to help them with homework, or just be there to talk to. At V they also emphasize the support from older youth.

Sometimes you need peace and quiet and so on. But V is like my second home; I can come here with only pants, a cardigan, newly awake—and just be here. (Girls, V)

The young people at V want to have influence and participate in decisions. Those who attend more often seem to take more responsibility. Girls show more engagement in different activities and take more responsibility. At T, some youth want to do this more than others, and the difference between genders is especially distinct. Not everyone is interested in taking responsibility and working for something they want. Some mention that they are in need of activities free from demands and obligations.

4. Discussion

This has been an explorative study. It fills a gap in the knowledge regarding who participates in NGO-run youth-centers in multicultural, socially deprived suburbs in Sweden.

Compared to a representative sample of Swedish youth, the participants in this study perceive their health as at least as good and see themselves as exercising a bit less, enjoying school a bit more, and being about as good at school as their classmates [12]. The youth also state that their parents know about their leisure activities and that they have a nice family environment. It is also an interesting finding of the study that the young people participating in the centers' activities do not use tobacco, and few have tried alcohol. Many of them state in the questionnaire that they feel safe in their neighborhood, especially girls. In the interviews, however, they talk about the unsafe neighborhood they live in, but it is also clear that they know how to handle the situation by accompanying each other home, as an example. Earlier studies by Persson, Kerr, and Stattin [34] and Mahoney and Stattin [23] showed a concentration of problem youth with poor relations with their parents in low-structured activities like Swedish youth-centers. In this study we find quite the opposite. Holder and colleagues [11] conclude that parents choose their children's leisure activities. It is hard to say if this is the case for these youth, but especially youth-center V has the policy always to meet with the parents of participants, unless staffs already have been in natural contact with the parents because they accompanied the participant as a young child. Some parents, especially of girls within certain ethnic groups, demand to meet the center leaders before allowing their children to participate. At youth-center T there is a pronounced trend that girls participate in structured activities and boys in unstructured activities. One explanation is that girls have fewer leisure activities overall, both because they think their schoolwork takes more time and because spending time with their families was important to them, which is in line with the study reported by the Swedish National Board of Health and Welfare [35]. In the past almost everyone was involved in sports, but now the girls in particular are not involved anymore. At T the unstructured activities seems to attract boys more, as Lindström and Öqvist [17] also concluded.

Youth-centers help young people who live nearby to participate in leisure activities. In these multi-cultural, socially deprived suburbs, young people often live together with many siblings and family members, and lack personal space. It is also mentioned that their parents do not give them rides into town to participate in other leisure-time activities—in this case for reasons of SES, e.g. having irregular working hours or not owning a car, rather than being uninvolved parents. The youth-centers offer the young people a sense of being in a place made for their own leisure activities, and often provide a living-room atmosphere. Immigrant youth living in disadvantaged neighborhoods perceive their schools as safe havens more than youths in advantaged neighborhoods [36]. In this study the youth in the same type of neighborhoods enjoy school as well, but also see their youth center as a safe haven.

Knowledge that was added from the interviews was that youth-centers' strategies for recruiting seems to have a large impact on who participates. Youth-center V, whose members often get involved in early childhood by coming with their parents, becomes part of the both boys' and girls' everyday life, and members view each other as friends or even family. At youth-center T, however, which involves youth from 12 years and up, it is more important that you bring your friends (often same sex) instead of considering everyone there to be your friends already. This makes youth-center T more sensitive to trends, causing it to attract different groups (gender or ethnicity) over time as friends become more important in early adolescence than they were in childhood [2]. It seems like the group of youth who visit youth-center V less than once a week are a special group when it comes to, for example, SES. They often live in another part of town and less often in a rented apartment. The young people at V who only come for weekend or holiday activities used to live close to the center or have friends who do so. At youth-center T there are few youth who visit less than once a week, but then the center does not offer weekend or holiday activities. Hertting and Kostenius [24] conclude that the adolescents who participated in organized leisure activities less than once a week were the most vulnerable from a socioeconomic perspective. This is not the case in our study, however this type of activity cannot strictly be regarded as organized leisure activity. The youth in our study are probably more socioeconomically vulnerable than Swedish youth in general.

Methodological Discussion

As in all studies we are struggling with some limitations. Collecting data from youth participating in a voluntary, partly unstructured activity can be tricky. Our approach was to get as many respondents as possible from the two participating youth-centers; therefore we set quite a long period for data collection. The data is self-reported and cross-sectional, which means that no causal relationships can be determined. However we think that the samples are representative of the participants at the youth-centers, because a quite large proportion of the regularly visiting youth took part. Due to some internal loss, only individuals with full information for all variables were included in the logistic regression analysis (not the unadjusted odds ratios), which affected the construction of models. We argue that the study's explorative character justifies including the large number of variables in the analysis. We are aware of the mass significance issue, which could make 5% of our tests significant although they were not.

One could discuss whether the focus-groups gave more or less information than individual interviews [37].

We argue that interaction between participants provided breadth in the answers, and that it was a cost-effective form of data collection. Interpreting interviews requires knowledge of the context in which a study is conducted [33]. The interviewers in this study were also the ones who analyzed the interviews and who analyzed the questionnaires. A strength is that staff and youth had concordant views on who participated at their youth-centers.

5. Conclusion

The participants in the youth-centers are Swedish born youths having foreign-born parents who live with both parents, often in crowded apartments with many siblings. Moreover they feel healthy, enjoy school and have good contact with their parents. It seems that strategies for recruiting youths to youth-centers have a large impact on who participate. One way to succeed in having a more equal gender and ethnicity distribution is to offer youth activities that are a natural step forward from children's activities. The youth-centers' proximity is also of importance for participation, in these types of neighborhoods. Good contact with parents is important for every youth activity, but is even more important to get youth to participate in a neighborhood with many immigrants with diverse views of society's institutions. Maintaining good contact with parents can also indirectly affect parents' networks and well-being.

Acknowledgements

The study could not have been conducted without the engaged and interested staff and young people at the two youth-centers.

Conflict of Interest

The authors declare that no conflict of interest exists.

Funding

The research was funded by a grant from the Swedish Public Health Agency.

References

[1]   United Nations (2003) World Youth Report 2003. The Global Situation of Young People.

[2]   Wiium, N. and Wold, B. (2009) An Ecological System Approach to Adolescent Smoking Behavior. *Journal of Youth and Adolescence*, **38**, 1351-1363. http://dx.doi.org/10.1007/s10964-008-9349-9

[3]   Persson, A. (2006) Leisure in Adolescence: Youths' Activity Choices and Why They Are Linked to Problems for Some and Not Others. Örebro University, Örebro.

[4]   Zick, C.D. (2010) The Shifting Balance of Adolescent Time Use. *Youth & Society*, **41**, 569-596. http://dx.doi.org/10.1177/0044118X09338506

[5]   Lehdonvirta, V. and Räsänen, P. (2010) How Do Young People Identify with Online and Offline Peer Groups? A Comparison between UK, Spain and Japan. *Journal of Youth Studies*, **14**, 91-108. http://dx.doi.org/10.1080/13676261.2010.506530

[6]   Larson, R.W. and Verma, S. (1999) How Children and Adolescents Spend Time across the World: Work, Play, and Developmental Opportunities. *Psychological Bulletin*, **125**, 701-36. http://dx.doi.org/10.1037/0033-2909.125.6.701

[7]   Reardon-Anderson, J., Capps, R. and Fix, M.E. (2002) The Health and Well-Being of Children in Immigrant Families. The Urban Institute, Series B, No. B-52.

[8]   Sletten, M.A. (2010) Social Costs of Poverty; Leisure Time Socializing and the Subjective Experience of Social Isolation among 13-16-year-old Norwegians. *Journal of Youth Studies*, **13**, 291-315. http://dx.doi.org/10.1080/13676260903520894

[9]   Statstics Sweden (2009) Barn i dag—En beskrivning av barns villkor med Barnkonventionen som utgångspunkt.

[10] Eriksson, L. and Bremberg, S. (2009) Fritidsaktiviteter bland unga—Hälsoeffekter. Swedish National Institute of Public Health, Stockholm.

[11] Holder, M.D., Coleman, B. and Sehn, Z.L. (2009) The Contribution of Active and Passive Leisure to Children's Well-Being. *Journal of Health Psychology*, **14**, 378-386. http://dx.doi.org/10.1177/1359105308101676

[12] Swedish National Institute of Public Health (2011) Svenska skolbarns hälsovanor 2009/10. Grundrapport, Stockholm.

[13] Commission on Social Determinants of Health (2008) Closing the Gap in a Generation: Health Equity through Action

on the Social Determinants of Health. Final Report of the Commission on Social Determinants of Health, Geneva.

[14] Swedish National Institute of Public Health (2011) Social Health Inequalities in Swedish Children and Adolescents—A Systematic Review. Second Edition, Stockholm.

[15] Blomfield, C.J. and Barber, B.L. (2011) Developmental Experiences during Extracurricular Activities and Australian Adolescents' Self-Concept: Particularly Important for Youth from Disadvantaged Schools. *Journal of Youth and Adolescence*, **40**, 582-594. http://dx.doi.org/10.1007/s10964-010-9563-0

[16] Feldman, A.F. and Matjasko, J.L. (2007) Profiles and Portfolios of Adolescent School-Based Extracurricular Activity Participation. *Journal of Adolescence*, **30**, 313-332. http://dx.doi.org/10.1016/j.adolescence.2006.03.004

[17] Lindström, L. and Öqvist, A. (2013) Assessing the Meeting Places of Youth for Citizenship and Socialization. *International Journal of Social Science & Education*, **3**, 446-462.

[18] Swedish National Board for Youth Affairs (2005) Unga och föreningsidrotten. En studie om föreningsidrottens plats, betydelser och konsekvenser i ungas liv. Stockholm.

[19] Thorlindsson, T. and Bernburg, J.G. (2006) Peer Groups and Substance Use: Examining the Direct and Interactive Effect of Leisure Activity. *Adolescence*, **41**, 321-339.

[20] Swedish National Institute of Public Health (2013) Barn och unga 2013—utvecklingen av faktorer som påverkar hälsan och genomförda åtgärder. Stockholm.

[21] Eccles, J.S., Barber, B.L., Stone, M. and Hunt, J. (2003) Extracurricular Activities and Adolescent Development. *Journal of Social Issues*, **59**, 865-889. http://dx.doi.org/10.1046/j.0022-4537.2003.00095.x

[22] Simpkins, S.D., Ripke, M., Huston, A.C. and Eccles, J.S. (2005) Predicting Participation and Outcomes in Out-of-School Activities: Similarities and Differences across Social Ecologies. *New Directions for Youth Development*, **2005**, 51-69. http://dx.doi.org/10.1002/yd.107

[23] Mahoney, J.L. and Stattin, H. (2000) Leisure Activities and Adolescent Antisocial Behavior: The Role of Structure and Social Context. *Journal of Adolescence*, **23**, 113-127. http://dx.doi.org/10.1006/jado.2000.0302

[24] Hertting, K. and Kostenius, C. (2012) Organized Leisure Activities and Well-Being: Children Getting It Just Right! *The Cyber Journal of Applied Leisure and Recreation Research*, **15**, 13-28.

[25] Trainor, S.J., Delfabbro, P.H., Anderson, S. and Winefield, A.H. (2010) Leisure Activities and Adolescent Psychological Well-Being. *Journal of Adolescence*, **33**, 173-186.

[26] Persson, A., Kerr, M. and Stattin, H. (2007) Staying in or Moving Away from Structured Activities: Explanations Involving Parents and Peers. *Developmental Psychology*, **43**, 197-207. http://dx.doi.org/10.1037/0012-1649.43.1.197

[27] Weiss, H.B., Little, P.M.D. and Bouffard, S.M. (2005) More than Just Being There: Balancing the Participation Equation. *New Directions for Youth Development*, **2005**, 15-31. http://dx.doi.org/10.1002/yd.105

[28] Eriksson, C., Geidne, S., Larsson, M. and Pettersson, C. (2011) A Research Strategy Case Study of Alcohol and Drug Prevention by Non-Governmental Organizations in Sweden 2003-2009. *Substance Abuse Treatment, Prevention, and Policy*, **6**, 8. http://dx.doi.org/10.1186/1747-597x-6-8

[29] Creswell, J.W. and Plano Clark, V.L. (2007) Designing and Conducting Mixed Methods Research. Sage Publications, Thousands Oaks.

[30] Statstics Sweden (2013) Vart femte barn har utländsk bakgrund 2013.

[31] Brunnberg, E., Lindèn Bostrom, M. and Berglund, M. (2008) Self-Rated Mental Health, School Adjustment, and Substance Use in Hard-of-Hearing Adolescents. *Journal of Deaf Studies and Deaf Education*, **13**, 324-335. http://dx.doi.org/10.1093/deafed/enm062

[32] Brunnberg, E., Lindén-Boström, M. and Berglund, M. (2008) Tinnitus and Hearing Loss in 15-16-Year-Old Students: Mental Health Symptoms, Substance Use, and Exposure in School. *International Journal of Audiology*, **47**, 688-694. http://dx.doi.org/10.1080/14992020802233915

[33] Graneheim, U.H. and Lundman, B. (2004) Qualitative Content Analysis in Nursing Research: Concepts, Procedures and Measures to Achieve Trustworthiness. *Nurse Education Today*, **24**, 105-112. http://dx.doi.org/10.1016/j.nedt.2003.10.001

[34] Persson, A., Kerr, M. and Stattin, H. (2004) Why a Leisure Context Is Linked to Norm-Breaking for Some Girls and Not Others: Personality Characteristics and Parent-Child Relations as Explanations. *Journal of Adolescence*, **27**, 583-598. http://dx.doi.org/10.1016/j.adolescence.2004.06.008

[35] Swedish National Board of Health and Welfare (2007) Frihet och ansvar. En undersökning om gymnasieungdomars upplevda frihet att själva bestämma över sina liv.

[36] Svensson, Y. (2012) Embedded in a Context: The Adaptation of Immigrant Youth. Örebro University, Örebro.

[37] Eriksson, C.-G. (1988) Focus Groups and Other Methods for Increased Effectiveness of Community Intervention—A Review. *Scandinavian Journal of Primary Health Care*, **1**, 73-80.

17

Comparison of the Length of Stay and Medical Expenditures among Japanese Hospitals for Type 2 Diabetes Treatments: The Box-Cox Transformation Model under Heteroscedasticity

Kazumitsu Nawata[1], Koichi Kawabuchi[2]

[1]Graduate School of Engineering, University of Tokyo, Tokyo, Japan
[2]Graduate School of Medical and Dental Sciences, Tokyo Medical and Dental University, Tokyo, Japan
Email: nawata@tmi.t.u-tokyo.ac.jp, kawabuchi.hce@tmd.ac.jp

Abstract

In this paper, we analyzed length of stay (LOS) in hospitals and medical expenditures for type 2 diabetes patients. LOS was analyzed by the power Box-Cox transformation model when variances differed among hospitals. We proposed a new test and consistent estimator. We rejected the homoscedasticity of variances among hospitals, and then analyzed the LOS of 12,666 type 2 diabetes patients hospitalized for regular medical treatments collected from 60 general hospitals in Japan. The variables found to affect LOS were age, number of comorbidities and complications, introduced by another hospital, one-week hospitalization, 2010 revision, specific-hospitalization-period (SHP), and principal diseases E11.5, E11.6 and E11.7. There were surprisingly large differences in ALOS among hospitals even after eliminating the influence of characteristics and conditions of patients. We then analyzed daily medical expenditure (DME) by the ordinary least squares methods. The variables that affected DME were LOS, number of comorbidities and complications, acute hospitalization, hospital's own outpatient, season, introduced by another hospital, one-week hospitalization, 2010 revision, SHP, time trend, and principal diseases E11.2, E11.4 and E117. The DME did not decrease after the SHP. After eliminating the influences of characteristics and conditions of patients, the differences among hospitals were relatively small, 12% of the overall average. LOS is the main determinant of medical expenditures, and new incentives to reduce LOS are needed to control Japanese medical expenditures. Since at least 99% of patients require medical care after leaving the hospital, systems that take proper care of patients for long periods of time after hospitalization are absolutely necessary for efficient treatment of diabetes.

Keywords

Type 2 Diabetes, Medical Expenditure, Length of Hospital Stay, Cox-Box Transformation, Heteroscedasticity

1. Introduction

In October 2015, the Ministry of Health, Labour and Welfare [1] announced that Japanese medical expenditures for fiscal year (FY, the Japanese fiscal year is April-March) 2013 exceeded 40 trillion yen (40.06 trillion yen), an increase of 0.85 trillion yen or 2.2% from previous years. Japan has had a mandatory insurance system since 1961. In FY 2013, public expenditures were 15.53 trillion yen (10.36 trillion from the central and 5.16 trillion from local governments), public insurance premiums were 19.52 trillion yen (8.12 trillion from employers and 11.40 trillion from the insured), and direct expenditures by patients were just 4.71 trillion yen or 11.7% of the total. Public expenditures increased by 0.39 trillion yen over the previous year, reaching 38.8% of total medical expenditure. Meanwhile, at the end of FY 2014, the Japanese long-term financial deficit reached 1009 trillion yen (809 trillion from central and 201 trillion from local governments) or 205% of the Japanese Gross Domestic Product (GDP) [2]. Thus, controlling medical expenditures by efficient use of medical resources is an urgent political issue for sustaining the medical insurance system.

Among various diseases, medical expenditure for cataract was 1.21 trillion yen, one of the most expensive disease [1]. The cost of diabetes, however, has become a worldwide problem. The International Diabetes Federation (IDF) [3] reported that total world health expenditure for this disease was $612 billion in 2014. Moreover, diabetes can cause serious complications such as vision loss, kidney disease (nephropathy), heart failure, and stroke [4] [5]. If the costs of taking care of the comorbidities and complications of diabetes were included, the medical costs of diabetes would likely be much higher. The Public Health Agency of Canada [6] has reported that the "direct health care costs may be as much as 4.5 times higher than when looking at diabetes alone". Lesniowska et al. [7] found that the costs of treating complications in Poland were more than five times those of hospital diabetes treatment. Chereches et al. [8] reported that comorbid depression increased diabetes-related costs in Romania. Yeaw [9] analyzed the costs of complications in the United States in cohorts based on age and diabetes type and found that the cost of renal diseases, lactic acidosis and peritoneal dialysis were highest. Zhuo et al. [10] estimated that the discounted excess lifetime medical costs for people with diabetes in the United States were $124,600, $91,200, $53,800 and $35,900 when diabetes was diagnosed at age 40, 50, 60 and 65, respectively. Condliffe, Parasuraman and Pollack [11] reported that medical expenditures for diabetes patients with comorbid hypertension and obesity were significantly higher than those of patients without these comorbidities. Yesudian et al. [12] summarized the literature about the economic burden of diabetes in India. In addition to the medical costs, diabetes reduces the labor supply and the productivity of patients. Dall et al. [13] reported that the national economic burden of pre-diabetes and diabetes in the United States reached $218 billion in 2007, $153 billion in higher medical costs and $65 billion in reduced productivity. More recently, the American Diabetes Association (ADA) [14] estimated that in 2012, the total cost of diabetes in the United States was $245 billion. Of this total, $69 billion were indirect costs related to reductions in productivity; this was broken down further as inability to participate in the labor force (2.7 billion), inability to work as a result of disease-related disability (21.6 billion), and lost productive capacity due to early mortality (18.5 billion). The Public Health Agency of Canada [6] found that the indirect costs of diabetes amounted to $1.7 billion (Canadian) in 2000. Other reports [15]-[19] suggest that diabetes and diabetes-related complications reduced employment, length of working days, and wage rates. All studies lead to the same conclusion: that the true cost of diabetes is much higher than the direct cost.

In Japan, a new inclusive payment system based on the Diagnosis Procedure Combination (DPC) was introduced in April 2003. The system is called the DPC/PDPS (per diem payment system). As of April 2015, it was estimated that a total of 1580 hospitals had joined the DPC/PDPS, and an additional 266 hospitals were preparing to join (hereafter DPC hospitals) [20]. The DPC hospitals have a total of 520,570 beds. This means that they comprise about 25% of the 7528 general hospitals and 58% of the total number of hospital beds (899,385) in Japan. Since DPC hospitals must computerize their medical information, we now have access to large-scale medical datasets.

The IDF [21] reported that 90% or more of diabetics have type 2 diabetes. (Diabetes can be classified as type 1 or type 2; for details, see ADA [22].) Nawata and Kawabuchi [23] [24] studied the length of stay (LOS) in hospitals for type 2 patients who joined educational programs for lifestyle improvement rather than treatment (hereafter educational hospitalization). They found a large variation among hospitals in average length of stay (ALOS), and that ALOS at some hospitals was unreasonably long even after eliminating the influence of patient characteristics. These researchers also evaluated the daily medical expenditure (DME) per patient [24]. Unlike ALOS, the variation in average daily medical expenditures (ADME) among hospitals were rather small, with the difference between the largest and smallest being just 15% of the overall average. However, in their study, type 2 diabetes patients who were hospitalized for regular medical treatments (hereafter, regular patients) were not analyzed. Since treatments for regular patients may vary depending on the conditions of patients, heterogeneity among regular patients is considered to be much larger than in the educational hospitalization cases. In our dataset, regular patients represented about two thirds of type 2 diabetes patients, and their treatment constituted over 70% of expenditures.

In this paper, we analyzed LOS and DME of regular patients. LOS was analyzed by the Box-Cox [25] transformation model (BC model), taking into account variance among hospitals. The maximum likelihood estimator (BC MLE), which maximizes the likelihood function under the normality assumption, has large biases of the BC MLE when heterogeneity exists in variances [26]. For LOS in particular, variances often differ greatly among hospitals, even after controlling for the characteristics of diseases, treatments and patients. Nawata [27] proposed a robust estimator that is consistent under heteroscedasticity. However, since the variance of the estimator is rather large, we sometimes failed to detect heteroscedasticity. Therefore, we propose a test and new estimator for heteroscedastic cases. Next, we analyzed the LOS of regular patients without any operations by the proposed methods. We used the DPC dataset of 12,666 patients with DPC code 10070xxxxx0x collected from 60 DPC hospitals in Japan. We then evaluated the daily expenditures by the ordinary least squares (OLS) method.

2. Models for the Analysis of LOS

For the analysis of cost-effectiveness in diabetes, cohort-study-type models are often used [28]. However, it is necessary to consider various risk factors for diabetes, including related complications and comorbidities. Watson *et al.* [29] reviewed over 100 studies and concluded that, "None of the identified papers included all of these features" ([29], p. 250). Therefore, we employed regression-type models. The distribution of LOS of regular patients is shown in **Figure 1**. The distribution shows a heavy tail on the right side. In analyzing medical costs with a multiple regression model, Sittig, Friedel and Wasem [30] also found that costs were not normally distributed and were skewed to the right, as in this study. They used the log transformation. In this paper, we used the BC model for the analysis of LOS. The BC transformation includes the log transformation. Since the distribution was not skewed, we used the OLS for the analysis of the DME.

2.1. BC Model and BC MLE

Suppose that the LOS of patient j in hospital i is given by the BC model:

$$z_{ij} = \left(t_{ij}^{\lambda} - 1\right)\big/\lambda \text{ if } \lambda \neq 0, \quad z_{ij} = \log\left(t_{ij}\right) \text{ if } \lambda = 0,$$
$$z_{ij} = x_{ij}'\beta + u_{ij} \quad i = 1, 2, \cdots, k, \ j = 1, 2, \cdots, n_i \tag{1}$$

where t_{ij} is LOS, λ is the transformation parameter, x_{ij} and β are the vectors of the explanatory variables and coefficients, k is the number of hospitals, n_i is the number of patients in hospital i, and $n = \sum_i n_i$. Here u_{ij} is assumed to follow the normal distribution with mean 0 and variance σ_{ij}^2. Let $\theta' = \left(\lambda, \beta', \sigma^2\right)$. The BC likelihood function under the normality assumption of the error terms is given by

$$\log L\left(\theta\right) = \sum_{i,j}\left[\log\phi\left\{\left(z_{ij} - x_{ij}'\beta\right)\big/\sigma\right\} - \log\sigma\right] + \left(\lambda - 1\right)\sum_{i,j}\log t_{ij}, \tag{2}$$

where ϕ is the probability density function of the standard normal assumption, and σ^2 is the variance of u_{ij} under homoscedasticity. The BC MLE maximizes the likelihood function given by Equation (2), and is consistent if the error terms are homoscedastic and the "small σ" assumption [31] is satisfied.

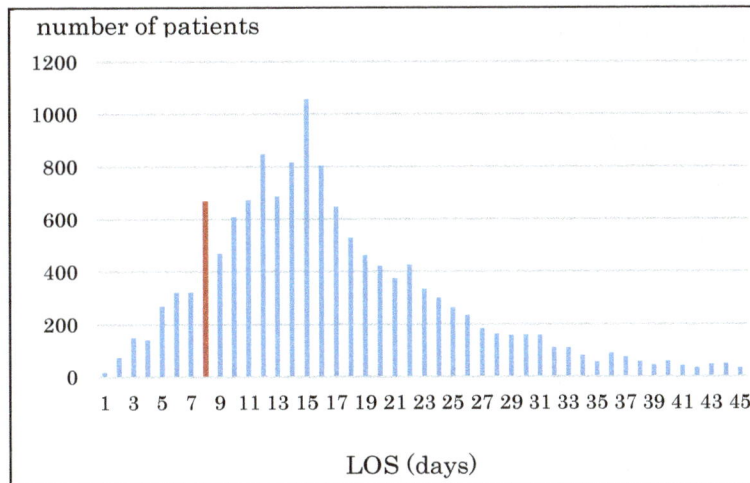

Figure 1. Distribution of LOS of regular patients.

2.2. Nawata's Estimator and the Test for the "Small σ" Assumption

Nawata [32] proposed a semiparametric estimator (hereafter, N-estimator), obtained by

$$G(\theta) = -\frac{1}{\sigma^2 \lambda} \sum_{i,j} \left[\left\{ \frac{\left(\lambda x'_{ij}\beta + 1 \right) \log\left(\lambda x'_{ij}\beta + 1 \right)}{\lambda} - x'_{ij}\beta \right\} \left(z_{ij} - x'_{ij}\beta \right) + \log\left(\lambda x'_{ij}\beta + 1 \right)\left(z_{ij} - x'_{ij}\beta \right)^2 + \frac{\lambda\left(z_{ij} - x'_{ij}\beta \right)^3}{\lambda x'_{ij}\beta + 1} \right]$$

$$+ \sum_{i,j} \left\{ \frac{1}{\lambda} \log\left(\lambda x'_{ij}\beta + 1 \right) + \frac{\left(z_{ij} - x'_{ij}\beta \right)}{\lambda x'_{ij}\beta + 1} \right\} = 0, \tag{3}$$

$$\sum_{i,j} x_{ij}\left(z_{ij} - x'_{ij}\beta \right) = 0, \quad \text{and} \quad \sigma^2 = \sum_{i,j} \frac{\left(z_{ij} - x'_{ij}\beta \right)^2}{n}.$$

These equations are available by the approximation of the $\partial \log L / \partial \theta$. Using the BC MLE and N-estimator, we can conduct the test for the "small σ" assumption (the null hypothesis is that the "small σ" assumption holds) by the Hausman test [33]. For details, see Nawata and Kawabuchi [23] [24].

2.3. A Test for Homoscedasticity

The N-estimator cannot be consistent under heteroscedasticity. Nawata [27] proposed a consistent estimator even under heteroscedasticity based on the third-moment restriction. However, as the result of a Monte Carlo study showed, the variances of the estimators were rather large [27], and we cannot sometimes reject the null hypothesis of homoscedasticity even if the error terms are heteroscedastic. In other words, the power of the Hausman test based on Nawata's [27] estimator may not be high in some cases. Here, we propose a new test. The advantage of the test is that the residuals of the BC model are directly used and we do not need an alternative estimator unlike the Hausman test. The null hypothesis is that the error terms are homoscedastic, and $\sigma_{ij}^2 = \sigma_0^2$ for any i and j. Note that we used the residuals of the BC MLE if the "small σ" assumption were accepted, and the N-estimator otherwise in the previous test. Let $\{e_i\}$ be residuals of the BC model and (λ_0, β'_0) be true parameter values. Then

$$e_{ij} = \hat{z}_{ij} - x'_{ij}\hat{\beta} = u_{ij} + \left(\frac{t_{ij}^{\hat{\lambda}} - 1}{\hat{\lambda}} - \frac{t_{ij}^{\lambda_0} - 1}{\lambda_0} \right) + x'_{ij}\left(\beta_0 - \hat{\beta} \right)$$

$$= u_{ij} + \psi_{ij}\left(\lambda_0 \right)\left(\hat{\lambda} - \lambda_0 \right) + x'_{ij}\left(\beta_0 - \hat{\beta} \right) + o_p\left(1/\sqrt{n} \right) \tag{4}$$

where $\hat{z}_{ij} = \left(t_{ij}^{\hat{\lambda}} - 1 \right) / \hat{\lambda}$ and $\psi_{ij}\left(\lambda \right) = \frac{dz_{ij}}{d\lambda} = \frac{1}{\lambda}\left(-z_{ij} + t_{ij}^{\lambda}\log t_{ij} \right)$. Therefore,

$$e_{ij}^2 = u_{ij}^2 + 2\psi_{ij}\left(\lambda_0\right)\left(\hat{\lambda} - \lambda_0\right)u_{ij} + x_{ij}'\left(\beta_0 - \hat{\beta}\right)u_{ij} + o_p\left(1/\sqrt{n}\right). \tag{5}$$

Under the null hypothesis,

$$\sqrt{n}\sum_{i,j}\left(f_{1ij} - f_{2ij}\right)e_{ij}^2 = \sqrt{n}\sum_{i,j}\left(f_{1ij} - f_{2ij}\right)\left(e_{ij}^2 - \sigma_0^2\right)$$

$$= \sqrt{n}\sum_{i,j}\left(f_{1ij} - f_{2ij}\right)\left(u_{ij}^2 - \sigma_0^2\right) + 2\sqrt{n}\left(\hat{\lambda} - \lambda_0\right)\sum_{ij}\left(f_{1ij} - f_{2ij}\right)\psi_{ij}\left(\lambda_0\right)u_{ij} + \sqrt{n}\left(\beta_0 - \hat{\beta}\right)'\sum_{i,j}x_{ij}'u_{ij} + o_p\left(1\right) \tag{6}$$

$$= \sqrt{n}\sum_{i,j}\left(f_{1ij} - f_{2ij}\right)\left(u_{ij}^2 - \sigma_0^2\right) + 2\sqrt{n}\left(\hat{\lambda} - \lambda_0\right)a + o_p\left(1\right)$$

where $f_{1ij} = \dfrac{\log\left(\lambda x_{ij}'\beta + 1\right)}{\sum_{i,j}\log\left(\lambda x_{ij}'\beta + 1\right)}$ and $f_{2ij} = \dfrac{1}{n}$. From Equation (6), we get

$$\sqrt{n}\sum_{i,j}\left(f_{1ij} - f_{2ij}\right)e_{ij}^2 \Big/ \sqrt{V_1} \to N\left(0,1\right) \tag{7}$$

$$V_1 = \lim_{n\to\infty}\left[n\sum_{i,j}\left(f_{1ij} - f_{2ij}\right)^2\left(Eu_{ij}^4 - \sigma^4\right) + 4a^2nV\left(\hat{\lambda}\right) + 4aE\left\{\sqrt{n}\left(\hat{\lambda} - \lambda_0\right)\sqrt{n}\sum_{i,j}\left(f_{1ij} - f_{2ij}\right)\left(u_{ij}^2 - \sigma_0^2\right)\right\}\right],$$

and

$$a = p\lim_{n\to\infty}\sum_{ij}\left(f_{1ij} - f_{2ij}\right)\psi_{ij}\left(\lambda_0\right)u_{ij},$$

under the null hypothesis, and we can use $t = \sqrt{n}\sum_{i,j}\left(f_{1ij} - f_{2ij}\right)e_{ij}^2\Big/\sqrt{\hat{V_1}}$ as the test statistic where $\hat{V_1}$ is the estimator of V_1. The calculation of V_1 may not be easy, and we get the following formula in the test

$$\left|\sqrt{V_2} - \sqrt{V_3}\right| \le \sqrt{V_1} \le \sqrt{V_2} + \sqrt{V_3}, \quad V_2 = n\sum_{i,j}\left(f_{1ij} - f_{2ij}\right)^2\left(Eu_{ij}^4 - \sigma^4\right), \quad V_3 = 4a^2nV\left(\hat{\lambda}\right). \tag{8}$$

When the BC MLE is used, $V_2 = \left(Eu_{ij}^4 - \sigma^4\right) = 2\sigma^4$ from the moment of the normal distribution.

2.4. A New Consistent Estimator under Heteroscedasticity

If the null hypothesis of homoscedasticity is accepted, we can use the BC MLE or N-estimator. When it is rejected, we modified Equation (3) and replaced $G\left(\theta\right)$ with

$$H\left(\theta\right) = -\frac{1}{\sigma^2\lambda}\sum_{i,j}\left[\left\{\frac{\left(\lambda x_{ij}'\beta + 1\right)\log\left(\lambda x_{ij}'\beta + 1\right)}{\lambda} - x_{ij}'\beta\right\}\left(z_{ij} - x_{ij}'\beta\right) + \frac{\lambda\left(z_{ij} - x_{ij}'\beta\right)^3}{\lambda x_{ij}'\beta + 1}\right] + \sum_{i,j}\frac{\left(z_{ij} - x_{ij}'\beta\right)}{\lambda x_{ij}'\beta + 1} = \sum_{i,j}h_{ij}\left(\theta\right) = 0. \tag{9}$$

$H\left(\theta_0\right)$ does not depend on the second moments of error terms, $E\left\{H\left(\theta_0\right)\right\} = 0$ even under heteroscedasticity where $\theta_0 = \left(\lambda_0, \beta_0, \bar{\sigma}^2\right)$ and $\bar{\sigma}^2 = \lim_{n\to\infty}\frac{1}{n}\sum_{i,j}\sigma_{ij}^2$. Therefore, from the same argument of Nawata [27] [32], there exists a consistent estimator of λ and β among the roots if $G\left(\theta\right)$ is replaced by $H\left(\theta\right)$ in Equation (3). Let $\hat{\theta}_M = \left(\hat{\lambda}_M, \hat{\beta}, \hat{\sigma}_M\right)$ be the consistent root. The asymptotic distribution of this estimator $\hat{\theta}_M$ is given by

$$\sqrt{n}\left(\hat{\theta}_M - \theta_0\right) \to N\left[0, A^{-1}B\left(A'\right)^{-1}\right], \tag{10}$$

where $A = -p\lim_{n\to\infty}\dfrac{1}{n}\dfrac{\partial\xi}{\partial\theta}\bigg|_{\theta_0}$, $\xi\left(\theta\right)' = \left[H\left(\theta\right), \sum_{i,j}\left(z_{ij} - x_{ij}'\beta\right)x_{ij}, \sum_{i,j}\left(z_{ij} - x_{ij}'\beta\right)^2 - n\bar{\sigma}^2\right]$,

$B = \lim_{n\to\infty}\dfrac{1}{n}\sum_{i,j}E\left[\dfrac{\partial\varsigma_{ij}}{\partial\theta}\bigg|_{\theta_0}\dfrac{\partial\varsigma_{ij}}{\partial\theta'}\bigg|_{\theta_0}\right]$, and $\varsigma_{ij}\left(\theta_0\right)' = \left[h_{ij}\left(\theta_0\right), x_{ij}'u_{ij}, \left(u_{ij}^2 - \bar{\sigma}^2\right)\right]$.

3. Evaluations of the LOS and DME

In this section, we analyze the LOS of regular type 2 diabetic patients by the proposed method and the DME per patient by the OLS method.

3.1. Data

The data used in this study were collected by the Department of Health Care Economics at the Tokyo Medical and Dental University from over 100 hospitals; the sample period was from July 2008 to March 2012. The data included patients' LOS, medical expenditures, age, gender, health-related conditions and medical treatments. For details, see Nawata and Kawabuchi [23]. The original dataset included 27,861 patients, and 22,430 patients (80%) were classified under the DPC code 100070xxxxxx0x (type 2 diabetes patient without diabetic ketoacidosis and secondary diseases). The ALOS and average medical expenditure (AME) for these patients were 17.4 days and 461,431 yen, respectively. This means that 77% of medical expenditures for diabetes were for these patients. As in the previous study [24], we only used the data of patients: 1) who were treated in clinical departments that mainly treat diabetes; and 2) whose principle disease was diabetes. Of the 21,603 patients who satisfied these criteria, 14,193 were regular patients. Diabetes can cause complications that require serious operations. It is natural that LOS would become longer and medical expenditures higher for these patients. Therefore, we excluded 932 patients who had received operations (ALOS and AME for patients with operations were 28.5 days and 882,378 yen, respectively). Finally, we used a data set of 12,666 patients in 60 hospitals (Hp1-60) with more than 60 regular patients to evaluate the effects of patients.

Table 1 shows LOS and medical expenditure by hospital. For all 12,666 patients, ALOS was 18.1 days with a standard deviation (SD) of 12.7 days. The AME was 461,680 yen with a SD of 273,253 yen. In the case of educational hospitalization, the ALOS was 13.7 days with a SD of 6.7 days, and the AME was 370,336 yen with a SD of 152,895 yen for 6,178 patients. Therefore, the ALOS was 4.4 days longer and AME was 91,344 yen higher for regular patients than for those with an educational hospitalization [24]. Moreover, the coefficients of variation (=SD/average) became 70% for LOS and 59% for medical expenditures. The coefficients of variation were 49% and 41% for the educational hospitalizations. This means that heterogeneity of regular patients was larger than that of educational hospitalization, as expected.

The maximum ALOS by hospital was 37.6 days (hp50) and the minimum was 10.0 days (hp42). The maximum was thus 3.8 times larger than the minimum, with a difference of 27.6 days. The maximum SD by hospital was 28.4 days (hp21), and the minimum was 4.7 days (hp52). This maximum was six times larger than the minimum and the variances were quite different among hospitals. This implies the importance of the proposed model, which takes into account the heteroscedasticity of the variances.

Figure 2 shows the relationship between the ALOS and AME by hospital. The correlation coefficient was 0.984, and there was an almost linear relation between these two variables. This implies that despite large heterogeneity among patients, ALOS was the largest determinant of AME.

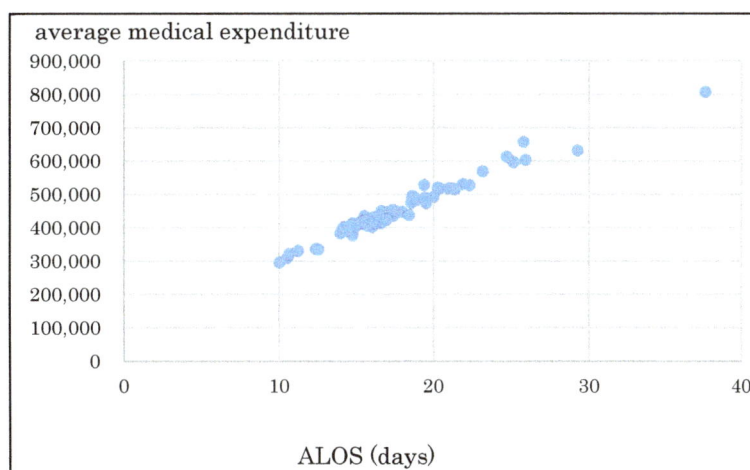

Figure 2. ALOS and average medical expenditures by hospital.

Table 1. Length of stay and medical expenditure by hospital.

HP	N	LOS (days)		ME (yen)		HP	N	LOS (days)		ME (yen)	
		ALOS	SD	AME	SD			ALOS	SD	AME	SD
HP1	582	14.79	5.85	413,632	144,371	HP32	192	16.85	9.83	442,586	219,745
HP2	137	18.55	13.83	474,460	301,932	HP33	149	15.17	8.55	412,000	185,321
HP3	85	17.94	15.11	449,164	317,935	HP34	149	10.67	4.96	322,364	143,331
HP4	63	15.54	8.99	435,237	206,362	HP35	62	17.40	8.98	436,615	181,931
HP5	89	25.72	20.51	658,025	439,181	HP36	212	14.38	8.90	391,749	193,203
HP6	254	14.70	6.31	406,213	141,270	HP37	259	15.81	6.46	413,243	146,484
HP7	99	25.10	25.15	597,842	555,042	HP38	304	17.35	9.21	453,310	207,938
HP8	252	16.63	9.43	450,692	334,735	HP39	294	23.15	14.77	569,587	358,668
HP9	148	21.22	9.92	517,550	209,554	HP40	341	12.52	7.75	335,680	175,104
HP10	70	18.40	11.62	438,506	224,096	HP41	357	22.31	10.70	527,369	232,023
HP11	102	15.35	12.71	421,123	292,665	HP42	653	15.71	5.84	424,447	137,315
HP12	302	16.11	6.93	431,296	162,428	HP43	89	14.98	6.42	404,746	154,791
HP13	149	16.03	7.36	402,396	133,737	HP44	186	16.04	7.35	416,456	161,017
HP14	429	24.67	11.59	612,452	245,115	HP45	330	19.99	10.29	493,362	217,380
HP15	193	14.77	6.69	377,203	140,015	HP46	136	19.41	13.63	489,587	299,087
HP16	98	18.64	12.41	489,848	271,582	HP47	229	15.66	10.30	407,329	232,307
HP17	542	10.54	7.43	309,743	164,012	HP48	177	16.47	10.60	435,584	234,179
HP18	124	14.20	6.04	402,431	148,693	HP49	603	16.97	8.78	423,653	181,434
HP19	70	16.59	12.18	414,280	233,975	HP50	557	37.57	24.83	807,833	484,304
HP20	79	12.37	7.40	337,624	158,109	HP51	179	21.88	19.35	531,286	422,577
HP21	80	29.24	28.35	632,467	622,123	HP52	240	10.03	4.74	297,370	115,368
HP22	138	13.94	4.95	383,960	123,768	HP53	268	20.38	10.94	518,470	243,989
HP23	64	18.63	8.37	496,006	187,280	HP54	196	14.55	6.23	406,779	152,333
HP24	181	16.96	13.57	447,201	299,459	HP55	102	21.37	10.05	515,697	211,656
HP25	177	18.94	11.72	485,520	261,974	HP56	229	15.34	10.05	416,528	228,015
HP26	244	15.55	7.33	410,726	168,783	HP57	177	20.24	9.40	520,557	280,607
HP27	269	16.53	12.87	421,123	284,123	HP58	70	11.21	6.08	331,358	152,516
HP28	93	14.11	8.31	398,494	200,704	HP59	208	25.86	13.25	604,269	313,967
HP29	75	19.37	20.51	528,224	555,561	HP60	99	19.49	14.71	473,631	314,834
HP30	254	17.51	10.07	451,452	223,114	All	12666	18.05	12.66	461,680	273,253
HP31	177	20.98	10.80	518,968	230,641						

N: Number of patients, ME: Medical expenditure per patient, AME: Average ME, SD: Standard deviation.

3.2. Evaluation of LOS

We chose the following as explanatory variables. The Female dummy (1: female, 0: male) was used for gender. The proportion of female patients was 42.3%. Since LOS tends to increase with patient age, we used Age as an explanatory variable. The average age of the patients was 63.8, and the standard deviation was 13.9 years. Japan has a mandatory health insurance system, and the percentage of medical fees paid by patients changed at age 70 in the sample period (30% for younger than 70; 10% for 70 or over). So, an Age 70 (1: 70 or over, 0: otherwise) dummy was also added. Other explanatory variables representing the conditions of patients included: Comorbidities (number of comorbidities), Complications (number of complications), Acute Hospitalization dummy (acute hospitalization: 1, otherwise: 0), Outpatient dummy (outpatient of the same hospital before hospitalization: 1, otherwise: 0), Introduction dummy (introduced by another hospital: 1, otherwise: 0), and Home dummy (1: returned to home: 1, otherwise: 0). Among our study subjects, 14.6%, 15.7%, 15.1% and 39.4% of patients had 1, 2, 3 and 4 comorbidities, respectively, while 16.1%, 10.6%, 7.0% and 10.2% of patients had 1, 2, 3 and 4 complications, respectively. The proportions of acute hospitalization patients, outpatients of the same hospital before hospitalization, patients introduced by another hospital, and patients who returned home were 18.9%, 80.1%, 38.2%, and 77.7%, respectively. To evaluate seasonal effects we added Winter (December to February) and Summer (July and August) dummies. Since the DPC/PDPS was revised in April 2010, an after 2010 dummy (after April, 2010: 1, otherwise: 0) was used. As shown in **Figure 1**, many patients were discharged from hospitals on the eighth day (after one week of hospitalization); hence, we added the One Week dummy (discharged on the eight day: 1, otherwise: 0). If the LOS exceeds the Specific-Hospitalization-Period (SHP, 29 days in this case) determined by the DPC/PDPS, the medical payment becomes a conventional fee-for-service system. Therefore, we added the Over SHP dummy (LOS is over the SHP: 1, otherwise: 0). For these variables, 55.0% of patients were after April 2010, 5.0% were discharged on the eighth day, and 11.0% stayed over the SHP.

To evaluate the time trend that may represent the progress of medical technologies, Time (number of months from July 2008) was used. For more specific classification of the principal disease, the International Disease Classification version 10 (ICD-10) was used. The ICD-10 classifies type 2 diabetes by complications. We used the E11.2-E11.7 dummies based on E11.9 (without complications). Among patients, 5.9% were classified under E11.2 (with kidney complications), 7.8% were classified under E11.3 (with ophthalmic complications), 5.2% were classified under E11.4 (with neurological complications), 0.8% were classified under E11.5 (with circulatory complications), 13.1% were classified under E11.6 (with other specified complications), and 32.1% were classified under E11.7 (with multiple complications). To evaluate the effects of hospitals, we added 60 hospital dummies and did not use the constant term.

As a result, Equation (1) becomes:

$$\begin{aligned} x'_{ij}\beta = {} & \beta_1 \text{Female} + \beta_2 \text{Age} + \beta_3 \text{Age } 70 + \beta_6 \text{Comorbidities} + \beta_5 \text{Complications} \\ & + \beta_6 \text{Acute Hospitalization} + \beta_7 \text{Outpatient} + \beta_8 \text{Introduction} + \beta_9 \text{Home} \\ & + \beta_{10} \text{One Week} + \beta_{13} \text{Over SHP} + \sum_\ell \beta_\ell \text{ICD-10 dummy} + \sum_i \beta_i i\text{-th Hospital dummy} \end{aligned} \qquad (11)$$

We first tested the "small σ" assumption. The estimates of λ were 0.3537 for the BC MLE and 0.3785 for the N-estimator. The value of the test statistic was $t = (0.3537 - 0.3785)/0.0338 = 1.775$ and the null hypothesis was accepted at the 5% level. Therefore, we used the residuals of the BC MLE in the test for heteroscedasticity. We got $\sqrt{n}\sum_{i,j}(f_{1ij} - f_{2ij})e_{ij}^2 = 0.0398$ and $\sqrt{V_1} \le \sqrt{V_2} + \sqrt{V_3} = 0.0121$, and the value of the test statistic was $t \ge 3.281$. The null hypothesis was rejected at the 1% level; thus, we could not use the BC MLE and had to use the newly proposed estimator.

The estimation results are presented in **Table 2**. The estimate of λ was 0.4824, which was sufficiently larger than that of the BC MLE. This coincides with the results of the Monte Carlo study [27], where the BC MLE underestimated λ under heteroscedasticity. The results of other variables were similar to those for educational hospitalization [23]. The estimates of Age, Comorbidities, Complications and Introduction dummy were positive and significant at the 1% level. This means that LOS was prolonged by age and complications. The LOS also became longer if patients came from another hospital. The estimate of After 2010 dummy was negative and significant at the 5% level, and it was admitted that the 2010 revision reduced LOS. The estimates of the Female,

Table 2. Results of estimation (LOS).

Variable	Estimate	SE	t-value	Variable	Estimate	SE	t-value
λ	0.4824	0.0010	485.31**	HP20	3.9390	0.2078	18.958**
Female	0.0286	0.0273	1.0477	HP21	5.5099	0.2978	18.502**
Age	0.0053	0.0015	3.6228**	HP22	4.2774	0.1450	29.509**
Age70	−0.0403	0.0411	−0.9807	HP23	4.8487	0.2142	22.635**
Comorbidities	0.1170	0.0107	10.885**	HP24	4.0421	0.1669	24.219**
Complications	0.1675	0.0109	15.372**	HP25	4.9755	0.1567	31.754**
Acute Hospitalization	0.0574	0.0421	1.3622	HP26	4.4978	0.1282	35.088**
Outpatient	0.0530	0.0432	1.2252	HP27	4.4246	0.1478	29.943**
Introduction	0.1490	0.0325	4.5833**	HP28	4.2511	0.1890	22.489**
Home	−0.0514	0.0373	−1.3785	HP29	4.5950	0.2458	18.692**
Winter	−0.0441	0.0339	−1.3034	HP30	3.9840	0.1428	27.904**
Summer	−0.0084	0.0333	−0.2512	HP31	5.2178	0.1451	35.956**
One Week	−1.3904	0.032809	−42.378**	HP32	4.3233	0.1518	28.489**
Over SHP	4.6233	0.0533	86.739**	HP33	4.5857	0.1435	31.946**
After 2010	−0.1137	0.0557	−2.0419*	HP34	3.5024	0.1309	26.765**
Time	0.0006	0.0023	0.2468	HP35	4.6768	0.1993	23.464**
ICD10 Dummies				HP36	4.2679	0.1424	29.973**
E112	0.0628	0.0594	1.0564	HP37	4.4344	0.1366	32.459**
E113	0.0634	0.0523	1.2118	HP38	4.6163	0.1378	33.505**
E114	0.0181	0.0748	0.2422	HP39	5.3361	0.1381	38.653**
E115	0.5088	0.1588	3.2028**	HP40	4.0143	0.1324	30.321**
E116	0.1200	0.0491	2.4432*	HP41	5.1711	0.1381	37.432**
E117	0.1296	0.0351	3.6976**	HP42	4.6685	0.1094	42.656**
Hospital Dummies				HP43	4.5198	0.2189	20.648**
HP1	4.4863	0.1169	38.367**	HP44	4.8467	0.1772	27.349**
HP2	4.4642	0.1731	25.783**	HP45	4.7989	0.1255	38.226**
HP3	4.5492	0.2039	22.316**	HP46	4.3817	0.1880	23.302**
HP4	4.6349	0.1832	25.306**	HP47	4.4592	0.1442	30.922**
HP5	4.8959	0.2677	18.288**	HP48	3.9485	0.1801	21.922**
HP6	4.5489	0.1352	33.644**	HP49	4.8959	0.1100	44.524**
HP7	4.9872	0.2066	24.134**	HP50	6.1109	0.1404	43.520**
HP8	4.5842	0.1304	35.143**	HP51	4.8743	0.1902	25.624**
HP9	5.0341	0.1516	33.214**	HP52	3.2377	0.1352	23.943**
HP10	4.5405	0.2328	19.501**	HP53	4.9419	0.1401	35.265**
HP11	4.0397	0.1738	23.238**	HP54	4.1868	0.1340	31.248**
HP12	4.8730	0.1175	41.478**	HP55	5.0853	0.1720	29.569**
HP13	4.5355	0.1493	30.379**	HP56	4.0793	0.1585	25.739**
HP14	5.2492	0.1279	41.043**	HP57	5.0209	0.1491	33.685**
HP15	4.6980	0.1367	34.365**	HP58	3.7117	0.1815	20.450**
HP16	4.6742	0.1888	24.755**	HP59	5.2332	0.1491	35.091**
HP17	3.6085	0.1212	29.764**	HP60	4.8338	0.1995	24.227**
HP18	4.0759	0.1557	26.174**	R2		0.5958	
HP19	4.4652	0.2330	19.161**				

SE: Standard Error, *Significant at the 5% level, **Significant at the 1% level.

age 70, Acute Hospitalization, Outpatient, Home, Winter and Summer dummies were not significant at the 5% level, and we could not find evidence that the LOS depended on these variables. The estimates of One Week and Over SHP dummies were positive and significant at the 1% level, showing that one-week hospitalization and exceeding the SHP affected LOS. With respect to the ICD-10 dummies, the estimates of E11.5 and E11.7 were positive and significant at the 1%, as was E11.6 at the 5% level; none of the other estimates was significant at the 5% level. For the hospital dummies, the maximum estimate was 6.111 (HP50), the minimum was 3.238 (HP52), and the difference was 2.873.

3.3. Evaluation of DME

Next, we evaluated daily medical expenditures (DME_{ij}) per patient. Since the distribution was not skewed, we used the OLS for the analysis of DME. Since heteroscedasticity of error terms might exist, the standard errors were obtained by the robust variance calculation method [34]. We considered the model given by

$$DME_{ij} = \beta_1 \text{Female} + \beta_2 \text{Age} + \beta_3 \text{Age } 70 + \beta_6 \text{Comorbidities} + \beta_5 \text{Complications}$$
$$+ \beta_6 \text{Acute Hospitalization} + \beta_7 \text{Outpatient} + \beta_8 \text{Introduction} + \beta_9 \text{Home} + \beta_{10} \text{LOS} \qquad (12)$$
$$+ \beta_{11} \text{Over SHP} + \beta_{12} \text{Over SHP*}\left(\text{LOS -SHP}\right) + \sum_\ell \beta_\ell \text{ICD-10 dummy} + \sum_i \beta_i \, i\text{-th Hospital dummy}$$

The medical expenditures of 129 patients were not available, and the DME of 42 were too low (below 10,000 yen). Excluding these patients, we used the dataset of 12,495 patients. The results of the estimation are presented in **Table 3**. The average daily medical expenditure (ADME) for regular patients was 27,375 yen, a little bit smaller than the ADME for educational hospitalization (27,983 yen) [24]. The estimates of Comorbidities and Complication were positive and significant at the 1% level. Thus, we found that comorbidities and complications not only made LOS longer but also DME higher. The estimates of Acute Hospitalization and Outpatients were significant at the 1% level but the signs were opposite. Acute hospitalization made DME higher but it were smaller if a patient was a hospital's own outpatient. The estimates of Winter and Summer were positive and significant at the 1% and 5% levels, respectively. In this case, we observed a seasonal effect. The estimate of After 2010 was positive and significant at the 1% level.

For the educational hospitalization case, the 2010 revision reduced DME, but we got the opposite result for regular patients. The estimate of LOS was negative and significant at the 1% level. Since daily payments to hospitals decrease as LOS becomes longer under the DPC/PDPS, this result is quite reasonable. On the other hand, estimates of Over SHP and Over SHP * (LOS - SHP) were positive and significant at the 1% level. After the SHP, payment is based on a conventional fee-for-service system, and we got the same result as for the educational hospitalization cases. The coefficient time was negative and significant at the 1% level, and there was a time trend that reduced DME. Among the ICD-10 dummies, E11.2, E11.4 and E11.7 were positive at the 1% or 5% levels, and the DME increased for these diseases. Among estimates of hospital dummies, the largest was 36,920 yen (HP28) and the smallest was 33,553 yen (HP49). The difference was 3368 yen or 12.3% of the ADME of all patients.

4. Discussion

The analyses in the previous section suggest that the large differences of medical expenditures among hospitals were mainly caused by the ALOS. Moreover, large differences existed among hospitals, and the influence of the hospital was much larger than that of other variables. For example, let us consider two male patients staying at the same hospitals. One patient is age 80, has 4 comorbidities and 4 complications, was introduced by another hospital, and has the ICD-10 code E11.7. The other patient is age 50, has no comorbidities or complications, was not introduced by another hospital, and has the ICD-10 code E11.9. (All other variables are set to the same values.) The former and later are the worst- and best-case scenario patients that we can consider. The difference of between these two patients is 1.534. The difference between the largest and smallest estimates of hospital dummies was 2.873, a much bigger number. Moreover, compared to the estimate of HP52 where the ALOS was the shortest, the estimates at 21 hospitals, more than one third of the total 60 hospitals, exceeded this criterion. This suggests that ALOS for some hospitals were unreasonably long, and it will be necessary for them to explain why and to revise their medical practices. It is difficult for the working generation to stay in a hospital for a long

Table 3. Results of estimation (daily medical expenditure).

Variable	Estimate	SE	t-value	Variable	Estimate	SE	t-value
Female	−63.3	64.4	−0.9822	HP20	34,964	465	75.223**
Age	4.7	3.5	1.3594	HP21	35,633	487	73.145**
Age70	−79.9	98.1	−0.8144	HP22	35,113	392	89.636**
Comorbidities	219.2	24.6	8.9076**	HP23	34,969	505	69.241**
Complications	196.7	26.3	7.4735**	HP24	34,820	364	95.705**
Acute Hospitalization	2464.7	88.3	27.897**	HP25	34,553	366	94.485**
Own Outpatient	−342.7	95.3	−3.5951**	HP26	33,963	341	99.735**
Another Hospital	−102.3	73.0	−1.4010	HP27	34,597	330	104.747**
Home	−3.5	83.5	−0.0419	HP28	36,920	443	83.270**
Winter	242.1	79.1	3.0612**	HP29	35,302	475	74.358**
Summer	168.3	79.9	2.1052*	HP30	33,617	336	100.148**
After 2010	823.5	131.9	6.2443**	HP31	34,284	364	94.135**
Over SHP	1308.3	150.4	8.7014**	HP32	34,841	356	97.771**
LOS	−443.2	6.0	−73.332**	HP33	35,537	382	93.087**
Over SHP * (LOS-SHP)	428.6	7.9	54.313**	HP34	35,817	378	94.847**
Time	−97.4	5.4	−18.117**	HP35	34,376	517	66.493**
ICD10 Dummies				HP36	34,825	352	98.883**
E112	474.0	133.2	3.5589**	HP37	34,371	366	93.966**
E113	−71.9	128.6	−0.5588	HP38	35,118	323	108.691**
E114	330.4	151.8	2.1767*	HP39	34,921	330	105.969**
E115	169.6	360.3	0.4706	HP40	33,847	315	107.344**
E116	32.8	114.2	0.2874	HP41	34,434	321	107.292**
E117	274.7	83.8	3.2764**	HP42	35,276	288	122.294**
Hospital Dummies				HP43	34,455	435	79.254**
HP1	35,750	294	121.678**	HP44	34,727	362	95.923**
HP2	34,623	396	87.377**	HP45	34,694	328	105.928**
HP3	35,780	459	77.946**	HP46	34,070	395	86.203**
HP4	35,643	515	69.228**	HP47	34,603	348	99.309**
HP5	36,026	448	80.364**	HP48	34,094	364	93.619**
HP6	35,961	341	105.558**	HP49	33,553	281	119.418**
HP7	34,220	438	78.150**	HP50	35,021	313	111.866**
HP8	34,820	340	102.329**	HP51	34,695	372	93.172**
HP9	33,968	392	86.757**	HP52	35,681	334	106.946**
HP10	35,554	495	71.846**	HP53	35,127	336	104.581**
HP11	34,862	425	81.970**	HP54	34,669	355	97.524**
HP12	34,361	308	111.477**	HP55	33,833	428	78.982**
HP13	34,518	383	90.128**	HP56	35,708	343	104.226**
HP14	35,810	310	115.561**	HP57	34,514	374	92.168**
HP15	34,792	364	95.640**	HP58	36,856	482	76.479**
HP16	36,048	435	82.873**	HP59	35,020	359	97.503**
HP17	36,121	290	124.763**	HP60	33,703	443	76.027**
HP18	35,510	404	87.805**	R2		0.4847	
HP19	34,072	489	69.699**				

S E: Standard Error, *Significant at the 5% level, **Significant at the 1% level.

period of time (two weeks or more). Therefore, long LOS might prevent working-age patients in the early stages of diabetes from getting proper treatments. The Japanese standard retirement age is 65, and the average age of patients was 64, with more than half of patients aged 65 or younger.

On the other hand, the differences of ADME among hospitals were relatively small. After eliminating the influence of patient characteristic and conditions, the differences between the maximum and minimum were only 12% of the overall average.

The estimate of Over SHP dummy was 4.623, very large compared to other non-hospital dummy variables. Once LOS exceeded the SHP, patients stayed in hospitals for long periods of time. Eleven percent of patients, not a small number, stayed over the SHP, and ALOS for these patients was 44.6 days. Payment is based on a conventional fee-for-service system after the SHP, and our analyses revealed that the DME did not decrease after the SHP. In other words, there is no incentive for hospitals to discharge patients earlier under the current DPC/PDPS. Therefore, new incentives for high and efficient quality medical services [35] [36] may be necessary to improve the DPC/PDPS in future revisions.

In our dataset, only 131 regular patients out of 14,193 were reported as complete recoveries; that is, at least 99% of patients required medical care after leaving the hospital. Moreover, a large number of patients do not follow prescribed therapies [37]. Dilla *et al.* [38] reported that it was possible to control medical expenses by reducing body mass index (BMI). Although compared to non-diagnosed individuals at risk for high blood sugar, diagnosed diabetics are more likely to improve their lifestyle, the effect diminishes and some behavioral responses to diabetes may be short-lived [39]. Therefore, systems that take proper care of patients for long periods of time after hospitalization are absolutely necessary for diabetes. However, such systems are not yet sufficiently established [22], and we need to institute them as soon as possible. For the development of new systems, adoption of health-information technologies [40] and proper budget allocation [41] are considered critically important. The differences of social and cultural factors should also be considered. Condliffe and Link [42] found that medical expenditures were different among races. Phelps, Hodgson and Lamson [43] suggested that it is necessary to consider ethnic group differences. Salois [44] pointed out that a "local" food economy might be an important factor in the prevention of obesity and diabetes. Finally, Pan and Ward [45] suggested the necessity of developing models to explain the relationship between self-related health and diabetes self-management in a non-Western context. In establishing desirable systems, these factors should also be considered.

5. Conclusions

In this paper, we consider an analysis of the LOS and daily medical expenditure (DME) for regular patients with type 2 diabetes. LOS was analyzed by the power Box-Cox transformation model when variances differed among hospitals. We proposed a new test and consistent estimator. We rejected the homoscedasticity of variances among hospitals, and the feasibility of the proposed model was strongly supported. We then analyzed the LOS of 12,666 type 2 diabetes regular patients collected from 60 DPC hospitals in Japan. The variables found to affect LOS were age, number of comorbidities and complications, introduced by another hospital, one-week hospitalization, 2010 revision, Specific-Hospitalization-Period (SHP), and principal diseases E11.5, E11.6 and E11.7. There were surprisingly large differences in ALOS among hospitals even after eliminating the influences of characteristics and conditions of patients.

We then analyzed the DME by the OLS method. The variables that affected DME were LOS, number of comorbidities and complications, acute hospitalization, hospital's own outpatient, season, introduced by another hospital, one-week hospitalization, 2010 revision, SHP, LOS, time trend, and principal diseases E11.2, E11.4 and E117. The DME did not decrease after the SHP. After eliminating the influence of characteristics and conditions of patients, the differences among hospitals were relatively small, 12% of the overall average. Since at least 99% of patients require medical care after leaving the hospital, systems designed to properly care for patients over long periods of time after hospitalization are absolutely necessary for diabetes.

Diabetes is a chronic disease and a long-term evaluation for medical expenditures and outcomes of treatments is necessary. Eggleston *et al.* [46] analyzed the data of 821 patients joining a self-funded health plan between 1999 and 2009 and concluded that the unit cost of treatment for diabetes, adjusting for the value of health outcomes, has been roughly constant over time. Thurecht and Brown [47] developed a diabetes simulation model that could provide a wide range of outputs to assess the current and projected impact of those with the disease in Australia. Such analyses are also necessary in Japan. Although type 1 diabetes was not analyzed in this study, it is also an important factor for controlling the costs of diabetes [48]. These are subjects to be analyzed in future studies.

Acknowledgements

The Institutional Review Boards of the University of Tokyo (number: KE12-7) and Tokyo Medical and Dental University (number: 839) approved the use of this dataset. We would like to thank an anonymous referee and Prof. Yoko Ibuka at the Tohoku University for their helpful comments and suggestions.

References

[1]   Ministry of Health, Labour and Welfare (2015) Hesiei 25 nendo kokumin iryouhi (National Medical Expenditures, Fiscal Year 2013, in Japanese).

[2]   Ministry of Finance (2015) Kuni oyobi chihou no chouki saimu sandaka (Long-Term Deficits of the Central and Local Governments, in Japanese).

[3]   International Diabetes Foundation (2014) DIABETES ATLAS. 6th Edition. http://www.idf.org/sites/default/files/Atlas-poster-2014_EN.pdf

[4]   American Diabetes Association ADA (2015) Complications. http://www.diabetes.org/

[5]   Alva, M., Gray, A., Mihayalov, B. and Clarke, P. (2014) The Effect of Diabetes Complications on Health-Related Quality of Life: The Longitudinal Data to Address Patient Heterogeneity. *Health Economics*, **23**, 487-500. http://dx.doi.org/10.1002/hec.2930

[6]   Public Health Agency of Canada (2015) The Health and Economic Impacts of Diabetes. Chapter 3, Diabetes in Canada: Facts from a Public Health Perspective. http://www.phac-aspc.gc.ca/cd-mc/publications/diabetes-diabete/facts-figures-faits-chiffres-2011/chap3-eng.php

[7]   Lesniowska, J., Schubert, A., Wojna, M., *et al.* (2014) Costs of Diabetes and Its Complications in Poland. *European Journal of Health Economics*, **15**, 653-660. http://dx.doi.org/10.1007/s10198-013-0513-0

[8]   Chereches, R.M., Litan, C.M., Zlati, A.M. and Bloom, J.R. (2012) Does Co-Morbid Depression Impact Diabetes Related Costs? Evidence from a Cross-Sectional Survey in a Low-Income Country. *Journal of Mental Health Policy and Economics*, **15**, 127-138.

[9]   Yeaw, J. (2014) Direct Medical Costs for Complications among Children and Adults with Diabetes in the US Commercial Setting. *Applied Health Economics and Health Policy*, **12**, 219-230. http://dx.doi.org/10.1007/s40258-014-0086-9

[10] Zhuo X., Zhang, P., Barker, L., *et al.* (2014) The Lifetime Cost of Diabetes and Its implications for Diabetes Prevention. *Diabetes Care*, **37**, 2557-2564. http://dx.doi.org/10.2337/dc13-2484

[11] Condliffe, S., Link, C.R., Parasuraman, S. and Pollack, M.F. (2013) The Effects of Hypertension and Obesity on Total Health-Care Expenditures of Diabetes Patients in the United States. *Applied Economics Letters*, **20**, 649-652. http://dx.doi.org/10.1080/13504851.2012.727966

[12] Yesudian, C.A.K., Grepstad, M., Visintin, E. and Ferrario, A. (2014) The Economic Burden of Diabetes in India: A Review of the Literature. *Globalization and Health*, **10**, 80. http://dx.doi.org/10.1186/s12992-014-0080-x

[13] Dall, T.M., Zhang, Y., Chen, Y.J., Quick, W.W., Yang, W.G. and Fogli, J. (2010) The Economic Burden of Diabetes. *Health Affairs*, **29**, 297-303. http://dx.doi.org/10.1377/hlthaff.2009.0155

[14] American Diabetes Association (ADA) (2013) Economic Costs of Diabetes in the U.S. in 2012. *Diabetes Care*, **36**, 1033-1046. http://dx.doi.org/10.2337/dc12-2625

[15] Minor, T. (2011) The Effect of Diabetes on Female Labor Force Decision: New Evidence from the National Health Interview Survey. *Health Economics*, **20**, 1468-1486. http://dx.doi.org/10.1002/hec.1685

[16] Minor, T. (2013) An Investigation into the Effect of Type I and Type II Diabetes Duration on Employment and Wages. *Economics and Human Biology*, **11**, 534-544. http://dx.doi.org/10.1016/j.ehb.2013.04.004

[17] Sørensen, J. and Ploug, U.J. (2013) The Cost of Diabetes-Related Complications: Registry-Based Analysis of Days Absent from Work. *Economic Research International*, **2013**, Article ID: 618039. http://dx.doi.org/10.1155/2013/618039

[18] Liu, X. and Zhub, C. (2014) Will Knowing Diabetes Affect Labor Income? Evidence from a Natural Experiment. *Economics Letters*, **124**, 74-78. http://dx.doi.org/10.1016/j.econlet.2014.04.019

[19] Seuring, T., Goryakin, Y. and Suhrcke, M. (2015) The Impact of Diabetes on Employment in Mexico. *Economics and Human Biology*, **18**, 85-100. http://dx.doi.org/10.1016/j.ehb.2015.04.002

[20] DPC Evaluation Division, Central Social Insurance Medical Council, Ministry of Health, Labour and Welfare (2015) DPC taishou byouin, junnbi byouin no kibo (heisei 27 nen 4 gatsu 1 nichi) mikomi [Estimated Numbers of DPC Hospitals and Preparing Hospitals by Sizes of Hospitals as of April 1st, 2015]. (In Japanese)

[21] IDF (2014) About Diabetes. http://www.idf.org/about-diabetes

[22] ADA (2015) Diabetes Basic. http://www.diabetes.org/

[23] Nawata, K. and Kawabuchi, K. (2015) Evaluation of Length of Hospital Stay Joining Educational Programs for Type 2 Diabetes Mellitus Patients: Can We Control Medical Costs in Japan? *Health*, **7**, 256-269. http://dx.doi.org/10.4236/health.2015.72030

[24] Nawata, K. and Kawabuchi, K. (2015) Financial Sustainability of the Japanese Medical Payment System: Analysis of the Japanese Medical Expenditure for Educational Hospitalization of Patients with Type 2 Diabetes. *Health* **7**, 1007-1021. http://dx.doi.org/10.4236/health.2015.78118

[25] Box, G.E.P. and Cox, D.R. (1964) An Analysis of Transformation. *Journal of the Royal Statistical Society B*, **26**, 211-252.

[26] Showalter, M.H. (1994) A Monte Carlo Investigation of the Box-Cox Model and a Nonlinear Least Squares Alternative. *Review of Economics and Statistics*, **76**, 560-570. http://dx.doi.org/10.2307/2109980

[27] Nawata, K. (2015) Robust Estimation Based on the Third-Moment Restriction of the Error Terms for the Box-Cox Transformation Model: An Estimator Consistent under Heteroscedasticity. *Economics Bulletin*, **3**, 1056-1064.

[28] Heinze, G., Hronsky, M., Reichardt, B., Baumgärtel, C., Müllner, M., Bucsics, A. and Winkelmayer, W.C. (2015) Potential Savings in Prescription Drug Costs for Hypertension, Hyperlipidemia, and Diabetes Mellitus by Equivalent Drug Substitution in Austria: A Nationwide Cohort Study. *Applied Health Economics and Policy*, **13**, 193-205. http://dx.doi.org/10.1007/s40258-014-0143-4

[29] Watson, P., Preston, L., Squires, H., Chilcott, J. and Brennan, A. (2014) Modelling the Economics of Type 2 Diabetes Mellitus Prevention: A Literature Review of Methods. *Applied Health Economics and Health Policy*, **12**, 239-253. http://dx.doi.org/10.1007/s40258-014-0091-z

[30] Sittig, D.T., Friedel, H. and Wasem, J. (2015) Prevalence and Treatment Costs of Type 2 Diabetes in Germany and the Effects of Social and Demographic Differences. *European Journal of Health Economics*, **16**, 305-311. http://dx.doi.org/10.1007/s10198-014-0575-7

[31] Bickel, P.J. and Doksum, K.A. (1981) An Analysis of Transformations Revisited. *Journal of the American Statistical Association*, **76**, 296-311. http://dx.doi.org/10.1080/01621459.1981.10477649

[32] Nawata, K. (2013) A New Estimator of the Box-Cox Transformation Model Using Moment Conditions. *Economics Bulletin*, **33**, 2287-2297.

[33] Hausman, J. (1978) Specification Tests in Econometrics. *Econometrica*, **46**, 1251-1272. http://dx.doi.org/10.2307/1913827

[34] White, H. (1980) A Heteroskedasticity-Consistent Covariance Matrix and Direct Test for Heteroskedasticity. *Econometrica*, **48**, 817-838. http://dx.doi.org/10.2307/1912934

[35] Kantarevic, J. and Kralj, B. (2013) Link between Pay for Performance Incentives and Physician Payment Mechanisms: Evidence from Diabetes Management Incentive in Ontario. *Health Economics*, **22**, 1417-1439. http://dx.doi.org/10.1002/hec.2890

[36] Iezzi, E., Bruni, M.L. and Ugolini, C. (2014) The Role of GP's Compensation Schemes in Diabetes Care: Evidence from Panel Data. *Journal of Health Economics*, **34**, 104-120. http://dx.doi.org/10.1016/j.jhealeco.2014.01.002

[37] Wilke, T., Groth, A., Mueller, S., Reese, D., Linder, R., Ahrens, S. and Verheyen, F. (2013) How to Use Pharmacy Claims Data to Measure Patient Nonadherence? The Example of Oral Diabetics in Therapy of Type 2 Diabetes Mellitus. *European Journal of Health Economics*, **14**, 551-568. http://dx.doi.org/10.1007/s10198-012-0410-y

[38] Dilla, T., Valladares, A., Nicolay, C., Salvador, J., Reviriego, J. and Costi, M. (2012) Healthcare Costs Associated with Change in Body Mass Index in Patients with Type 2 Diabetes Mellitus in Spain: The ECOBIM Study. *Applied Health Economics and Policy*, **10**, 417-430. http://dx.doi.org/10.1007/BF03261876

[39] Slade, A.N. (2012) Health Investment Decisions in Response to Diabetes Information in Older Americans. *Journal of Health Economics*, **31**, 502-520. http://dx.doi.org/10.1016/j.jhealeco.2012.04.001

[40] Daim, T.U., Basoglu, N. and Topacan, U. (2013) Adoption of Health Information Technologies: The Case of a Wireless Monitor for Diabetes and Obesity Patients. *Technology Analysis & Strategic Management*, **25**, 923-938. http://dx.doi.org/10.1080/09537325.2013.823150

[41] Mehrotra, S. and Kim, K. (2011) Outcome Based State Budget Allocation for Diabetes Prevention Programs Using Multi-Criteria Optimization with Robust Weights. *Health Care Management Science*, **14**, 324-337. http://dx.doi.org/10.1007/s10729-011-9166-7

[42] Condliffe, S. and Link, C.R. (2014) Racial Differences in the Effects of Hypertension and Obesity on Health Expenditures by Diabetes Patients in the US. *Applied Economics Letters*, **21**, 280-283. http://dx.doi.org/10.1080/13504851.2013.856990

[43] Phelps, K.W., Hodgson, J.L. and Lamson, A.L. (2012) Satisfaction with Life and Psychosocial Factors among Underserved Minorities with Type 2 Diabetes. *Social Indicators Research*, **106**, 359-370. http://dx.doi.org/10.1007/s11205-011-9811-z

[44] Salois, M.J. (2012) Obesity and Diabetes, the Built Environment, and the "Local" Food Economy in the United States, 2007. *Economics and Human Biology*, **10**, 35-42. http://dx.doi.org/10.1016/j.ehb.2011.04.001

[45] Pan, X. and Ward, R.M. (2015) Self-Management and Self-Rated Health among Middle-Aged and Older Adults with Type 2 Diabetes in China: A Structural Equation Model. *Social Indicators Research*, **120**, 247-260. http://dx.doi.org/10.1007/s11205-014-0575-0

[46] Eggleston, K.N., Shah, N.D., Smith, S.A., Berndt, E.R. and Newhouse, J.P. (2011) Quality Adjustment for Health Care Spending on Chronic Disease: Evidence from Diabetes Treatment, 1999-2009. *American Economic Review: Papers & Proceedings*, **101**, 206-211. http://dx.doi.org/10.1257/aer.101.3.206

[47] Thurecht, L. and Brown, L. (2011) Economic Modelling of the Prevention of Type 2 Diabetes in Australia—The Diabetes Model. *International Journal of Microsimulation*, **4**, 71-80.

[48] Kruger, J. and Brennan, A. (2013) The Cost of Type 1 Diabetes Mellitus in the United Kingdom: A Review of Cost-of-Illness Studies. *European Journal of Health Economics*, **14**, 886-899. http://dx.doi.org/10.1007/s10198-012-0433-4

18

Role of Breastfeeding in Promoting Maternal & Child Health and Policy Implications in New Zealand

Adhikari Ramil

Massey University, Wellington, New Zealand
Email: dr_ramils@yahoo.com

Abstract

Worldwide researches over infant's health have generally focused and aimed on understanding the complex factors (both positive and negative) affecting the infant's health which further had ultimately helped them to frame policies nationally as well as internationally. Out of these factors, breastfeeding is one of the vital concerns for research related to infant mortality and morbidity. The World Health Organization recommends that infants should be exclusively breastfed until first six months and receive nutritionally adequate and safe complementary foods thereafter while breastfeeding continues for up to two years of age or beyond. In New Zealand (NZ), only 12% of 6 months old children were exclusively breastfed in 2006. The Ministry of Health plays a leading role for the protection, promotion and supporting breastfeeding in NZ. There are a number of areas/implications that NZ need to focus at such as providing antenatal and postpartum education, training of health professionals, community and workplace support, policy frameworks, breastfeeding statistics and intersectoral approach. These measures mainly focus at the initiation but less has been done to continue and support breastfeeding in NZ. In order to achieve this, all of these areas should be given prime and equal consideration. Hence, there is a strong need to develop strategies that maintain and promote breastfeeding at 6 months or beyond in NZ taking into considerations of various barriers and enabling factors.

Keywords

Breastfeeding, Benefits, Barriers, Policy Implications

1. Introduction

Worldwide researches over infant's health have generally focused and aimed on understanding the complex factors (both positive and negative) affecting the infant's health which further had ultimately helped them to frame policies nationally as well as internationally. Out of these factors, breastfeeding is one of the vital concerns for research related to infant mortality and morbidity [1]. Globally, the rate for exclusive breastfeeding up to 6 months of age was 20% for Central and European countries as compared to 44% for South Asia. Breastfeeding (BF) is defined as the transfer of the human milk from the mother to the child that is the infant receives milk directly from mother's breast [2]. And Exclusive Breastfeeding (EBF) refers to that the infant receives no other form of milk or liquid for the first four months and that breast milk be used until one year of infant's age [3].Human milk is considered as tailor-made (well-suited) for the baby. It is believed to be the best start of infant's life because of its nutritional, immunological and psychological benefits to both mother and infant. Apart from the numerous health benefits of breast milk for mother and child, like in other developed countries, to promote breastfeeding as an optimum infant feeding practice has become an important and integral aspect of the New Zealand (NZ) public health agenda [4].In order to achieve this goal, it is very crucial to understand and increase awareness regarding the role of breastfeeding for both mother and child and also to minimize and control various barriers for the same. The objective of this research paper is to highlight the role of breastfeeding in promoting mother and child health followed by the discussion of policy implications in New Zealand.

2. Background

2.1. International Breastfeeding Status

No doubt, good nutrition in infancy promotes and strengthens optimum growth and development of the child. Infant feeding is not only providing nutrition to an infant but also is a psychological, social and educational interaction between parent and infant [2]. There had been significant evidence over the past decades that breast milk provides all the essential nutrients in well-balanced proportion thereby fostering growth and development of an infant which is impossible to mimic or replace with any other kind of food [5].

Globally, in the developing countries like Philippines, Zimbabwe and Nepal, overall 96.6% (birth to 6 months)and 87.9% (6 to 12 months) of infants were currently breast-fed, 87.4% of 6 to 12 months old infants consumed water, 29.6% had other milk products, infant formula (15.1%) and 41.0% of other liquids respectively [1]. In addition to this, the rate for EBF up to 6 months of age was 20% for Central and European countries as compared to 44% for South Asia [6]. In United Kingdom, according to Baby Friendly Initiative Statistics, 81% of babies were breastfed at birth. This figure got dramatically reduced to 69% by one week and 17% at 3 months, 12% and 1% at 4 and 6 months (EBF) respectively. The World Health Organization (WHO), American Academy of Pediatrics (AAP) and American Academy of Family Physicians recommends EBF for the first 6 months of infant's life and thereafter to start with nutritionally adequate and safe complementary foods along with the continuation of breastfeeding up to 2 years or more. Also, Healthy People 2010 (national health promotion and disease prevention initiative in the United States) aims to increase BF rates as 75% of all mothers to start BF at birth, 50% of them to continue till 6 months, 25% forEBF for 6 months and 25% of mothers to continue breastfeed until 1 year of age [7].

2.2. Breastfeeding Status in New Zealand

Despite of these global targets, only 12% of babies were EBF for 6 months in New Zealand. In the year 2005, it was found that the EBF rate on discharge into the baby friendly hospitals was about 80.5%. This rate was 50% by the 6weeks and got further dropped by less than 40% till 3 months of age. In other words, the EBF rates were much higher at the time of birth or discharge from hospital but however there was a decline for the same up to 6 months thus highlighting a need for policy implications for promoting breastfeeding as a public health agenda and improving BF rates specifically at 6 weeks, 3and 6 months in New Zealand. Also, these BF rates had ethnic disparities and were very low among Maori, Pacific and Asian populations as compared to New Zealanders [8]. The current data from Plunket indicated that the EBF rates were higher but when they got combined with full BF rates, there was no much difference hence indicating this area as a highest need of concern. The full BF rates at 6 weeks and 3 months was 66% and 55% respectively in the year 2006 [9].

3. Benefits of Breastfeeding to

a) Infant
Moving further, scientific evidence had acknowledged that BF is considered as a gold standard for the infant.

It is believed to be the best start of infant life because of its nutritional, immunological and psychological benefits to both mother and infant. In terms of nutrition, human milk is considered as tailor-made (well-suited) for the baby. In other words, it provides the exact amount of correct nutrients in a well-balanced proportion at a right temperature as required by body of the infant [10].For instance, low amount of protein (Whey) and sodium content in the human milk prevents from overloading on the immature kidneys of the infant. It also provides essential minerals such as iron, zinc and calcium in order to meet the infant growth demands [11].

In addition to this, infant is born with immature immune system as well as the organs that may require a period of time to function at optimum level. Breast milk contains prebiotics (substances that enhance the growth of beneficial microflora), free fatty acids (FFA), mono glycerides, antimicrobial peptides, human milk glycans, bifidus factor, lysozyme, lacto peroxidase, lacto ferrin, lipoprotein lipase and epidermal growth factors (stimulate the gastrointestinal epithelium as a barrier) that are all responsible for developing and enhancing infant's innate immune system [12]. The presence of these antimicrobial, anti-inflammatory and immunologic stimulating agents protect the baby from diarrhea and other various infectious diseases such as respiratory and urinary tract infections, otitis media, necrotizing enterocolitis, bacterial meningitis and bacteremia [13]-[15]. Not only in the development of the immune system but the presence of essential and saturated fatty acids, medium chain triglycerides and long chain polyunsaturated fatty acids helps in the development of central nervous system (CNS) of the infant [11]. Overall breast milk is considered as the baby's first immunization. Breast milk gets more easily digested by the infant as compared to formula or any other milk and colostrum produced during the first 4 days of pregnancy helps in smoothing the passage of meconium (sticky dark stool in the bowels of baby during pregnancy) through the intestine [16].

The mechanic of sucking the breast milk directly from mother's breast helps in the development of jaw muscles and oral cavity. Sucking along with proper positioning of the infant during breastfeed promotes better jaw alignment and shaping of the hard palate that further results in straight and brace free smile. In addition to this, appropriate development of craniofacial structures helps in effective speech and communication patterns for the child in his/her later life [10]. Moving ahead, sudden infant death syndrome (SIDS) is drastically prevalent in New Zealand especially among Maori. During the period 2003-2007, 61.6% of infants who died from SIDS were Maori. Now, though the research for the causes and prevention of SIDS is ongoing but BF with benefit of proper jaw and oral cavity formation can reduce the risk and incidence of SIDS [17]. EBF for the first six months of life protect the infant from various food allergies and asthma and also provides time for the infant's immune system to develop. Frequency and duration of breastfeeding matters a lot. The more and for longer duration the baby gets fed, lesser are the chances of getting infections and allergies [14].

Apart from the above mention benefits, breastfeeding may have several other minor benefits too. Breastfeed babies have fewer rashes from the diapers or nappies because of the low pH of bowels. It may also prevent picky eater syndrome that may occurs later in life as babies who are breastfeed for longer periods accept different taste more easily than who are not. Last but not the least, breastfeeding the infant, reduces the chances of lymphoma, leukemia and obesity which further prevents the risk of developing complications in later life such as heart diseases, stroke, high blood pressure, diabetes and many more and also have a positive effect on cognitive development and skills [18]. In other words, studies had shown that children who were ever breastfeed had more intelligence quotients (IQ) as compared to those who did not received [10].

b) Mother

Moving ahead, the considerable beneficial effects of breastfeeding on the health of the mother had been paid less attention in the past. Probably, this could be one of the reasons that had affected the overall breastfeeding rates too in the olden times. Currently number of researches have been conducted for the same and had proven plentiful amounts of beneficial effects for the mother in terms of physical, general health perception, mental health scores and mother's parity. Breastfeeding women are able to produce sufficient amount of milk even if the calorie intake is low. This increase caloric demand with breastfeeding helps the mother to be nutritionally sound and return to its pre-pregnant state far more quickly than those mothers who do not breastfeed. In addition to this, breastfeeding releases oxytocin into the body that helps in the uterine contractions and shrinking of the uterus. Also, breastfeeding women experience greater weight loss and fat reduction ultimately helping them to return to the pre-pregnant state [19]. Exclusive breastfeeding suppresses the ovulation that further delays mensuration for about 4 - 6 months of post partum period thus providing spacing and acting as a natural method for family planning. This method is known as Lactation Amenorrhea Method, LAM [7].

Not only this, there is significant evidence that breastfeeding reduces the risk of breast and ovarian cancers in the mothers [20]. Studies have proven that there is 4.3% reduction in the risk of developing breast cancer for each year a woman breastfeeds in her lifetime. In other words, women who had developed breast cancer, the average lifetime of breastfeeding duration in them is much shorter as compared to those in which the disease is absent [21]. One of the case control study of Sri Lankan women showed that increased duration of breastfeeding dramatically reduces the risk of developing breast cancer and there was a dose-response relationship between the two [22]. With regard to breastfeeding and ovarian cancer, agency of healthcare research and quality (AHRQ) performed a meta-analysis on 9 studies and found a reduction in the risk of ovarian cancer by 21% in breastfeeding women as compared to those who had never breastfeed [7].

Moreover, the increased time duration of lifetime breastfeeding has also been found to be associated with low risk of developing diabetes (Type 2) and hip fractures in postmenopausal women. Studies have also indicated that women who do not breastfeed are at higher risk of developing post partum depression (the cause for which is likely unclear), hypertension, hyperlipidemia and cardiovascular diseases. In other terms, breastfeeding has a positive impact on systolic and diastolic blood pressure of the mothers [23].

Apart from the physiological benefits, breastfeeding provides psychological support to both mothers and babies. Oxytocin is a hormone that passes form the mother to the baby through the breast milk. Both oxytocin and prolactin, known as "mothering" hormones plays a vital role in providing the sense of completion, satisfaction, well being, relaxation and mothering. Furthermore, going through a positive and supportive breastfeeding experience further helps the mothers to gain confidence, self-esteem and ego [19]. In a quasi-experimental study of Australian primipara's views about breastfeeding, mothers reported that after 6 weeks of time they feel like they "got into right" and had a wonderful and pleasurable feeling of increased determination of breastfeeding their child and described breastfeeding as a magical experience overall. Not only this, mothers identified the advantages of breastfeeding for their infant, for instance, enhancing their attachment, providing comfort, giving them something they loved, increasing their immunity and contributing to their babies blooming [24].

In another study to explore the maternal perceptions of early breastfeeding experiences and breastfeeding outcomes at 6 weeks, it concluded for the same. Mothers had explained positive feelings regarding breastfeeding experiences that included feelings of enhanced attachment, enjoyment of breastfeeding and a sense of pride and personal fulfillment [25]. Therefore, breastfeeding the baby not only helps the mothers physically but also provides a greater sense of psychological, intimate and emotional bonding with the infant. Breastfeeding nurtures both the mother and infant [26]. Even the baby feels warmth, identifies mother and her love which in turn in the later stages teaches him the lesson of love, sacrifice, friendship and relations. This has been proved in one of the study that aims to clarify or explore the role of breastfeeding in the mother-infant relationship. The results of the study concluded that a positive correlation exists between breastfeeding and mother-infant bonding [27].

Now, surprisingly breastfeeding has some societal and economic benefits, too. It is not only good for the mother and baby but is also beneficial for the environment and mother earth. One study showed that if each baby is bottle-fed, in the US, it might produce more than 86,000 tons of waste into the landforms in the form of cans and packaging [10]. Breastfeeding is cheap, money and time saving. It saves the costs of purchasing formulae milk and bottles. The US department of agriculture, published in 2001, estimated that a minimum of 3.6 billion could be saved if the breastfeeding rates met the goals of Healthy People 2010 [19].

4. Breastfeeding Barriers to Mothers in NZ

One of the main breastfeeding barrier for mothers is their early return to work. In NZ, The Parental Leave and Employment Protection Act of 1987 entitles 14 weeks of paid parental leave to the mother or either of the parent in a joint adoption in order to promote and improve breastfeeding rates in NZ [8]. The Department of Labor (DOL) had conducted a survey on the effect of paid parental leave and breastfeeding rates with the results of 84% of participants believed that paid parental leave does play a significant role however 20% of them thought that 14 weeks were insufficient to improve breastfeeding rates. This directly suggests that the short duration of paid parental leave is one of the major factor that contribute to many mothers returning to work much earlier than they would prefer ultimately having dropped breastfeeding rates at 3 and 6 months in NZ [28].

Societal norms and cultural beliefs also create hindrance for mothers to breastfeed. The Ministry of Health, 2003 maternity service consumer satisfaction survey found that 89% of women intend to breastfeed their babies and 94% of women breastfeed their babies either exclusively, fully or partially. In spite of this positive attitude, New Zealand women reported their concern with regard to lack of support from their partner/family members to continue breastfeeding. In addition, various cultural practices, such as cigarette smoking, obesity, sense of guilt, use of bottle-feeding and availability of infant formulae milk, low socio economic status especially with regard to Maori and Pacific communities all adds into the barriers list of breastfeeding in NZ [29].

5. Policy Implications in NZ

No doubt, the discussion above has provided a clear evidence of the beneficial role of breastfeeding in promoting maternal and child health and also regarding the dropped breastfeeding rates globally as well as in NZ. Now, with regard to policy implications in NZ for the same, the Ministry of Health (MOH) provides the leadership for breastfeeding strategies and policies and thus has set the following breastfeeding targets for NZ. Firstly, to increase the exclusive and full breastfeeding prevalence rate at 6 weeks to 74% by 2005 and 90% by 2010. Secondly, to increase the exclusive and full breastfeeding prevalence rate at 3 months to 57% by 2005 and 70% by 2010 and thirdly, to increase the exclusive and full breastfeeding prevalence rate at 6 months to 21% by 2005 and 27% by 2010 [30].

In order to achieve these targets, a number of interventions had been taken at the national, regional and local levels within NZ that can further be explained under three broad headings, that is practices or implications to protect, promote and support breastfeeding. First of all, under the protection, there are 3 main legislative framework and policies that have been formed and timely reviewed in order to protect breastfeeding in NZ. The Human Right Act 1993 protects the right to breastfeed by stating that a women has the right to breastfeed and the child to be breastfed, wherever mother and her child is otherwise permitted to and is protected from discrimination for breastfeeding. The Parental Leave and Employment Protection Act of 1987 is an other legislative measure that entitles 14 weeks of paid parental leave to the mother or either of the parent in a joint adoption in order to promote and improve breastfeeding rates in NZ [8]. Along with this, other employment or work related measures such as allowing breastfeeding breaks for mother who wish to breastfeed the infant at work, flexible working hours, onsite crèches and provision of appropriate facilities for expressing and storing breast milk were also included under the Employment Relations Act 2007. Another framework is Corrections Regulations 2005 that protect the right to breastfeed for the imprisoned mothers and to promote mother infant bonding by providing them the opportunity to stay with their babies for a minimum of six months and beyond up to 2 years [29].

Internationally and nationally, studies have indicated that there is a positive relationship between paid maternity leave and breastfeeding rates. In NZ, the Department of Labor (DOL) had conducted a survey on the effect of paid parental leave and breastfeeding rates with the results of 84% of participants believed that paid parental leave does play a significant role however 20% of them thought that 14 weeks were insufficient to improve breastfeeding rates. This directly suggests that the short duration of paid parental leave is one of the major factor that contribute to many mothers returning to work much earlier than they would prefer ultimately having dropped breastfeeding rates at 3 and 6 months in NZ [28]. Recently, there have been proposals made in the parliament of NZ in the year 2014 to increase paid parental leave from 14 to 26 weeks. This will definitely have a huge impact as of dose-response relationship and will provide a new direction towards the success and meeting MOH breastfeeding targets for NZ.

Moving further, there is a seven-point action plan which includes establishing a national inter-sectoral breastfeeding committee, implementing Baby Friendly Hospitals throughout New Zealand, gaining active participation of Maori and Pacific whanau, establishing consistent breastfeeding reporting and statistics, increasing breastfeeding promotion, advocacy and coordination, ensuring that pregnant women can access prenatal education and ensuring high quality and ongoing postpartum care for improving the initiation, promotion and maintenance of breastfeeding in New Zealand [8]. In other words, providing antenatal and postpartum education, training of health professionals, community and workplace support, policy frameworks, breastfeeding statistics and intersectoral approach are the main key areas or interventions that NZ should focus for promoting breastfeeding. All of these areas should be given prime and equal consideration for achieving MOH breastfeeding targets.

Breastfeeding is a learned experience. Hence, educating the mothers and family members play a vital role in the promotion and support for breastfeeding. Providing antenatal education to the mothers will not only helps with their decision to breastfeed but also prepare them mentally to start breastfeeding soon after the birth which is also widely supported by the baby friendly initiative into the hospitals [31]. This clinical practice of breastfeeding soon after birth is a strong support for the initiation of breastfeeding and as a result the breastfeeding rates are highest at birth within NZ. However, these interventions concentrate much on the initiation and less has been done to maintain the exclusive continuation of it up to 6 months or beyond [9]. Thus, supporting breast-feeding is very important within NZ so as to meet MOH breastfeeding targets.

Now, in context to supporting BF, various interventions like conducting workshops, seminars, public aware-ness campaigns must be addressed especially with regard to Maori and Pacific populations due to prevalence of lower breastfeeding rates among them. At present, there are two programs for improving breastfeeding rates in Maori known as B4Baby in South Auckland and Mum4Mum (peer support program) in the Hutt Valley [8]. There are other breastfeeding support organizations such as lead maternity cares (LMC), general practitioner services, Royal NZ Plunket Society, New Zealand Breastfeeding Authority (NZBA), Well Child services and other community health workers that aims to support and promote breastfeeding in NZ. For example, the NZ maternity care system had established Lead Maternity Carer (LMC) the role of which is to conduct home visits, provide continuity of care during and after pregnancy and educating the mothers and families [30]. It is of pa-ramount importance that these multiple organizations need to work hand-in-hand (adopt intersectoral approach) both among themselves and with the mothers and families especially with Maori and Pacific communities. This will not only promote coordination, communication and collaboration but will also result in the maximum utili-zation of available services and minimize any duplication. Furthermore, there are lactation support groups with-in district health boards (DHB's) for providing free advise and support and people should be made aware of it so as to make maximum benefit out of them [32].

Next, for imparting best quality education, the training of health professionals such as nurses, midwives and general practitioners is the next main key area that can hugely affect breast feeding rates. They should be trained in such a way that they are able to provide clear, effective and clinical or evidence based information [29]. Last but not the least, research is one of the crucial component in addressing the effectiveness of any intervention. Thus, breastfeeding statistics including rates (initiation, duration, intensity, ethnicity), health practices in the hospitals and communities, policies and frameworks, should be collected accurately and timely as this will help to make comparisons between the past and present and also to set future targets. Data regarding various enabling factors and barriers (like smoking, plunked visits, cultural beliefs, clinical-poor antenatal education, breast sur-gery and breast diseases and societal barriers-returning to work early, low socio economic status, unawareness, poor family support) of breastfeeding should also be collected and the above mentioned interventions to promote the enabling factors and minimizing the barriers ultimately will result in good breastfeeding outcomes [33]. On the whole, societal encouragement and acceptance of breastfeeding along with mass media and policy frame-works together will have a huge impact on breastfeeding rates.

6. Conclusion

In a conclusion, it can be concluded that NZ has high breastfeeding rates at the time of birth but these slowly decline till 3 and 6 months of age thereby arising the need to address it as one of the public health agenda. The MOH play a leading role for the protection, promotion and supporting breastfeeding in NZ. There are a number of interventions that had been taken at national, regional and local levels. These measures mainly focus at the in-itiation but less has been done to continue and support breastfeeding in NZ. Hence, there is a strong need to de-velop strategies such as establishing a national inter-sectoral breastfeeding committee, implementing Baby Friendly Hospitals throughout New Zealand, gaining active participation of Maori and Pacific whanau, estab-lishing consistent breastfeeding reporting and statistics, increasing breastfeeding promotion, advocacy and coor-dination, ensuring that pregnant women can access prenatal education and ensuring high quality and ongoing postpartum care for improving the initiation, promotion and maintenance of breastfeeding in New Zealand [8]. All of the above mention implications will contribute towards both maintaining and promoting breastfeeding at 6 months or beyond taking into consideration various barriers and enabling factors.

References

[1]   Marriot, M.B., Campbell, L., Hirsch, E. and Wilson, D. (2007) Preliminary Data from Demographic and Health Sur-veys on Infant Feeding in 20 Developing Countries. *The Journal of Nutrition*, **137**, 518-523.

[2]   Lowdermilk, L.D., Perry, E.S., Cashion, K. and Alden, R.K. (2012) Maternity and Women's Health Care. 10th Edition, Elsevier Incorporate, St. Louis.

[3]   Kotch, B.J. (2005) Maternal and Child Health: Programs, Problems and Policy in Public Health. 2nd Edition, Jones &

Bartlett Publishers, Burlington.

[4]   Dykes, F. (2006) Breastfeeding in Hospital: Mothers, Midwives and the Production Line. Routledge, London.

[5]   Lonnerdal, B. (2000) Breast Milk: A Truly Functional Food. *Nutrition*, **16**, 509-511.
      http://dx.doi.org/10.1016/S0899-9007(00)00363-4

[6]   Imdad, A., Yakoob, Y.M. and Bhutta, A.Z. (2011) Effect of Breastfeeding Promotion Interventions on Breastfeeding
      Rates, with Special Focus in Developing Countries. *BMC Public Health*, **11**, 1471 2458.
      http://dx.doi.org/10.1186/1471-2458-11-s3-s24

[7]   Eglash, A., Montgomeery, A. and Wood, J. (2008) Breastfeeding. *DM*, **5**, 343-411.
      http://dx.doi.org/10.1016/j.disamonth.2008.03.001

[8]   National Breastfeeding Advisory Committee of New Zealand. (2009) National Strategic Plan of Action for Breast-
      feeding 2008-2012: National Breastfeeding Advisory Committee of New Zealand's Advice to the Director-General of
      Health. Ministry of Health, Wellington.

[9]   Royal New Zealand Plunket Society (2010) Breastfeeding Data: Analysis of 2004-2009 Data. Royal New Zealand
      Plunket Society, Wellington.

[10] Perkins, S. and Vannais, C. (2004) Breastfeeding for Dummies. Wiley Publishing Incorporation, Hoboken.

[11] Ying, W.S. (2005) Breastfeeding: Laws and Societal Impact. Nova Science Publishers, New York.
      http://dx.doi.org/10.1097/00000446-200505000-00005

[12] Lawrence, M.R. and Pane, A.C. (2007) Human Breast Milk: Current Concepts of Immunology and Infectious Diseases.
      Current Problem Pediatric Adolescent Health Care, **37**, 7-36. http://dx.doi.org/10.1016/j.cppeds.2006.10.002

[13] Newburg, D. (2009) Neonatal Protection by Innate Immune System of Human Milk Consisting of Milk Oligosacchia-
      rides and Glycans. *Journal of Animal Science*, **87**, 26-34. http://dx.doi.org/10.2527/jas.2008-1347

[14] Ogbuanu, I.U., Karmaus, W., Arshad, S.H., Kurukulaaratchy, R.J. and Ewart, S. (2009) Effect of Breastfeeding Dura-
      tion on Lung Function at Age 10 Years: A Prospective Birth Cohort Study. *Thorax*, **64**, 62-66.
      http://dx.doi.org/10.1136/thx.2008.101543

[15] Hanson, L. (2004) Protective Effects of Breastfeeding against Urinary Tract Infection. *Acta paediatrica*, **93**, 154-156.
      http://dx.doi.org/10.1111/j.1651-2227.2004.tb00695.x

[16] Trotter, S. (2004) Breastfeeding: The Essential Guide. Circa Print Solutions Limited, Renfrewshire.

[17] McKenna, J.J. and McDade, T. (2005) Why Babies Should Never Sleep Alone: A Review of the Co-Sleeping Contro-
      versy in Relation to SIDS, Bed Sharing and Breastfeeding. *Paediatric Respiratory Reviews*, **6**, 134-152.
      http://dx.doi.org/10.1016/j.prrv.2005.03.006

[18] Johnston, P., Flood, K. and Spinks, K. (2004) The Newborn Child. 9th Edition, Elsevier Science, London.

[19] Lauwers. J. and Swisher, A. (2011) Counseling the Nursing Mother: A Lactation Consultant Guide. 5th Edition, Jones
      and Bartlett Learning, Burlington.

[20] Galson, K.S. (2008) Mothers and Children Benefits From Breastfeeding. *Journal of American Dietetic Association*,
      108, 1106. http://dx.doi.org/10.1016/j.jada.2008.04.028

[21] La Leche League International (2004) The Womanly Art of Breastfeeding. 7th Edition, La Leche League International
      Incorporation, New York.

[22] Silvia, D.M., Senarath, U., Gunatilake, M. and Lokuhetty, D. (2010) Prolonged Breastfeeding Reduces Risk of Breast
      Cancer in Sri Lankan Women: A Case-Control Study. *Cancer Epidemiology*, **34**, 267-273.
      http://dx.doi.org/10.1016/j.canep.2010.02.012

[23] American Dietetic Association (2009) Position of the American Dietetic Association: Promoting and Supporting
      Breastfeeding. *Journal of the American Dietetic Association*, **109**, 1926-1942.
      http://dx.doi.org/10.1016/j.jada.2009.09.018

[24] Hall, A.W. and Hauck, Y. (2005) Getting It Right: Australian Primiparas' View about Breastfeeding: A Quasi Experi-
      mental Study. *International Journal of Nursing Studies*, **44**, 786-795. http://dx.doi.org/10.1016/j.ijnurstu.2006.02.006

[25] Wojnar, D. (2004) Maternal Perceptions of Early Breastfeeding Experiences and Breastfeeding Outcomes at 6 Weeks.
      Clinical Effectiveness in Nursing, **8**, 93-100. http://dx.doi.org/10.1016/j.cein.2004.08.001

[26] The National Health Committee (1999) Review of Maternity Health Services in New Zealand. National Health Com-
      mittee, Wellington.

[27] Jansen, J., Weerth, D.C. and Walraven, R.M.J. (2008) Breastfeeding and the Mother-Infant Relationship—A Review.
      Developmental Review, **28**, 503-521. http://dx.doi.org/10.1016/j.dr.2008.07.001

[28] Department of Labor (2007) Parental Leave in New Zealand: 2005-2006 Evaluation. Department of Labor, Wellington.

[29] National Breastfeeding Advisory Committee of New Zealand (2008) Background Report: Protecting, Promoting and Supporting Breastfeeding in New Zealand. Ministry of Health, Wellington.

[30] Ministry of Health (2002) Breastfeeding: A Guide to Action. Ministry of Health, Wellington.

[31] New Zealand Breastfeeding Authority (2007) Baby Friendly Hospital Initiative and Baby Friendly Communities Initiative. New Zealand Breastfeeding Authority, New Zealand.

[32] Ministry of Health. (2008) Food and Nutrition Guidelines for Healthy Infants and Toddlers (Aged 0-2): A Background Paper. Ministry of Health, Wellington.

[33] Butler, S., Williams, M., Tukuitonga, C. and Paterson, J. (2004) Factors Associated with Not Breast Feeding Exclusively among Mothers of a Cohort of Pacific Infants in New Zealand. *New Zealand Medical Journal*, **117**, U908.

19

Prevalence of Chronic Pain, Especially Headache, and Relationship with Health-Related Quality of Life in Middle-Aged Japanese Residents

Junko Mitoma[1], Masami Kitaoka[1], Hiroki Asakura[1], Enoch Olando Anyenda[1], Daisuke Hori[1], Nguyen Thi Thu Tao[1], Toshio Hamagishi[1], Koichiro Hayashi[1], Fumihiko Suzuki[1], Yukari Shimizu[1], Hiromasa Tsujiguchi[1], Yasuhiro Kambayashi[1], Yuri Hibino[1], Tadashi Konoshita[2], Takiko Sagara[1], Aki Shibata[1], Hiroyuki Nakamura[1]

[1]Department of Environmental and Preventive Medicine, Graduate School of Medical Science, Kanazawa University, Ishikawa, Japan
[2]Third Department of Internal Medicine, Fukui University School of Medicine, Fukui, Japan
Email: mitoma@stu.kanazawa-u.ac.jp

Abstract

The aim of this study was to evaluate the prevalence of chronic pain (CP) and the relationship between CP, especially headache adjusted for CP at other sites, and health-related quality of life (HRQoL) in middle-aged Japanese residents. We examined the prevalence of CP (defined as pain persisting for 3 months or more) and HRQoL (SF-36) in 1117 middle-aged residents of Japan. We assessed the eight dimensions of health status and the 3 component SF-36 summary score to evaluate HRQoL. The prevalence of CP was 15.3% among men and 15.1% among women. Multiple linear regression analysis demonstrated that lumbar pain ($p < 0.001$, $\beta = -0.132$), knee pain ($p < 0.001$, $\beta = -0.115$), foot pain ($p = 0.042$, $\beta = -0.065$), and age ($p < 0.001$, $\beta = -0.154$) were independently correlated with a lower physical component score (PCS). Older age ($p < 0.001$, $\beta = 0.221$) showed a significant positive correlation with mental component score (MCS), while neck/shoulder pain ($p < 0.01$, $\beta = -0.096$), knee pain ($p < 0.001$, $\beta = -0.109$), upper limb pain ($p < 0.01$, $\beta = -0.098$), and lumbar pain ($p = 0.022$, $\beta = -0.077$) all showed a significant negative correlation with MCS. The presence of chronic headache ($p = 0.011$, $\beta = -0.082$) was the only factor significantly correlated with a lower role component score (RCS). We identified a negative correlation between chronic headache and RCS, unlike the relation between musculoskeletal pain and PCS or MCS, suggesting that RCS was an independently influenced by CP differently from PCS or MCS in Japanese residents.

Keywords

Quality of Life, Chronic Pain, Headache, SF-36, Pain

1. Introduction

The International Association for the Study of Pain (IASP) defines pain as an unpleasant sensory and emotional experience associated with actual or potential tissue damage, or described in terms of such damage [1]. In addition, the IASP defines chronic pain (CP) as pain without an apparent biological cause that persists beyond the normal time for tissue healing (usually 3 months) [2].

Some of the previous studies have been hospital-based [3] or focused on the elderly persons [4], and few studies have investigated CP in the general Japanese population. In a telephone survey study, among the general population in European countries and Israel shows a variation in prevalence of CP that ranges from 12% to 30% depending on the geographical area and age [5]. Previous survey shows that 9% to 28% of the Japanese population have CP, and that it is less frequent in people under 40 years old than in other age groups, whereas it appears to be higher in the 41 - 60 age group than in the others [6] [7]. Also there is a higher prevalence among elderly persons and in women [6]-[8]. A study performed in Japan reports aging as part of reason for increase of persons suffering from CP, however, it still remains unclear [9]. CP is usually musculoskeletal pain, such as lumbar pain, shoulder pain, or knee pain [6]-[8]. It is common for people with CP to be on long-term therapy and to be dissatisfied with their current treatment [10].

CP causes deterioration of HRQoL because it not only affects the physical condition and ability to function, but also the person's mental health and daily activities [7], which can lead to exacerbation of symptoms. CP restricts the ability to work and is responsible for substantial health care costs, resulting in it being a major public health problem worldwide [5]. Considering that the health effects of CP are multi-dimensional, it is important to elucidate the involvement of physical, mental, and social factors, as well as how role factors are related to CP.

Among the various body sites affected by CP, headache is reported to cause marked impairment of daily activities, such as family and social activities [11]. Chronic headache results in substantially greater disability than other types of headache [12], and is often combined with other chronic pain disorders [13]. To measure the disability caused by headache itself, we need to adjust for the impact of chronic pain at other sites. Therefore, we examine the prevalence of both headache and CP at other sites, as well as the impact on HRQoL, in middle-aged Japanese residents.

2. Methods

2.1. Subjects and Methods

We performed this study from October to December 2012. The target population was all of the middle-aged persons legally residing in the two elementary school districts in a rural area (Shika, Isikawa prefecture). This study was supported by the Shika Municipal Government, which provided a list of all residents aged 40 to 65 years in this area. The eligible population was 1291 persons and almost all of them were Japanese citizens.

We provided self-administered questionnaire to the residents. After they filled in the answers, participants were asked to return the questionnaires in sealed envelopes to members of the health promotion team employed by Shika Municipal Government.

The self-administered questionnaire was designed to obtain demographic data such as the age, gender, height and weight, as well as self-reported information on medical conditions such as cerebrovascular disease, cardiovascular disease, hypertension, dyslipidemia, diabetes mellitus, history of fracture over 10 years, osteoarthritis, depression, osteoporosis, insomnia, rheumatoid arthritis, CP at up to 3 sites, and HRQoL.

We asked the subjects to rate the severity of CP on a 10-point scale (0 = no pain to 10 = most severe pain ever experienced). We defined CP as pain persisting for 3 months or longer (in agreement with the IASP) at a severity of more than 5 so that we could compare our data with other surveys performed in Europe and Japan [5] [6]. We asked about the presence of pain affecting the head, neck, shoulder, upper limb, back, lumbar, hip, knee, foot, chest, and abdomen. We classified the site of pain as follows: head, neck/shoulder, upper limb, lumbar region, hip, knee, foot, and other (including back, hip, chest, and abdomen).

To measure HRQoL, we used the SF-36, Japanese version 2. The SF-36 is used worldwide to measure HRQoL, especially in general populations. It has been translated into Japanese and validated for use in Japan [14]. SF-36 measures eight dimensions of health over four weeks, which are physical functioning (PF), role physical (RP), bodily pain (BP), general health (GH), vitality (VT), social function (SF), role emotional (RE), and mental health (MH). We used a norm-based scoring (NBS) system, in which all scores were converted to the values relative to the Japanese population (mean = 50 and standard deviation = 10 with a normal distribution; higher scores indicate better HRQoL) [15]. These eight scores were further summarized into three component summary scores, which were the physical component summary (PCS), mental component summary (MCS), and role component summary (RCS). The factor structures of SF-36 reported in Japan [16], China [17] [18], Taiwan [19], and Singapore [20] are considered to differ from those found in western countries [21]. A previous study on validation of component models supported a three-component model as superior to a two-component model in Japan [22]. A three-component model was demonstrated to provide "purer" factor-loading patterns in the physical and mental components, with the mental component showing greater improvement [22]. Therefore, we employed a three-component model in this study.

2.2. Statistics

We used the unpaired t-test and analysis of variance (ANOVA) for continuous data. The chi-square test was employed for categorical data, except when the expected number of cells was less than 5 in which case we used Fisher's exact test. We used analysis of covariance (ANCOVA) for continuous data adjusted for age and gender. Multiple linear regression analysis was performed with a forward stepwise approach to estimate the impact of each variable on the component summary scores. The independent variables assessed included the age, gender (male 0, female 1), and each site of pain (no pain 0, with pain 1). All tests were 2-tailed, with differences reported as significant at $p < 0.05$. Analyses were conducted using IBM SPSS Statistics version19 for Windows.

2.3. Study Protocol Approval and Consent

This study was conducted with the approval of the ethics review board of Kanazawa University (Kanazawa, Japan). All participants provided written informed consent by signing a form that described the purpose and procedures of the study, the potential risks and benefits associated with participation, the strictly voluntary nature of participation, the right to withdraw from the study without prejudice or penalty, and the guaranteed confidentiality and security of personal data.

3. Results

We excluded persons who did not give consent (n = 111), who could not be contacted (n = 52), and who were hospitalized or institutionalized (n = 11) from the 1291 residents, and obtained responses from 1117 people (86.0%; 556 men and 561 women, mean age: 54.7 ± 7.73 in male, 54.7 ± 7.66 in female).

The prevalence of CP was 15.3% among men and 15.1% among women. In the male subjects, the site of pain (in decreasing order) was neck/shoulder pain in 6.86%, lumbar pain in 6.69%, foot pain in 3.43%, knee pain in 2.88%, upper limb pain in 1.98%, and headache in 0.899%, while the site of pain in the female subjects was neck/shoulder pain in 7.16%, lumbar pain in 5.92%, knee pain in 3.58%, foot pain in 2.85%, upper limb pain in 1.96%, and headache in 1.43%. There was one site of CP in 8.76% of male subjects and 7.94% of female subjects, two sites in 4.20% and 4.69%, and three sites in 2.92% and 2.71% (**Table 1**).

While VT, MH, and MCS were significantly higher, PCS was lower in the older subjects compared with the younger subjects among both males and females. PF was significantly lower in older subjects compared with younger subjects among females only (**Table 2**).

ANCOVA with covariates of age and gender showed that PF, RP, BP, GH, VT, SF, RE, MH, PCS, and MCS were all significantly lower in the subjects with CP compared to those without CP. Only RCS showed no significant difference between subjects with and without CP (**Table 3**).

To evaluate the impact of pain at different sites on HRQoL, we performed stratified analysis by pain site. The subjects with CP affecting the neck/shoulder, lumbar, knee, foot, and other sites had a significantly lower PCS than those without CP. In subjects with CP at all sites, MCS was significantly lower than in those without CP. In subjects with chronic headache, RCS was significantly lower than in those without CP (**Table 4**).

Table 1. Characteristics of the participants (N = 1117).

Gender	Male (n = 556)	Female (n = 561)	P value
Age: mean (SD)	54.7 (7.73)	54.7 (7.66)	0.340
Height (cm): mean (SD)	168.8 (6.14)	155.4 (5.49)	0.018
Weight (kg): mean (SD)	67.8 (10.4)	54.4 (8.01)	<0.001
BMI: mean (SD)	23.8 (3.12)	22.6 (3.25)	0.246
Diseases			
Cerebrovascular disease (%)	1.80	0.535	0.055
Cardiovascular disease (%)	2.70	1.60	0.208
Hypertension (%)	22.5	19.3	0.184
Dyslipidemia (%)	10.4	16.4	<0.01
Diabetes mellitus (%)	10.3	5.35	<0.01
Fracture within 10 years (%)	4.86	3.39	0.217
Osteoarthritis (%)	1.80	3.39	0.095
Depression (%)	1.62	1.96	0.666
Osteoporosis (%)	0.540	2.14	0.034
Insomnia (%)	1.44	1.60	0.821
Rheumatoid arthritis (%)	0.719	0.891	1.000
Prevalence of pain			
Any (%)	15.3	15.1	0.919
Head (%)	0.899	1.43	0.412
Upper-limb (%)	1.98	1.96	0.980
Neck/Shoulder (%)	6.86	7.16	0.846
Lumbar (%)	6.69	5.92	0.600
Knee (%)	2.88	3.58	0.508
Foot (%)	3.43	2.85	0.580
Others (%)	2.89	2.32	0.553
Number of chronic pain site			
One site (%)	8.76	7.94	0.935
Two sites (%)	4.20	4.69	
Three sites (%)	2.92	2.71	
SF-36 score			
PF: mean (SD)	49.9 (11.0)	49.5 (9.97)	0.306
RP: mean (SD)	51.2 (9.22)	50.6 (9.29)	0.397
BP: mean (SD)	49.9 (10.7)	50.3 (10.2)	0.536
GH: mean (SD)	48.0 (9.04)	48.4 (9.24)	0.481
VT: mean (SD)	50.3 (10.2)	50.1 (10.1)	0.907
SF: mean (SD)	51.5 (9.23)	50.7 (9.56)	0.157
RE: mean (SD)	51.8 (8.93)	50.7 (9.34)	0.026
MH: mean (SD)	50.3 (9.31)	50.3 (9.52)	0.191
PCS: mean (SD)	48.5 (10.6)	49.0 (9.96)	0.684
MCS: mean (SD)	49.1 (9.74)	49.6 (9.80)	0.659
RCS: mean (SD)	53.0 (10.1)	51.8 (10.1)	0.376

SD: Standard Deviation; PF: Physical Functioning; RP: Role Physical; BP: Bodily Pain; GH: General Health; VT: Vitality; SF: Social Function; RE: Role Emotional; MH: Mental Health; PCS: Physical Component Summary; MCS: Mental Component Summary; RCS: Role Component Summary; Others include chest, abdomen, hip, and back pain. We used the unpaired t-test for continuous data and the χ^2 test for categorical data.

Table 2. SF-36 scores of subjects in each age group.

	Male										Female										
	40 - 49			50 - 59			60 - 65			P value		40 - 49			50 - 59			60 - 65			P value
	N	Mean	SD	N	Mean	SD	N	Mean	SD		N	Mean	SD	N	Mean	SD	N	Mean	SD	
PF	136	50.3	(12.9)	164	50.8	(8.23)	179	48.9	(11.5)	0.272	140	51.5	(8.75)	195	49.6	(8.95)	178	47.9	(11.6)	<0.01
RP	135	52.0	(8.93)	163	51.1	(8.24)	179	50.6	(10.2)	0.410	141	51.8	(8.79)	193	50.8	(8.90)	177	49.4	(9.98)	0.061
BP	136	49.4	(10.8)	164	50.3	(11.0)	180	49.8	(10.5)	0.767	142	50.3	(9.42)	195	50.1	(10.7)	178	50.6	(10.3)	0.899
GH	136	48.2	(8.38)	164	47.2	(9.33)	178	48.6	(9.25)	0.311	141	48.8	(8.81)	193	47.7	(9.77)	177	48.8	(8.97)	0.447
VT	136	48.4	(10.2)	164	48.9	(9.80)	177	53.1	(9.91)	<0.001	141	47.6	(9.80)	194	49.4	(10.2)	176	53.0	(9.75)	<0.001
SF	136	51.4	(8.65)	163	51.2	(8.86)	180	51.8	(10.0)	0.858	142	49.5	(10.8)	193	50.7	(9.68)	178	51.5	(8.22)	0.182
RE	135	52.5	(8.27)	162	51.2	(8.96)	179	51.8	(9.37)	0.439	141	50.9	(9.51)	193	50.7	(9.34)	176	50.6	(9.27)	0.955
MH	136	48.6	(8.88)	164	49.3	(9.48)	177	52.5	(9.09)	<0.001	141	48.4	(10.2)	192	50.2	(9.18)	176	51.9	(9.04)	<0.01
PCS	134	49.7	(12.2)	161	49.6	(8.14)	176	46.7	(11.1)	0.018	140	51.7	(8.69)	188	48.9	(9.39)	173	47.0	(11.0)	<0.001
MCS	134	47.0	(9.39)	161	47.6	(9.72)	176	52.0	(9.36)	<0.001	140	47.0	(9.54)	188	48.9	(10.3)	173	52.4	(8.74)	<0.001
RCS	134	53.9	(9.26)	161	52.5	(10.1)	176	52.8	(10.7)	0.439	140	51.6	(11.4)	188	52.3	(9.63)	173	51.4	(9.59)	0.676

SD: Standard Deviation; PF: Physical Functioning; RP: Role Physical; BP: Bodily Pain; GH: General Health; VT: Vitality; SF: Social Function; RE: Role Emotional; MH: Mental Health; PCS: Physical Component Summary; MCS: Mental Component Summary; RCS: Role Component Summary; ANOVA was employed for categorical data.

Table 3. SF-36 scores of participants with or without chronic pain.

	With chronic pain			Without chronic pain			P value
	N	Mean	SD	N	Mean	SD	
PF	150	44.9	12.4	831	50.6	9.72	<0.001
RP	149	45.4	12.6	828	51.8	8.17	<0.001
BP	150	38.8	9.43	834	52.2	9.22	<0.001
GH	150	42.2	8.89	828	49.3	8.79	<0.001
VT	151	43.0	9.72	827	51.6	9.64	<0.001
SF	150	47.9	11.2	832	51.6	8.91	<0.001
RE	148	47.1	11.8	827	51.9	8.43	<0.001
MH	150	45.4	9.68	826	51.2	9.08	<0.001
PCS	145	41.7	11.9	817	50.1	9.38	<0.001
MCS	145	42.7	9.83	817	50.5	9.27	<0.001
RCS	145	52.5	13.4	817	52.3	9.48	0.838

SD: Standard Deviation; PF: Physical Functioning; RP: Role Physical; BP: Bodily Pain; GH: General Health; VT: Vitality; SF: Social Function; RE: Role Emotional; MH: Mental Health; PCS: Physical Component Summary; MCS: Mental Component Summary; RCS: Role Component Summary; ANCOVA was done with adjustment for age and gender.

Table 5 shows the results of multiple linear regression analysis with a forward stepwise approach to select independent variables for the three component summary scores. In this analysis, the independent variables included gender, age, and the site of pain. A lower PCS was independently correlated with CP at other sites ($p < 0.001$, $\beta = -0.172$), lumbar CP ($p < 0.001$, $\beta = -0.132$), age ($p < 0.001$, $\beta = -0.154$), knee CP ($p < 0.001$, $\beta = -0.115$), and foot CP ($p = 0.042$, $\beta = -0.065$). Older age ($p < 0.001$, $\beta = 0.221$) showed a significant positive correlation with MCS, while neck/shoulder CP ($p < 0.01$, $\beta = -0.096$), CP at other sites ($p < 0.001$, $\beta = -0.108$), knee CP ($p < 0.001$, $\beta = -0.109$), upper limb CP ($p < 0.01$, $\beta = -0.098$), and lumbar CP ($p = 0.022$, $\beta = -0.077$) all showed a significant negative correlation with MCS. Chronic headache ($p = 0.011$, $\beta = -0.082$) only showed a significant correlation with a lower RCS (**Table 5**).

Table 4. SF-36 component summary scores for subjects with or without chronic pain at different sites.

Chronic pain site		N	PCS			MCS			RCS		
			Mean	SD	P value	Mean	SD	P value	Mean	SD	P value
Head	(−)	962	48.8	10.3	0.171	49.4	9.77	0.013	52.5	10.0	0.013
	(+)	10	45.1	10.5		41.2	6.05		44.3	19.9	
Upper-limb	(−)	955	48.9	10.3	0.050	49.5	9.74	<0.001	52.4	10.0	0.365
	(+)	17	43.5	7.68		40.4	7.23		50.2	14.0	
Neck-shoulder	(−)	898	49.1	10.2	<0.001	49.8	9.59	<0.001	52.5	9.87	0.195
	(+)	70	44.0	10.8		43.1	9.70		50.9	13.0	
Lumbar	(−)	905	49.4	9.85	<0.001	49.8	9.66	<0.001	52.4	10.0	0.653
	(+)	61	40.9	12.4		43.4	9.31		51.9	12.5	
Knee	(−)	940	49.1	10.0	<0.001	49.6	9.68	<0.001	52.3	10.0	0.195
	(+)	30	39.2	12.5		42.2	10.2		54.7	13.0	
Foot	(−)	939	49.0	10.2	<0.001	49.5	9.77	<0.01	52.4	9.94	0.396
	(+)	31	40.7	11.0		44.9	8.69		50.9	14.9	
Others	(−)	946	49.1	10.0	<0.001	49.6	9.66	<0.001	52.4	10.0	0.835
	(+)	24	35.8	13.2		40.8	9.90		52.8	14.6	

SD: Standard Deviation; PCS: Physical Component Summary; MCS: Mental Component Summary; RCS: Role Component Summary; Others include chest, abdomen, hip, and back pain. ANCOVA was performed with adjustment for age and gender.

Table 5. Multiple regression analysis of the relations between 3 component summary score and the pain site, gender.

Criterion	Variables	B	SE	Beta Standardized	t	P	95.0% Confidence Interval for B	
							Lower Bound	Upper Bound
PCS	(Constant)	61.02	2.25		27.18	<0.001	56.6	65.4
	Others	−11.29	2.03	−0.172	−5.57	<0.001	−15.3	−7.31
	Lumbar	−5.55	1.35	−0.132	−4.12	<0.001	−8.19	−2.90
	Age	−0.21	0.04	−0.154	−5.03	<0.001	−0.285	−0.125
	Knee	−6.78	1.86	−0.115	−3.65	<0.001	−10.4	−3.13
	Foot	−3.78	1.86	−0.065	−2.03	0.042	−7.44	−0.133
MCS	(Constant)	34.94	2.15		16.28	<0.001	30.7	39.2
	Age	0.28	0.04	0.221	7.23	<0.001	0.205	0.357
	Neck-shoulder	−3.60	1.24	−0.096	−2.90	<0.01	−6.03	−1.17
	Others	−6.72	1.93	−0.108	−3.48	<0.001	−10.5	−2.93
	Knee	−6.11	1.74	−0.109	−3.51	<0.001	−9.52	−2.70
	Upper-limb	−7.22	2.30	−0.098	−3.14	<0.01	−11.7	−2.71
	Lumbar	−3.06	1.33	−0.077	−2.29	0.022	−5.68	−0.440
RCS	(Constant)	52.47	0.33		159.78	<0.001	51.8	53.1
	Head	−8.16	3.22	−0.082	−2.54	0.011	−14.5	−1.84

PCS; $R^2 = 0.117$, Adjusted $R^2 = 0.112$; MCS; $R^2 = 0.119$, Adjusted $R^2 = 0.113$; RCS; $R^2 = 0.07$, Adjusted $R^2 = 0.006$; SE: Standard Error; PCS: Physical Component Summary; MCS: Mental Component Summary; RCS: Role Component Summary; Others include chest, abdomen, hip, and back pain. Multiple linear regression analysis was performed with a forward stepwise approach, including gender, age, and site of pain.

4. Discussion

In previous reports, prevalence rates of CP have varied [6]-[8], possibly due to bias related to different collection rates of questionnaires and selection bias. Participants in other studies were selected from internet volunteers and mail survey panels, so there were relatively low response rates, such as 72.2% for internet research [6] and 55% for the mail survey [7] In addition, there have been few investigations into the prevalence of CP or the relationship between CP and HRQoL involving an epidemiological survey of all residents in a region. One of our aim was to clarify more accurate prevalence rate of CP and its relationship with and HRQoL. In this study, we defined CP as an NRS score of more than 5 so that we could perform comparison with previous studies. Our results indicated that the prevalence of CP was 15.3% among men and 15.1% among women. In addition, CP was more prevalent in the lumbar and neck/shoulder regions of our working age subjects. According to previous population-based surveys, the prevalence of CP was 19% in Europe and 13.6% in Japan [5] [6]. Our survey method agreed with the previous population-based finding that the prevalence of CP is about 15.0%, suggesting that our data were reliable.

The prevalence of chronic headache differs depending on the gender, age and geographic region [23]. Takeshima *et al.* examined the prevalence of headache in Daisen, a rural community in Japan, and reported that the prevalence of migraine was 2.3% in men and 9.1% in women [24]. An epidemiologic study performed by Sakai *et al.* revealed that the prevalence of migraine during the past year was 8.4% [25]. However, these studies assessed migraine and not chronic headache. Our study showed that the prevalence of chronic headache was 0.899% among men and 1.43% among women, suggest that there was no significant gender difference. Unfortunately, few data on chronic headache are available in Japan, different from migraine. Previous research has been performed in Spain [26], the Netherlands [27], the United States [28], and Korea [29], showing that the prevalence of chronic headache was 1.8% - 4.2%, with the lowest rate of 1.8% in Korea. These studies have suggested that the prevalence of chronic headache is lower in Asia than in western countries. Our results for a rural Japanese population support the concept that there is a lower prevalence of CP in Asia compared with Europe.

Suzukamo demonstrated that, among the 3 components of SF-36, RCS is strongly associated with the RP, SF, and RE subscales in specific social activities such as the number of times work, school, or housework missed for health-related reasons, and that this model was more appropriate than a two-component model for Japan and other Asian countries [22] [30]. It has been reported that social activities have independent health benefits [31], while the WHO has claimed that activity and participation involve factor structures in the international classification of functioning, disability, and health (ICF), in the same way as body function and structure [32].

We found that the influence of chronic headache on MCS and RCS, and not on PCS, whereas of musculoskeletal pain had a significant influence on PCS and MCS. Taken together with our identification of significant difference in PCS and MCS, but not in RCS between age categories, it seems that RCS is independent and distinct from either PCS or MCS in Japan.

It is noteworthy that our study demonstrated a relationship between chronic headache and RCS, because this has not been reported previously. Sakai *et al.* examined chronic tension headache and showed impairment of daily activities in 40.5% by this type of headache [33]. Bigal *et al.* reported that the impact of chronic headache is significantly greater than that of migraine, e.g. with regard to missing work and reducing productivity [11] [12]. In addition, Wang found lower SF-36 scores than normal in outpatients with headache and a lower score in those with chronic headache rather than migraine [34]. However, the influence of pain at other sites on HRQoL was not considered in previous studies. Holroyd *et al.* demonstrated that HRQoL scores were lower in chronic tension headache than in healthy controls, along with lower scores for back pain and arthritis [35]. In addition to our finding of a lower HRQoL in the present study population with chronic headache, we analyzed the effect of chronic headache after adjusting for pain at other sites which may have an impact on HRQoL. Therefore, our finding of a relationship between headache and RCS, which is supported by the above methods of analysis, provides convincing evidence for involvement of chronic headache in HRQoL (probably a different etiology from that at the other sites).

5. Conclusion

In conclusion, we demonstrated a relationship between RCS and chronic headache, but no relationships between RCS and musculoskeletal pain, while there was relationship between musculoskeletal pain and PCS or MCS. It suggested that RCS was independent component distinct from PCS and MCS in Japan. These results also suggested the influence of headache on HRQoL, probably because it had a different etiology from pain at other sites.

Acknowledgements

This study was supported by a Health Labour Sciences Research Grant for "Study on elucidation of the actual situation of intractable pain and development of countermeasures" (Principal Researcher: Takahiro Ushida, 2011-2012) and the fund for Priority Research Systems from Kanazawa University (No. 22,608) 2011-2012.

Limitations

There were some limitations of the present study. For example, it was a cross-sectional study with no clinical assessment. Causation cannot be inferred from a cross-sectional study, and prospective studies are needed to confirm causation. Also, we could not identify the etiology of pain, which would require objective investigations such as neurological examination or magnetic resonance imaging. Despite these limitations, we believe this study provides some useful insights for medical and public health practitioners because of the systematic method and high return rate of questionnaires.

References

[1]   Merskey, H. and Bogduk, N. (1994) Classification of Chronic Pain. 2nd Edition, IASP Task Force on Taxonomy. IASP Press, Seattle. http://www.iasp-pain.org/Education/content.aspx?ItemNumber=1698

[2]   Harstall, C. and Ospina, M. (2003) PAIN Clinical Updates 2003, XI, 7-9. http://iasp.files.cms-plus.com/Content/ContentFolders/Publications2/PainClinicalUpdates/Archives/PCU03-2_1390265 045864_38.pdf

[3]   Gureje, O., Von Korff, M., Simon, G.E. and Gater, R. (1998) Persistent Pain and Well-Being. *Jama*, **280**, 147. http://dx.doi.org/10.1001/jama.280.2.147

[4]   Dawson, J., Linsell, L., Zondervan, K., Rose, P., Carr, A., Randall, T., *et al.* (2005) Impact of Persistent Hip or Knee Pain on Overall Health Status in Elderly People: A Longitudinal Population Study. *Arthritis Rheum*, **53**, 368-374. http://dx.doi.org/10.1002/art.21180

[5]   Breivik, H., Collett, B., Ventafridda, V., Cohen, R. and Gallacher, D. (2006) Survey of Chronic Pain in Europe: Prevalence, Impact on Daily Life, and Treatment. *European Journal of Pain*, **10**, 287-333. http://dx.doi.org/10.1016/j.ejpain.2005.06.009

[6]   Hattori, S. (2006) The Prevalence of Chronic Pain in Japan. *Nihon Yakurigaku Zasshi*, **127**, 176-180. http://dx.doi.org/10.1254/fpj.127.176

[7]   Nakamura, M., Nishiwaki, Y., Ushida, T. and Toyama, Y. (2011) Prevalence and Characteristics of Chronic Musculoskeletal Pain in Japan. *Journal of Orthopaedic Science*, **16**, 424-432. http://dx.doi.org/10.1007/s00776-011-0102-y

[8]   Matsudaira, K., Takeshita, K., Kunogi, J., Yamazaki, T., Hara, N., Yamada, H., *et al.* (2011) Prevalence and Characteristics of Chronic Pain in the General Japanese Population. *Pain Clin*, **32**, 1345-1356.

[9]   Suka, M. and Yoshida, K. (2009) The National Burden of Musculoskeletal Pain in Japan: Projections to the Year 2055. *Questionnaire Survey on Musculoskeletal Pain*, **25**, 313-319.

[10]   Nakamura, M., Nishiwaki, Y., Ushida, T. and Toyama, Y. (2014) Prevalence and Characteristics of Chronic Musculoskeletal Pain in Japan: A Second Survey of People with or without Chronic Pain. *Journal of Orthopaedic Science*, **19**, 339-350. http://dx.doi.org/10.1007/s00776-013-0525-8

[11]   Bigal, M.E., Rapoport, A.M., Lipton, R.B., Tepper, S.J. and Sheftell, F.D. (2003) Assessment of Migraine Disability Using the Migraine Disability Assessment (MIDAS) Questionnaire: A Comparison of Chronic Migraine with Episodic Migraine. *Headache*, **43**, 336-342. http://dx.doi.org/10.1046/j.1526-4610.2003.03068.x

[12]   Bigal, M.E., Serrano, D., Reed, M. and Lipton, R.B. (2008) Chronic Migraine in the Population: Burden, Diagnosis, and Satisfaction with Treatment. *Neurology*, **71**, 559-566. http://dx.doi.org/10.1212/01.wnl.0000323925.29520.e7

[13]   Buse, D.C., Manack, A., Serrano, D., Turkel, C. and Lipton, R.B. (2010) Sociodemographic and Comorbidity Profiles of Chronic Migraine and Episodic Migraine Sufferers. *Journal of Neurology, Neurosurgery & Psychiatry*, **81**, 428-432. http://dx.doi.org/10.1136/jnnp.2009.192492

[14]   Fukuhara, S., Bito, S., Green, J., Hsiao, A. and Kurokawa, K. (1998) Translation, Adaptation, and Validation of the SF-36 Health Survey for Use in Japan. *Journal of Clinical Epidemiology*, **51**, 1037-1044. http://dx.doi.org/10.1016/S0895-4356(98)00095-X

[15] Fukuhara, S. and Yoshimi, S. (2011) Manual of SF-36v2 Japanese Version. Institute for Health Outcome and Process Evaluation Research.

[16] Fukuhara, S., Ware, J.E., Kosinski, M., Wada, S. and Gandek, B. (1998) Psychometric and Clinical Tests of Validity of the Japanese SF-36 Health Survey. *Journal of Clinical Epidemiology*, **51**, 1045-1053. http://dx.doi.org/10.1016/S0895-4356(98)00095-X

[17] Li, L., Wang, H.M. and Shen, Y. (2003) Chinese SF-36 Health Survey: Translation, Cultural Adaptation, Validation, and Normalisation. *Journal of Epidemiology & Community Health*, **57**, 259-263. http://dx.doi.org/10.1136/jech.57.4.259

[18] Yu, J., Coons, S.J., Draugalis, J.R., Ren, X.S. and Hays, R.D. (2003) Equivalence of Chinese and US-English Versions of the SF-36 Health Survey. *Quality of Life Research*, **12**, 449-457. http://dx.doi.org/10.1023/A:1023446110727

[19] Fuh, J.L., Wang, S.J., Lu, S.R., Juang, K.D., Lee, S.J. (2000) Psychometric Evaluation of a Chinese (Taiwanese) Version of the SF-36 Health Survey amongst Middle-Aged Women from a Rural Community. *Quality of Life Research*, **9**, 675-683. http://dx.doi.org/10.1023/A:1008993821633

[20] Thumboo, J., Fong, K.Y., Machin, D., Chan, S.P., Leon, K.H., Feng, P.H., *et al.* (2001) A Community-Based Study of Scaling Assumptions and Construct Validity of the English (UK) and Chinese (HK) SF-36 in Singapore. *Quality of Life Research*, **10**, 175-188. http://dx.doi.org/10.1023/A:1016701514299

[21] Ware Jr., J.E., Kosinski, M., Bayliss, M.S., McHorney, C.A., Rogers, W.H. and Raczek, A. (1995) Comparison of Methods for the Scoring and Statistical Analysis of SF-36 Health Profile and Summary Measures: Summary of Results from the Medical Outcomes Study. *Medical Care*, **33**, AS264-AS279.

[22] Suzukamo, Y., Fukuhara, S., Green, J., Kosinski, M., Gandek, B. and Ware, J.E. (2011) Validation Testing of a Three-Component Model of Short Form-36 Scores. *Journal of Clinical Epidemiology*, **64**, 301-308. http://dx.doi.org/10.1016/j.jclinepi.2010.04.017

[23] Jensen, R. and Stovner, L.J. (2008) Epidemiology and Comorbidity of Headache. *The Lancet Neurology*, **7**, 354-361. http://dx.doi.org/10.1016/S1474-4422(08)70062-0

[24] Takeshima, T., Ishizaki, K., Fukuhara, Y., Ijiri, T., Kusumi, M., Wakutani, Y., *et al.* (2004) Population-Based Door-to-Door Survey of Migraine in Japan: The Daisen Study. *Headache*, **44**, 8-19. http://dx.doi.org/10.1111/j.1526-4610.2004.04004.x

[25] Sakai, F. and Igarashi, H. (1997) Prevalence of Migraine in Japan: A Nationwide Survey. *Cephalalgia*, **17**, 15-22. http://dx.doi.org/10.1046/j.1468-2982.1997.1701015.x

[26] Castillo, J., Mu-oz, P., Guitera, V. and Pascual, J. (1999) Kaplan Award 1998. Epidemiology of Chronic Daily Headache in the General Population. *Headache*, **39**, 190-196. http://dx.doi.org/10.1046/j.1526-4610.1999.3903190.x

[27] Russell, M.B. (2005) Tension-Type Headache in 40-Year-Olds: A Danish Population-Based Sample of 4000. *The Journal of Headache and Pain*, **6**, 441-447. http://dx.doi.org/10.1007/s10194-005-0253-3

[28] Scher, A.I., Stewart, W.F., Liberman, J. and Lipton, R.B. (1998) Wolff Award 1998 Prevalence of Frequent Headache in a Population Sample. *Headache*, **38**, 497-506. http://dx.doi.org/10.1046/j.1526-4610.1998.3807497.x

[29] Park, J., Moon, H., Kim, J., Lee, K. and Chu, M.K. (2014) Chronic Daily Headache in Korea: Prevalence, Clinical Characteristics, Medical Consultation and Management. *Journal of Clinical Neurology*, **10**, 236-243. http://dx.doi.org/10.3988/jcn.2014.10.3.236

[30] Nezu, S., Okamoto, N., Morikawa, M., Saeki, K., Obayashi, K., Tomioka, K., *et al.* (2014) Health-Related Quality of Life (HRQOL) Decreases Independently of Chronic Conditions and Geriatric Syndromes in Older Adults with Diabetes: The Fujiwara-Kyo Study. *Journal of Epidemiology*, **24**, 259-266. http://dx.doi.org/10.2188/jea.JE20130131

[31] Glass, T.A., de Leon, C.M., Marottoli, R.A. and Berkman, L.F. (1999) Population Based Study of Social and Productive Activities as Predictors of Survival among Elderly Americans. *BMJ*, **319**, 478-483. http://dx.doi.org/10.1136/bmj.319.7208.478

[32] World Health Organization (2001) International Classification of Functioning, Disability and Health (ICF). Geneva. http://www.who.int/classifications/icf/en/

[33] Sakai, F. and Igarashi, H. (1997) Prevalence of Migraine in Japan: A Nationwide Survey. *Cephalalgia*, **17**, 15-22. http://dx.doi.org/10.1046/j.1468-2982.1997.1701015.x

[34] Wang, S.J., Fuh, J.L., Lu, S.R. and Juang, K.D. (2001) Quality of Life Differs among Headache Diagnoses: Analysis of SF-36 Survey in 901 Headache Patients. *Pain*, **89**, 285-292. http://dx.doi.org/10.1016/S0304-3959(00)00380-8

[35] Holroyd, K.A., Stensland, M., Lipchik, G.L., Hill, K.R., O'Donnell, F.S. and Cordingley, G. (2000) Psychosocial Correlates and Impact of Chronic Tension-Type Headaches. *Headache*, **40**, 3-16. http://dx.doi.org/10.1046/j.1526-4610.2000.00001.x

20

Controlling Dengue: Effectiveness of Biological Control and Vaccine in Reducing the Prevalence of Dengue Infection in Endemic Areas

Bryan Paul[1]*, Wai Liang Tham[2]

[1]Faculty of Science, University of Alberta, Edmonton, Canada
[2]Faculty of Medicine, University of British Columbia, Vancouver, Canada
Email: *bpaul@ualberta.ca, *bryanpaul.ian@gmail.com

Abstract

With the increased prevalence of dengue infection in tropical countries, concerned members of the public are now pressing their local health ministries to act immediately and effectively in managing the rising numbers of reported cases. This includes reviews of the methodologies and the effectiveness of current combative systems to find other possible novel approaches that might yield better results. One of those novel approaches is the integration of a parasite into mosquito vector, manipulating the parasite-host interaction to reduce the transmission of dengue in endemic hotspots. Another alternative is by Sanofi-Pasteur's dengue vaccine that showed over 60.8% success rate in reducing severe dengue infection in children aged 9 - 16 during its final clinical implementation phase. This report will compare and contrast these two novel ideas to determine which of the approaches are more likely to be effective in the long run. The aspects covered will include the application, effectiveness, functionality, and problems with these approaches. The results could then be utilised by governments or organizations to select precise and effective methods in reducing the prevalence of dengue infections in their countries.

Keywords

Dengue, Pathogenesis, Pathology, Immunology, Biological Control, Vaccine

---

*Corresponding author.

1. Introduction

Dengue, which uses arthropods and other mosquitoes as vectors, is common in tropical and sub-tropical climates, and is often associated with other diseases such as malaria, chikungunya, yellow fever, St. Louis encephalitis, West Nile virus, Japanese encephalitis, and Tick-borne encephalitis [1] [2]. Commonly transmitted by the mosquitoes *Aedes aegypti* and *Aedes albopictus*, dengue is considered one of the fastest growing hemorrhagic viruses worldwide [1]-[4]. It is less well-known due to the localisation of the disease, which is uncommon outside of tropical and sub-tropical regions [4]. Recently, increased travelling to and from endemic countries has resulted in the spread of dengue in new regions [2] [4] [5]. From 2010 to 2013, dengue outbreaks have been reported in several European countries and in the United States [4] [5]. The outbreaks are believed imported via travellers that visited endemic regions such as the Caribbean, Asia, and Latin America [4] [5]. Closer to home, Canadian authorities issued warning for travellers to be alert on dengue fever including what to do and to look for if they get infected [6].

Factors such as rapid population growth and the ease of migration also compound the problems of endemic nations. Close contact between human and vectors coupled with an increased size of the host population often increases the chances of contracting dengue [7]-[9]. The widespread occurrence of such population networks plays significant roles in distributing the disease, and pathologically, this condition often provide excellent room for disease to continue developing and growing [8] [10]. Additionally, global economic trade from endemic countries such as the shipment of used tires and changing weather patterns also contributes to the expansion of dengue infections beyond the vector's niche [7] [11] [12].

According to May 2015 update, the World Health Organisation (WHO) estimated that over 3.9 billion people worldwide are at risk of contracting dengue and there are roughly 284 - 528 million infections every year [13]. 500,000 people are hospitalised with severe dengue annually and 2.5% of them succumb to the infection [13]. Of all reported cases, most of the patients with severe infection of dengue are children [13]. With high numbers of infections and mortality rates, the dengue endemic can no longer be ignored.

As an example, dengue cases in Malaysia alone show an astonishing increment towards the end of 2014 with 43,346 cases reported from January to September 2013, while 76,700 cases were reported within the same window in 2014 [14]. Out of all these reported cases, another major increase of death toll was observed from 43 cases in 2013 to 146 cases in 2014 [14]. With an estimated increase of 76.9% sufferers, dengue has become a major health issue in Malaysia, with local news media and the public criticizing their health ministry for failing to curb the increase in the prevalence of the disease [15]. According to Paul and Tham (2015), in January 2015, the numbers of infected individuals keep increasing by 59% when compared to similar statistic of the same month in 2014 [16].

Several combative measures across all endemic countries have been applied and tested to suppress the prevalence of dengue over the years and most common one is the heavy use of *Aedes* larvicide [7] [14]. Others include education on dengue pathogenesis and pathology for public and active extermination of mosquito breeding sites, which include all bodies of stagnant water [7] [14].

In this study, the use of vaccines and biological control will be discussed. Current research and experimental results of these dengue protective ideas will be discussed and evaluated in terms of their functionality, confidence, and application in endemic areas. In addition, problems that may arise upon the application of both measures once they are introduced indefinitely will be evaluated. The pathogenesis and pathology of dengue will also be discussed to provide strong arguments to support the use of vaccines and biological control in preventing dengue infection.

2. Pathogenesis and Pathology of Dengue

Transmitted by the mosquito vectors *A. aegypti* and *A. albopictus*, dengue is a viral type disease (arbovirus) and is categorised as viral hemorrhagic fevers (VHF) [1]-[4]. Common dengue serotypes called DENV (dengue virus) that are found globally are DENV-1, DENV-2, DENV-3, and DENV-4 [1]-[4] [7] [11] [13] [17]. Recently, dengue researchers have also found a new serotype of dengue, DENV-5, from infected patients in Borneo [18]. Out of this five serotypes, DENV-3 and DENV-4 have been associated with the Dengue Shock Syndrome (DSS) stage, whereby the infection deemed severe and often leads to fatalities [17]. As seen in **Figure 1**, DENV1 and DENV 3 are found to be highly associated with a 95% species similarity, while DENV2 is closely related to a

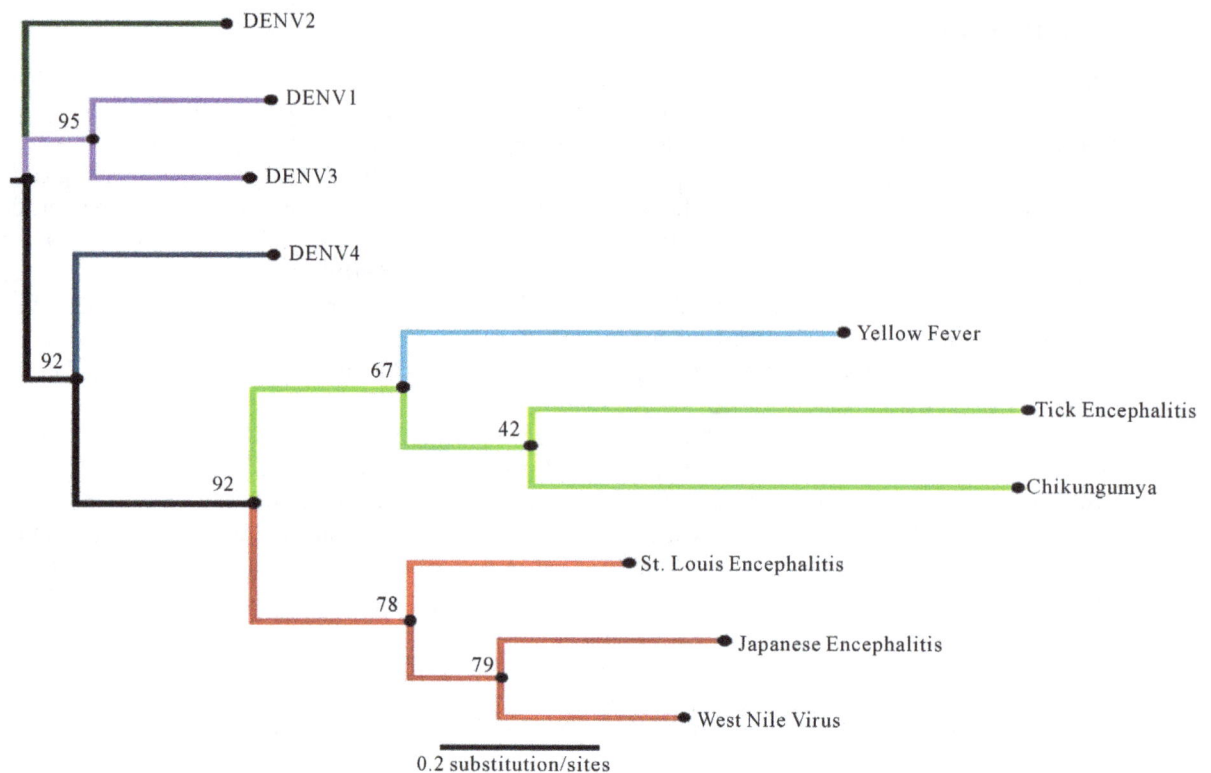

Figure 1. Phylogenetic Tree of Viral Hemorrhagic Fever (VHF) viruses of family *Flaviviridae*. Tree is made using complete genomic sequences obtained from National Center for Biotechnology Information (NCBI) of which accession numbers are given. Bootstrap values are illustrated between most nodes and based on calculation of 100 possible combinations. Higher bootstrap value signifies higher similarity between species of viruses. Phylogenetic illustration is made using the software Geneious and FigTree v1.4.2.

flaviviridae ancestor, and DENV4 is closely related to other *flaviviridae* viruses. The accession numbers of all serotypes used to construct the phylogenetic tree are M87512.1 (DENV1), M29095.1 (DENV2), AY662691.1 (DENV3), AF326825.1 (DENV4), NC_001672.1 (Tick-borne Encephalitis), AY 508813.1 (Japanese Encephalitis), NC_007580.2 (St. Louis Encephalitis), HM147824.1 (West Nile Virus), NC_ 004162.2 (chikungunya) and NC_002031.1 (Yellow Fever) [19]-[28].

Classified as a flavivirus, dengue is composed of a single positive-stranded RNA virus of the *Flaviviridae* family [4] [29]. Immunologically, viruses of RNA origin have proved to be difficult to treat due to their ability to rapidly change their genomic structures, or because pathogenicity islands may favour their development [18]. These factors have made these viruses highly successful in maintaining their reservoir and may become infectious in any environment or host they occupy. DENV is known to be equipped with three main protein structures and as many as seven non-structural proteins that encode for its pathogenicity [30]. These three main proteins; E-protein, prM/M protein, and C proteins are thought to be responsible for the component of the virus including attachment while the NS1, NS2A/B, NS3, NS4A/B, and NS5 non-structural proteins are deemed essential for its replication mechanism [30].

Jain *et al.* (2014) argue that DENV can infect a diverse range of insect or mammalian cells due to its structure [31]. This is typical for mosquito vector diseases in which a virus can 'hop' in from the arthropod host to an intermediate host [32].When inoculated into humans, DENV will deliver itself to the liver cells (hepatocytes) and to the intestinal cells (enterocytes) for further development and replication [31] [33]. In severe infection, this virus can cause necrosis of these hepatocytes and enterocytes which often leads to tissues loss and blood loss [33].

Early detection of dengue infection can often save lives [3] [4]. Due to its latency within the first few days post infection, an infected person will not know he or she is infected until specific symptoms are expressed, as seen in **Figure 2** [3] [4]. Normal symptoms of early infection are documented as headache, retro-orbital pain, muscle aches, joint pain, fever, and rashes [2]-[4]. These symptoms are often observed during the Dengue

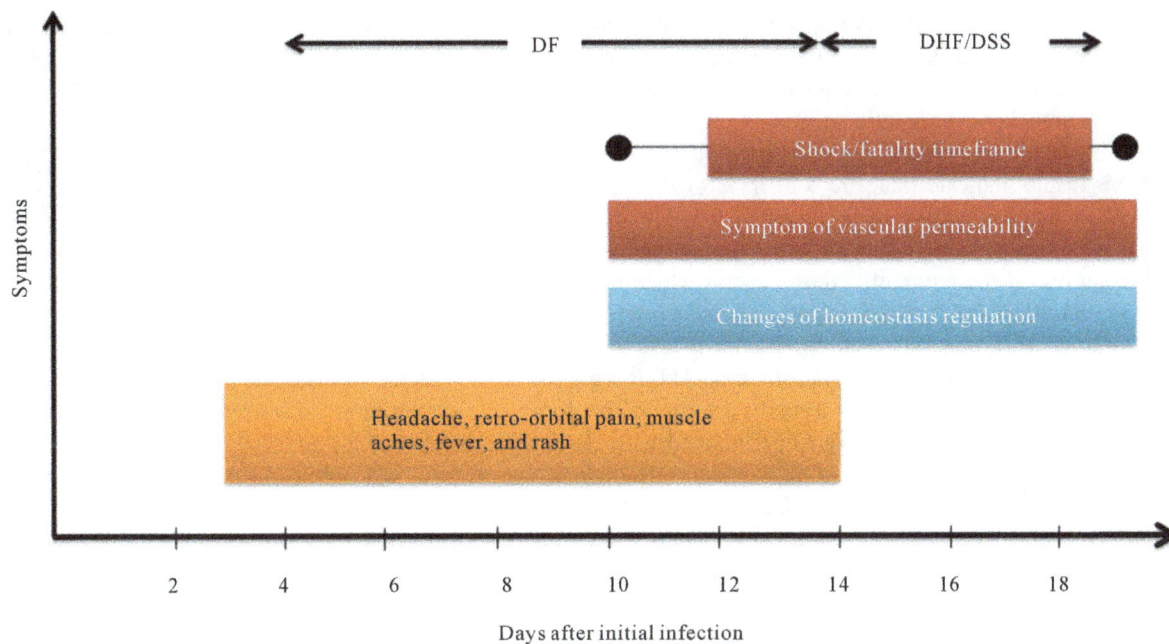

Figure 2. Adaptation of generalised timescale of dengue infection within a patient. Figure illustrates generalised symptoms of dengue including major infection stages. Symptoms according to collection literatures only exist after initial infection in a host. Figure is a summary of symptoms taken from various studies on dengue infections and pathologies.

Fever (DF) stage which is between 3 to 14 days post infection [2]-[4] [34]. About 10 days post infection, dengue will start to progress into a new phase called Dengue Haemorrhagic Fever (DHF) stage and is often coupled with the lethal DSS stage [2]-[4]. Within the DHF/DSS period, dengue infection can lead to shock, thus causing fatalities if left unattended and untreated [2]-[4]. In DSS stage, patients are often observed showing changes in the homeostatic regulation and vascular permeability coupled with appearance of bleeding out as their cell integrity is compromised and start to haemolyse [3] [9] [33] [35].

Although countless of researches had been conducted on dengue over the past 50 years of its discovery, the pathogenesis of dengue (specifically) is not yet entirely known and our understanding of this disease is limited [31] [36]. This will later influence our discussions on the choice of combative measures and their effectiveness when dealing with DENV.

3. Dengue Vectors Biological Control

The simplest concept of biological control is defined as a method to reduce pests using their natural antagonists to maintain equilibrium in a disrupted population [37] [38]. Dengue researchers have therefore developed the idea of using the *Aedes* mosquito's natural parasites or predators to supress the transmission of DENV and disrupt the life-cycle of the arthropod vector. These include utilising extensive studies of parasite-host interaction in *Aedes* vectors by the use of parasitic bacteria and more traditional method such as introducing predatory fishes into mosquito breeding sites [39]-[45]. The concept of introducing insect parasites as a means of suppressing dengue will be specifically discussed.

As humans, we harbour millions of other organisms in our body that live either as symbionts or parasites [46]. Similarly, insects of various classes and orders also have other organisms living freely within them. Specific parasites in dengue vectors can be manipulated to fight these vectors [41]-[45]. However, it is imperative that we look for the parasites that are present in all of the vector's life stages to increase the effectiveness and efficacy of biological control.

Marimuthu *et al.* (2013) discussed the idea of introducing "eco-friendly" bacteria parasites in mosquitoes because of the increasing resistance of mosquito larvae to commonly used larvicide. *Bacillus thuringiensis* was found to be highly specific and a common parasite in mosquitoes of the Diptera order, such as *Aedes* and *Anopheles* (Malaria) [39] [40]. The specificity is due to *B. thuringiensis* ability to produce a specific toxin (δ-toxin) that is toxic to mosquito larva, thus reducing the amount of emerging adults mosquitoes in the environment [39]. This however is no longer the case as recently there are reports indicating that mosquito's larva develop resistance against their bacterial parasites thus rendering useless the application of inoculating wild-type *B. thuringiensis* into larva population [39] [47]. However, if *B. thuringiensis* is inoculated with cobalt nanoparticles (Co-NPs), the effectiveness of bacteria toxicity is increased, thus reducing the resistance issues faced earlier [39]. Their results indicate that 100% of *A. aegypti* larva died after introduction of an 8 - 10 fold concentration of Co-NPs into the larval population whereas wild-type *B. thuringiensis* required a 20-fold concentration to achieve the same results [39]. Although with promising results, there are no indications that the result of the study is being applied at the moment. Other bacteria which had been studied as bacterial parasites for the mosquitoes include *Bacillus cereus*, *Streptomyces* sp., and *Paecilomyces* sp. [39].

Similar to *B. thuringiensis*, *Wolbachia* is also a species of insects' bacteria but is classified more as a symbiont rather than a parasite of mosquitoes [41]. *Wolbachia* is not species specific and it possesses symbiotic diversity towards other insects within the arthropod kingdom [41]. It is estimated that 25% to 70% of insects in the phylum Arthropoda are known to be infected with *Wolbachia* and become hosts [41]. *Wolbachia* targets adult mosquitoes instead of the larva and is found residing in the mid-gut and ovaries [42] [45]. Other locations of *Wolbachia* within the insect host include salivary glands and the brain, which may be correlated with reduced DENV transmission and replication [45]. The first observed pathology of *Wolbachia* in *Aedes* is that the bacteria induced restrictions on the reproduction process in infected female mosquitoes by changing their reproduction cycle and life-span, thus reducing their ability to produce progeny [48]. *Wolbachia* will modulate high iron level in the mosquito during blood meals, especially within the ovaries, thus disrupting the mosquito's reproduction cycle [45]. In addition, shorter life-spans are observed within affected populations, thus reducing the chances of female mosquito obtaining blood meals from their preferred host and to mate with male mosquito [42]. Other studies conducted also illustrate that infected female mosquito are less likely to produce offspring when mating with non-infected male mosquito and vice versa [43]. Results indicated mixed outcomes as one study illustrates that the prevalence of dengue transmission is discovered to be much lower if male *Aedes* is infected with *Wolbachia* while another study indicates lower dengue transmission with infected female *Aedes* [43] [44].

The parasite-host idea of using *Wolbachia* infected mosquitoes to control transmission of dengue was then tested in the field by releasing these mosquitoes into the environment to mate with the wild mosquito population. Field studies conducted in Australia show that the *Wolbachia* strain ωMel managed to colonize most of the wild-type *Aedes* mosquitos' population and that the results correlate with significant reduction of DENV infection in a specific area [45]. In addition, the study also concluded that other RNA viruses transmitted by *Aedes* species such as malaria, chikungunya, yellow fever, and West Nile viruses are greatly reduced in *Wolbachia*-infected mosquito population [45]. Other similar studies had been conducted in other endemic areas globally and their results also show a significant reduction in DENV transmission by *Wolbachia* infected mosquitoes [15].

4. Dengue Virus (DENV) Vaccine

One of the popular choices in medicine to eradicate a disease is to use vaccines. Vaccines have demonstrated the ability to produce a major reduction in disease-related mortality and prevalence in a human population [49]. The first flavivirus vaccine successfully developed is Max Theiler's YFD (yellow fever disease) vaccine in 1951 [50]. The vaccine was created using attenuated live virus in which has saved more than 500 million people globally since its introduction in 1937 [50].

From an immunological perspective, the usage of live-attenuated virus in vaccine is considered to be an effective way of inducing immune responses since attenuated virus can "teach" our immune system to readily recognize antigen molecular patterns upon subsequent infections [51]. The end product of this inoculation is the production of "licensed" memory cells during the humoral and adaptive immune stages, in which these cells will readily fight against further viral invasion [51].

The development of DENV vaccines should encompass all the serotypes present in order for it to be successful [2] [4] [18] [31] [36] [50]. A multivalent vaccine is important in dengue virus treatment as a vaccine that targets one serotype will only be specific to that serotype viral structures but not others [11] [36] [50] [52]. In an endemic area, a person can be infected with either one serotype or multiple serotypes of DENV [11] [36] [50] [52]. Targets of vaccines should encompass all the main protein structures as well as the non-structural proteins as discussed in the previous section. At the moment, available DENV vaccines produced or on production only target four out of five serotypes presence (mainly because DENV5 is new and a vaccine is yet to be developed) and is known as tetravalent vaccine [50] [52].

The idea of tetravalent vaccine, a concocted mixture containing all live-attenuated DENV serotypes to teach human immune response to recognize and target them, was first developed in the early 2000s at Mahidol University, Thailand as a novel way to combat the prevalence of DENV1-4 that affected many individuals in Southeast Asia [48]. Similarly as YFV vaccine, the dengue tetravalent vaccine is made by using live-attenuated virus of dengue of which serotypes DENV1, DENV2, and DENV4 attenuated viruses are developed using dog kidney cells and serotype DENV3 attenuated virus developed using African green monkey kidney cells [48] [53]. Attenuated viruses are subjected to bio-marker testing in the kidney cells of tested animals and follow procedures outline in **Figure 3** prior to manufacturing a vaccine [53]. This early tetravalent vaccine was not deemed successful as the patient vaccinated with the vaccine showed occurrence of dengue-like symptoms after clinical testing [48]. The reason of the failure can be caused by different factors, and a plausible explanation is that the attenuated virus might regain its pathogenicity after inoculation. Further improvement is then made with the vaccine by other organizations in which it is renovated using a recombinant live-attenuated virus using mixture of live YFV virus with live dengue virus [48] [53]-[55]. The results differ significantly since the first clinical trial of a vaccinated patient showed immuno-competency on all four DENV serotypes and did not show any sign of dengue-like symptoms [48].

Thailand was the first country to test the redesigned tetravalent vaccine of TDEN (Tetravalent Dengue) that targeted all four serotypes, and clinical results indicate symptoms and clinical signs of dengue were greatly reduced to mild, or moderate, and or transient stages [52]. Additionally, the team of researchers had also given promising review that the TDEN vaccine does not result in serious vaccines-related side-effects [52]. In Malaysia, another tetravalent vaccine called CYD-TDV (tetravalent candidate dengue vaccine) is utilised [56]. The target comprises of healthy children aged 2 - 11 years and clinical results are satisfactory, whereby the humoral immune system, responsible for antigen-viral recognition, respond to all four DENV serotypes [56]. Similar studies in Thailand and their clinical results indicate that the CYD-TDV vaccine protected those vaccinated against all four serotypes and volunteers did not express side-effects after vaccination [56].

Recently, Sanofi-Pasteur announced that they have managed to develop a successful dengue vaccine in which their final clinical trial shows a tremendous reduction of 60.8% of dengue infection in vaccinated volunteers [57] [58]. These volunteers comprised of more than 20,000 children aged 9 - 16 from countries in Latin America, and were observed to be highly protected against dengue infection, specifically in the DHF stages [57]. In addition, it is estimated that roughly around 80% of these volunteers escaped the risk of hospitalisation and over 90% are protected against severe dengue symptoms [58]. The vaccine used for this clinical trial is of CYD-TDV similar to that utilised in clinical trials in Thailand and Malaysia. The method of administering the vaccine is done in three-dose vaccinations over 25 months [58]. Although promising, the published study involved only volunteers from one geographical region. However, Sanofi-Pasteur's head of research and development assured the public

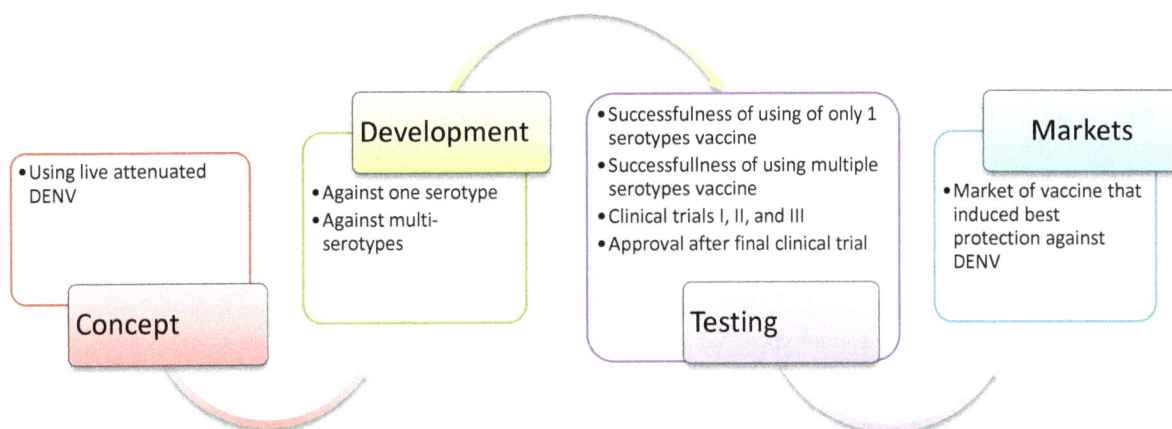

Figure 3. Step in utilising concept to develop effective vaccine. Model illustrates the simplified pathway in creating effective vaccines before being introduced permanently to publics.

that the vaccine could work effectively given the outstanding and consistent results [58]. Overall, Sanofi's clinical trials had involved more than 40,000 volunteers across the globe and these volunteers are predominantly those that live in endemic areas of Asia and Latin America [59].

5. Discussion

Both biological control and vaccination present outstanding results in managing the prevalence of dengue in their experimental areas. We are now left with a choice between the aforementioned combative measures in order to assure maximum effectiveness and towards reducing dengue.

Biological control enables the manipulation of the parasite-host interaction or symbiont to reduce dengue transmission in endemic areas. Two studies that we looked into were the use of parasitic bacteria *B. thuringiensis* and symbiotic bacteria *Wolbachia*. Although both produced outstanding results, we encountered several problems related to the manipulation of the relationship between these bacteria and *Aedes* mosquitoes. First, the mosquitoes' populations inoculated with *B. thuringiensis* are shown to develop resistance towards *B. thuringiensis* after period of time, signifying that the *Aedes* mosquito might possess immunity against its parasitic tenants [39] [47]. Secondly, mosquitos inoculated with *Wolbachia* shows preference in shutting down transmission of certain serotype of DENV rather than all serotypes. Frentiu *et al.* (2014) illustrate that *Wolbachia*-infected mosquitoes shut down the transmission of DENV1 but continued transmitting DENV2 and DENV 3 [45]. It is mentioned that the DENV3 serotype is one of the two severe serotypes of DENV that may induce shock and death. *Aedes* may also develop resistance towards *Wolbachia* symbiont as illustrated by the case of *B. thuringiensis*. Thus, studies concerning mosquito immunology are important in preventing the possibility of mosquito developing resistance. Other concerns are the environmental impact on the overall ecosystem. In Malaysia for example, environmentalists are against the introduction of *Wolbachia* infected mosquitoes into the wild for reason that it may pollute Malaysia's pristine rainforest condition [15]. However several studies conducted on usage of treated mosquito assured the public that introduction of these mosquitoes does not risk any potential damage to the environment and the existing food chain.

In vaccination, the main problem that may arise is the issue of resistance towards the vaccine itself. Viruses are known to have rapid replication and can interchange genomes depending on whether the viruses benefit from the changes or not. This creates a situation in which the development of new vaccines tends to become obsolete due to the fast changes in viruses' genomics structures. This inevitable issue creates another problem in which pharmaceutical companies completely stop producing new vaccine as they do not see the incentives in continuing as it is deemed economically unprofitable [60]. Next is the issue of using live-attenuated viruses in vaccine. Although attenuated, small percentage of these viruses may revert back to their original pathology, thus resulting in accidental secondary DENV infection towards those vaccinated [52] [61]. As shown in the study of first tetravalent vaccine, vaccinated patients show a recurrence in dengue-like infection post vaccination [48]. Method of delivery and stability of the vaccine might also pose an issue for a vaccine to effectively work. In major endemic areas, most of the vulnerable individuals live beyond reach of modernization and this creates the problem of accessing electricity needed to cool live attenuate virus in order to keeping them stable [61]. In addition, an effective dengue vaccine needs to encompass all serotypes in existence for optimal effectiveness. Although Sanofi-Pasteur successfully created the functional tetravalent dengue vaccine, they would need to factor in the emergence DENV5 in Southeast Asia. Another possible problem with vaccine is that it cannot be used to treat immuno-competent patient as it may lead to other secondary infections in that patient [60]. The suggestions to improve the efficacy of vaccine are to develop new vaccines to target specific sites in DENV that cannot be interchanged, creating stabilised vaccines that can be delivered at any temperature without the chances of reversion, and continual research and study of drugs efficient enough against the virus but do not adversely affect the intended host [61].

Overall, biological control approach seems to be a viable option at the moment as it deals with the issue of transmission at its root and is inexpensive to cultivate [42]-[45]. Although it may be slightly problematic, the approach tends to be an excellent and effective combative measure in long-term protection against dengue transmission in any endemic areas. Note that for added protection, vaccination should also be considered as this approach can help induce a stronger immune response against dengue infection. Education about dengue's pathology could also help to reduce dengue transmission, since everyone will feel responsible for maintaining the cleanliness of his or her environment [3]. However, as mentioned previously, we still do not know much about this disease and a lot is still needed to be done to understand it. Therefore, more research is still needed on these two combative measures to make them impenetrable to dengue replication and reproduction. Suggestion of researches in the future are to create novel vaccine that directly target main proteins that are essential for DENV attachment regardless of serotypes whilst weakening its non-structural proteins and finding a sustainable ecological approach to weaken DENV transmission via introduction of a novel parasite-symbiont bacteria that is counter-resistant to mosquitos and larvae capabilities of manipulating their genome to resist bacterial infections.

Acknowledgements

Writing is conducted by B.P and T.W.L. Editing and proofreading is conducted by W.L.T. Research, data collections, and analysis is conducted by B.P. Data and statistic on Malaysia's Dengue can be obtained from World Health Organisation (WHO) at http://www.who.int/mediacentre/factsheets/fs117/en/. Article is produced by undergraduates, B.P (UAlberta) and T.W.L. (UBC).

References

[1] (2014) Mosquito-Borne Diseases. American Mosquito Control Association.
http://www.mosquito.org/mosquito-borne-diseases

[2] McFee, R.B. (2013) Viral Hemorrhagic Fever Viruses. *Disease-a-Month*, **59**, 410-425.
http://dx.doi.org/10.1016/j.disamonth.2013.10.003

[3] (2014) Sign and Symptom of Dengue Virus. http://www.denguevirusnet.com/signs-a-symptoms.html

[4] Mangold, K. and Reynolds, S. (2013) Review of Dengue Fever. *Pediatric Emergency Care*, **29**, 665-669.
http://dx.doi.org/10.1097/PEC.0b013e31828ed30e

[5] Wilson, M.E., Weld, L.H., Boggild, A., Keystone, J.S., Kain, K.C., Sonnenburg, F. and Schwartz, E. (2007) Fever in Return Travellers: Result from the Geosentinel Surveillance Network. *Clinical Infectious Diseases*, **44**, 1560-1568.
http://dx.doi.org/10.1086/518173

[6] Government of Canada (2014) Dengue Fever. http://travel.gc.ca/travelling/health-safety/diseases/dengue

[7] Sizmur, C. (2014) Malaysia Steps up Campaign against Dengue.
http://www.publichealth.basf.com/agr/ms/public-health/en_GB/content/public-health/our-partners/Dengue/dengue_in_malaysia

[8] Hu, H., Nigmatulina, K. and Eckhoff, P. (2013) The Scaling of Contact Rates with Population Density for the Infectious Disease Models. *Mathematical Biosciences*, **244**, 125-134. http://dx.doi.org/10.1016/j.mbs.2013.04.013

[9] Tam, J.S., Barbeschi, M., Shapovalova, N., Briand, S., Memish, Z.A. and Kieny, M.P. (2012) Research Agenda for Mass Gatherings: A Call to Action. *Lancet Infection*, **12**, 231-239. http://dx.doi.org/10.1016/s1473-3099(11)70353-x

[10] Miller, J.C. and Voltz, E.M. (2013) Incorporating Disease and Population Structure into Models of SIR Disease in Contact Networks. *PloS One*, **8**, 1-14. http://dx.doi.org/10.1371/journal.pone.0069162

[11] Wongkoon, S., Jaroensutasinee, M. and Jaroensutasinee, K. (2013) Distribution, Seasonal Variation & Dengue Transmission Prediction in Sisaket, Thailand. *Indian Journal of Medical Research*, **138**, 347-353.

[12] Colon-Gonzalez, F.J., Fezzi, C., Lake, I.R. and Hunter, P.R. (2013) The Effects of Weather and Climate Change on Dengue. *PLoS Neglected Tropical Diseases*, **7**, 1-9. http://dx.doi.org/10.1371/journal.pntd.0002503

[13] WHO (2015) Dengue Fever Fact Sheet No 117. Updated January 2015.
http://www.who.int/mediacentre/factsheets/fs117/en/

[14] Malaysia Remote Sensing Agency (2014) http://idengue.remotesensing.gov.my/.

[15] Sue-Chern, L. (2014) As Dengue Death Rise, Will Malaysia Try Breeding Out "Bad" Aedes? The Malaysian Insider.
http://www.themalaysianinsider.com/malaysia/article/as-dengue-deaths-rise-will-malaysia-try-breeding-out-bad-aedes

[16] Paul, B. and Tham, W.L. (2015) Interrelation between Climate and Dengue in Malaysia. *Health*, **7**, 672-678.
http://dx.doi.org/10.4236/health.2015.76080

[17] Yacouba, S., Mongkolsapayaa, J. and Screatona, G. (2013) Pathogenesis of Dengue. *Current Opinion of Infectious Disease*, **26**, 284-289. http://dx.doi.org/10.1097/QCO.0b013e32835fb938

[18] Normile, D. (2014) Surprising New Dengue Virus Throws a Spanner in Disease Control Efforts. *Science*, **342**, 415.
http://dx.doi.org/10.1126/science.342.6157.415

[19] Fu, J., Tan, B.H., Yap, E.H., Chan, Y.C. and Tan, Y.H. (1992) Full-Length cDNA Sequence of Dengue Type 1 Virus (Singapore Strain S275/90). *Virology*, **188**, 953-958. http://dx.doi.org/10.1016/0042-6822(92)90560-C

[20] Putnak, J.R., Charles, P.C., Padmanabhan, R., Irie, K., Hoke, C.H. and Burke, D.S. (1988) Functional and Antigenic Domains of the Dengue-2 Virus Nonstructural Glycoprotein NS-1. *Virology*, **163**, 93-103. http://dx.doi.org/10.1016/0042-6822(88)90236-X

[21] Lim, S.P., Ooi, E.E. and Vasudevan, S.G. (2004) Full Length Genomic Sequence of a Dengue Virus of Serotype 3 from Singapore. (Unpublished)

[22] Durbin, A.P., Karron, R.A., Sun, W., Vaughn, D.W., Reynolds, M.J., Perreault, J.R., Thumar, B., Men, R., Lai, C.J., Elkins, W.R., Chanock, R.M., Murphy, B.R. and Whitehead, S.S. (2001) Attenuation and Immunogenicity in Humans of a Live Dengue Virus Type-4 Vaccine Candidate with a 30 Nucleotide Deletion in Its 3'-Untranslated Region. *Annual Journal of Tropical Medicine Hygiene*, **65**, 405-413.

[23] Wallner, G., Mandl, C.W., Kunz, C. and Heinz, F.X. (1995) The Flavivirus 3'-Noncoding Region: Extensive Size Heterogeneity Independent of Evolutionary Relationships among Strains of Tick-Borne Encephalitis Virus. *Virology*, **213**, 196-178. http://dx.doi.org/10.1006/viro.1995.1557

[24] Shah, P.S., Tanaka, M., Khan, A.H., Mathenge, E.G., Fuke, I., Takagi, M., Igarashi, A. and Morita, K. (2006) Molecular Characterization of Attenuated Japanese Encephalitis Live Vaccine Strain ML-17. *Vaccine*, **24**, 402-411. http://dx.doi.org/10.1016/j.vaccine.2005.10.048

[25] Ciota, A.T., Lovelace, A.O., Ngo, K.A., Le, A.N., Maffei, J.G., Franke, M.A., Payne, A.F., Jones, S.A., Kauffman, E.B. and Kramer, L.D. (2007) Cell-Specific Adaptation of Two Flaviviruses Following Serial Passage in Mosquito Cell Culture. *Virology*, **357**, 165-174. http://dx.doi.org/10.1016/j.virol.2006.08.005

[26] McMullen, A.R., Albayrak, H., May, F.J., Davis, C.T., Beasley, D.W. and Barrett, A.D. (2013) Molecular Evolution of Lineage 2 West Nile Virus. *Journal of General Virology*, **94**, 318-325. http://dx.doi.org/10.1099/vir.0.046888-0

[27] Rice, C.M., Lenches, E.M., Eddy, S.R., Shin, S.J., Sheets, R.L. and Strauss, J.H. (1985) Nucleotide Sequence of Yellow Fever Virus: Implications for Flavivirus Gene Expression and Evolution. *Science*, **229**, 726-733. http://dx.doi.org/10.1126/science.4023707

[28] Khan, A.H., Morita, K., Parquet, M., Parquet, M. del C., Mathenge, E.G. and Igarashi, A. (2002) Complete Nucleotide Sequence of Chikungunya Virus and Evidence for an Internal Polyadenylation Site. *Journal of General Virology*, **83**, 3075-3084. http://dx.doi.org/10.1099/0022-1317-83-12-3075

[29] Rodenhuis-Zybert, I.A., Wilschut, J. and Smit, J.M. (2010) Dengue Virus Life Cycle: Viral and Host Factors Modulating Infectivity. *Cellular and Molecular Life Sciences*, **67**, 2773-2786. http://dx.doi.org/10.1007/s00018-010-0357-z

[30] Perera, R. and Kuhn, R.J. (2008) Structural Proteomics of Dengue Virus. *Current Opinion in Microbiology*, **11**, 169-178. http://dx.doi.org/10.1016/j.mib.2008.06.004

[31] Jain, B., Chaturvedi, U.C. and Jain, A. (2014) Role of Intracellular Events in the Pathogenesis of Dengue: An Overview. *Microbial Pathogenesis*, **69-70**, 45-48. http://dx.doi.org/10.1016/j.micpath.2014.03.004

[32] Belosovic, M. (2014) *Plasmodium* sp. Zoology 352 Lecture Series, University of Alberta, Edmonton.

[33] Buret, A.G. (2014) Pathogenesis of Parasitic Disease. Zoology 352 Lecture Series, University of Alberta, Edmonton.

[34] Gubler, D.J. (2010) Dengue Viruses. In: Mahy, B.W.J. and Van Regenmortel, M.H.V., Eds., *Desk Encyclopedia of Human and Medical Virology*, Academic Press, Boston, 372-382.

[35] Povoa, T.F., Alves, A.M.B., Oliveira, C.A.B., Nuovo, G.J., Chagas, V.L.A. and Paes, M.V. (2014) The Pathology of Severe Dengue in Multiple Organs of Human Fatal Cases: Histopathology, Ultrastructure and Virus Replication. *PloS ONE*, **9**, 1-16. http://dx.doi.org/10.1371/journal.pone.0083386

[36] Ishikawaa, T., Yamanakab, A. and Konishi, E. (2014) A Review of Successful Flavivirus Vaccines and the Problems with Those Flaviviruses for Which Vaccines Are Not Yet Available. *Vaccine*, **32**, 1326-1337. http://dx.doi.org/10.1016/j.vaccine.2014.01.040

[37] Hoffmann, M.P. and Frodsham, A.C. (1993) Natural Enemies of Vegetable Insect Pests. Cooperative Extension, Cornell University, Ithica, 63 p.

[38] Bellows, T.S. (2001) Restoring Population Balance through Natural Enemy Introductions. *Biological Control*, **21**, 199-205. http://dx.doi.org/10.1006/bcon.2001.0936

[39] Marimuthu, S., Rahuman, A.A., Kirthi, A.V., Santhoshkumar, T., Jayaseelan, C. and Rajakumar, G. (2013) Eco-Friendly Microbial Route to Synthesize Cobalt Nanoparticles Using *Bacillus thuringiensis* against Malaria and Dengue Vectors. *Parasitology Resources*, **112**, 4105-4112. http://dx.doi.org/10.1007/s00436-013-3601-2

[40] Lee, H.L., Chen, C.D., Masri, S.M., Chiang, Y.F., Chooi, K.H. and Benjamin, S. (2008) Impact of Larvaciding with a *Bacillus thuringiensis isrealensis* Formulation, VectoBac WG, on Dengue Mosquito Vectors in a Dengue Endemic Site in Selangor State Malaysia. *Southeast Asian Journal Tropical Medicine Public Health*, **39**, 601-609.

[41] Kozek, W. and Rao, R. (2007) The Discovery of *Wolbachia* in Arthropods and Nematodes—A Historical Perspective. *Issues in Infectious Diseases*, **5**, 1-14. http://dx.doi.org/10.1159/000104228

[42] Turley, A.P., Moreira, L.A., O'Neill, S.L. and McGraw, E.A. (2009) *Wolbachia* Infection Reduces Blood-Feeding Success in the Dengue Fever Mosquito, *Aedesaegypti*. *PLoS Neglected Tropical Diseases*, **3**, 1-7. http://dx.doi.org/10.1371/journal.pntd.0000516

[43] Hancock, P.A., Sinkins, S.P. and Godfray, H.C.J. (2011) Strategies for Introducing *Wolbachia* to Reduce Transmission of Mosquito-Borne Diseases. *PLoS Neglected Tropical Diseases*, **5**, 1-10. http://dx.doi.org/10.1371/journal.pntd.0001024

[44] Hoffmann, A.A., Iturbe-Ormaetxe, I., Callahan, A.G., Phillips, B.L., Billington, K., Axford, J.K., Montgomery, B., Turley, A.P. and O'Neill, S.L. (2014) Stability of the wMel *Wolbachia* Infection Following Invasion into *Aedesaegypti* Populations. *PLoS Neglected Tropical Diseases*, **8**, 1-9. http://dx.doi.org/10.1371/journal.pntd.0003115

[45] Frentiu, F.D., Zakir, T., Walker, T., Popovici, J., Pyke, A.T., Van Der Hurk, A., McGraw, A.E. and O'Neill, S.L. (2014) Limited Dengue Virus Replication in Field-Collected *Aedesaegypti* Mosquitoes Infected with *Wolbachia*. *PLoS Neglected Tropical Disease*, **8**, e2688. http://dx.doi.org/10.1371/journal.pntd.0002688

[46] Baron, S., Ed. (1996) Medical Microbiology. 4th Edition, The University of Texas Medical Branch at Galveston, Galveston.

[47] Chatterjee, S., Ghosh, T.S. and Das, S. (2010) Virulence of *Bacillus cereus* as Natural Facultative Pathogen of *Anopheles subpictus* Grassi (Diptera: Culicidae) Larvae in Submerged Rice-Fields and Shallow Ponds. *African Journal of Biotechnology*, **9**, 6983-6986.

[48] Dayan, G.H., Thakur, M., Boaz, M. and Johnson, C. (2013) Safety and Immunogenicity of Three Tetravalent Dengue Vaccine Formulations in Healthy Adults in the USA. *Vaccine*, **31**, 5048-5055. http://dx.doi.org/10.1016/j.vaccine.2013.08.088

[49] McNeil, M.M., Gee, J., Weintraub, E.S., Belongia, E.A., Lee, G.M., Glanz, J.M., Nordin, J.D., Klein, N.P., Baxter, R., Naleway, A.L., Jackson, L.A., Omer, S.B., Jacobsen, S.J. and DeStefano, F. (2014) The Vaccine Safety Datalink: Successes and Challenges Monitoring Vaccine Safety. *Vaccine*, **32**, 5390-5399. http://dx.doi.org/10.1016/j.vaccine.2014.07.073

[50] Heinz, F.X. and Stiasny, K. (2012) Flaviviruses and Flavivirus Vaccines. *Vaccine*, **30**, 4301-4307. http://dx.doi.org/10.1016/j.vaccine.2011.09.114

[51] Hemming, D. (2014) Immune Regulation to Post 2014. Immunology 371 Lecture Series, University of Alberta, Edmonton.

[52] Watanaveeradej, V., Gibbons, R.V., Simasathien, S., Nisalak, A., Jarman, R.G., Kerdpanich, A., Tournay, E., De La Barrerra, R., Dessy, F., Toussaint, J.F., Eckels, K.H., Thomas, S.J. and Innis, B.L. (2014) Safety and Immunogenicity of a Rederived, Live-Attenuated Dengue Virus Vaccine in Healthy Adults Living in Thailand: A Randomized Trial. *American Journal of Tropical Medicine and Hygiene*, **91**, 119-128. http://dx.doi.org/10.4269/ajtmh.13-0452

[53] Bhamarapravati, N. and Sutee, Y. (2000) Live Attenuated Tetravalent Dengue Vaccine. *Vaccine*, **18**, 44-47. http://dx.doi.org/10.1016/S0264-410X(00)00040-2

[54] Guirakhoo, F., Weltzin, R., Chambers, T.J., Zhang, Z.-X., Soike, K., Ratterree, M., Arroyo, J., Georgakopoulos, K., Catalan, J. and Monath, T.P. (2000) Recombinant Chimeric Yellow Fever-Dengue Type 2 Virus Is Immunogenic and Protective in Nonhuman Primates. *Journal of Virology*, **74**, 5477-5485. http://dx.doi.org/10.1128/JVI.74.12.5477-5485.2000

[55] Guirakhoo, F., Kitchener, S., Morrison, D., Forrat, R., McCarthy, K., Nichols, R., Yoksan, S., Duan, X., Ermak, T.H., Kanesa-Thasan, N., Bedford, P., Lang, J., Quentin-Miller, M.J. and Monath, T.P. (2006) Live Attenuated Chimeric Yellow Fever Dengue Type 2 (ChimeriVax-DEN2) Vaccine: Phase I Clinical Trial for Safety and Immunogenicity: Effect of Yellow Fever Pre-Immunity in Induction of Cross Neutralizing Antibody Responses to All 4 Dengue Serotypes. *Human Vaccine*, **2**, 60-67. http://dx.doi.org/10.4161/hv.2.2.2555

[56] Hss, A.-S., Koh, A.-T., Tan, K.K., Chan, L.G., Zhou, L., Bouckenooghe, A., Crevat, D. and Hutagalung, Y. (2013) Safety and Immunogenicity of a Tetravalent Dengue Vaccine in Healthy Children Aged 2-11 Years in Malaysia: A Randomized, Placebo-Controlled, Phase III Study. *Vaccine*, **31**, 5814-5822. http://dx.doi.org/10.1016/j.vaccine.2013.10.013

[57] Huet, N. (2014) Final Trial Confirms Efficacy of Sanofi's Dengue Vaccine. Reuters. http://www.reuters.com/article/2014/09/03/us-sanofi-dengue-idUSKBN0GY0C520140903

[58] Villar, L., Dayan, G.H., Arredondo-García, J.L., Rivera, D.M., Cunha, R., Deseda, C., Reynales, H., Costa, M.S., Morales-Ramírez, J.O., Carrasquilla, G., Rey, L.C., Dietze, R., Luz, K., Rivas, E., Montoya, M.C.M., Supelano, M.C., Zambrano, B., Langevin, E., Boaz, M., Tornieporth, N., Saville, M. and Noriega, F. (2015) Efficacy of a Tetravalent Dengue Vaccine in Children in Latin America. *The New England Journal of Medicine*, **372**, 113-123. http://dx.doi.org/10.1056/NEJMoa1411037

[59] Bernal, A. (2014) The World's First, Large-Scale Dengue Vaccine Efficacy Study Successfully Achieved Its Primary

Endpoint. Sanofi Pasteur Media.
http://www.sanofipasteur.com/en/articles/theworld-s-first-large-scale-dengue-vaccine-efficacy-study-successfully-achi
eved-its-primary-clinical-endpoint.aspx

[60] Belosevic, M. (2014) Concept of Integrated Control against Parasites. Zoology 352 Lecture Series, University of Al-
      berta, Edmonton.

[61] Buret, A. (2014) Drugs and Parasites. Zoology 352 Lecture Series, University of Alberta, Edmonton.

21

Comparison of Contraceptive Methods Chosen by Breastfeeding, and Non-Breastfeeding, Women at a Family Planning Clinic in Northern Nigeria

A. Mohammed-Durosinlorun[1*], A. Abubakar[1], J. Adze[1], S. Bature[1], C. Mohammed[1], M. Taingson[1], A. Ojabo[2]

[1]Department of Obstetrics and Gynaecology, Faculty of Medicine, Kaduna State University, Kaduna, Nigeria
[2]Department of Obstetrics and Gynaecology, College of Health Sciences, Benue State University, Makurdi, Nigeria
Email: *ababdaze@yahoo.com

Abstract

Introduction: Breast feeding may pose a further challenge to uptake of contraception by possibly restricting use of certain methods for real or perceived risks of side effects. **Methodology:** A retrospective study was done at the Barau Dikko Teaching Hospital, Kaduna. Available family planning clinic client cards from January 1st, 2000 to March 31st, 2014 were retrieved and information collected on demographics, reproductive and menstrual history, contraceptive choices and breast feeding status. Data were analyzed using the statistical package for social sciences (SPSS) version 15. Missing responses were stated and excluded from analysis. Chi square was used as a test of association with significance level established at *p* value, 0.05. **Results:** A total number of 5992 client cards were retrieved. All clients were female and married, and majority of clients aged between 25 - 34 years (53.1%), had either completed their secondary education or gone further (56%) and were Muslims (52.3%). Only 2924 women stated that they were currently breastfeeding (48.8%), 1828 women were not breastfeeding (30.5%) and 1240 women (20.7%) did not state their breastfeeding status. Younger and more educated women were more likely to be breastfeeding than older women and less educated ones (*p* < 0.05). Only 4636 cards (77%) had correctly filled data on the choice of contraceptives chosen by breastfeeding status with 2854 women breast feeding and 1302 (45.6%) chose injectable hormonal contraception, 888 (31.1%) chose intrauterine contraceptive devices, 484 (17%) chose oral contraceptive pills and 180 (6.3%) chose contraceptive implants. There was no record of condom use or use of permanent methods of contra-

---

*Corresponding author.

ception. **Conclusion:** Breastfeeding rates were high among women seeking contraception. The pattern of contraception is similar among both breastfeeding and non-breastfeeding women, with injectable contraception being the preferred choice. Awareness should be raised on the safety of a wider variety of contraception available for breastfeeding women.

Keywords

Contraceptive Methods, Breastfeeding, Northern Nigeria

1. Introduction

Every year, more than five hundred thousand women lose their lives from complications of pregnancy and childbirth, with more than half of these deaths occurring in the postnatal period, and in sub-Saharan Africa [1]. Nigeria is among countries with high maternal mortality rates, yet contraceptive uptake rates are still relatively low in the country. Only about 10% of currently married Nigerian women use modern forms of contraception including the lactational amenorrhea method (LAM) [2] [3]. Breast feeding may pose a further challenge to the uptake of contraception by possibly restricting use of certain methods for either real, or perceived risks of possible side effects.

Breast feeding is a widespread and culturally acceptable practice in Nigeria which has undisputed benefits for both the infant and mother [4]. For the baby, the milk has anti-infective properties, ideal nutritional characteristics facilitating infant survival [5] and encourages bonding. For the mother, breastfeeding promotes a quicker recovery after childbirth, and offers some protection from ovarian cancer, breast cancer and type II diabetes [6]. Exclusive breastfeeding is also an effective contraceptive method but food supplementation, the resumption of menstrual bleeding, and reaching the sixth postpartum month while breastfeeding are all associated with increased fertility [4]. The current Nigerian demographic and health survey shows that only 17 percent of children are exclusively breastfed for six months, with early introduction of complementary feeds [3].

In the Philippines, Rous [7] found that some women may actually substitute modern contraception for breast-feeding, leading to the unintended consequence of reducing the rate of breast-feeding. However, others feel that women will usually wean children off breast milk when they get pregnant, so better spacing with modern contraception may actually allow women to breast-feed longer. Hence, contraceptive counseling during breastfeeding extends beyond issues of efficacy, because the selected method must be appropriate for a woman's breastfeeding expectations [8]. In choosing contraceptive methods other than LAM, the non-hormonal methods of contraception such as reversible barrier methods or the copper intrauterine device (IUD), or permanent surgical methods, are usually preferred for breastfeeding mothers. This is because they avoid transfer of hormones into milk which poses a theoretical risk to the infant [9] [10].

Evidence from some systematic reviews suggests that progestogen-only methods of contraception do not adversely affect breastfeeding performance when used during lactation, or adversely affect infant growth, health, or development [11]. A single study of a desogestrel pill, however reported two cases of gynecomastia in exposed infants [11]. Overall, systematic reviews investigating the effects of hormonal contraception (COC, POPs and injectables) on breast milk concluded that there is insufficient evidence to establish if hormonal contraception indeed has any effect on breast milk quantity or quality, and provide some reassurance that hormonal contraception does not have an adverse effect on infant growth or development [10].

Timing is also important when initiating hormonal contraception. The WHO recommends that if combined hormonal methods are going to be utilized, they should not be initiated until at least 6 months postpartum after breastfeeding skills and patterns are already well established [12]. However, progesterone only methods may be initiated after 6 weeks [12]. Hormonal methods maybe discouraged in circumstances where there is already existing low milk supply or history of lactation failure, history of breast surgery, multiple births (twins, triplets), preterm birth or compromised health of mother and/or baby [8].

This study was done to determine how breastfeeding affects the contraceptive choices of women in this environment and to make relevant recommendations on how to increase uptake of appropriate methods of contraception in this group of women, also to see if there are any differences in the contraceptive uptake by breastfeeding status.

2. Methodology

This was a retrospective study done at the Barau Dikko Teaching Hospital (BDSH), a 240-bed secondary/tertiary Care hospital located in Kaduna and catering for the metropolis and its environs. We retrieved all available client cards from the family planning clinic from January 1st, 2000 to March 31st, 2014. Information was collected to determine the contraceptive choices of breastfeeding women at first visit and subsequently, as well as data on demographics, reproductive and menstrual history. Approval for the study was gotten from hospital authorities and there was no risk to clients whose information was kept confidential. Data was analyzed using the statistical package for social sciences (SPSS) version 15. Missing responses were stated as such and excluded from analysis. Chi square was used as a test of association with significance level established at p value, 0.05.

3. Results

A total number of 5,992 client cards were retrieved and all clients were female and married. Majority of clients were aged between 25 - 34 years (53.1%), had either completed their secondary education or gone further (56%) and were Muslims (52.3%). Demographic characteristics are shown in **Table 1**.

Table 1. Demographic characteristics of family planning clients.

Variable Age in years	Frequency	Percent (%)
<20	131	2.2
20 - 24	985	16.4
25 - 29	1501	25.1
30 - 34	1680	28.0
35 - 39	1053	17.6
40 - 44	455	7.6
45 - 49	139	2.3
≥50	47	0.8
Missing	1	0.0
Education		
None	595	9.9
Some secondary	685	11.4
Some primary	409	6.8
Completed secondary		
or more	3410	56.9
Completed primary	861	14.4
Missing	32	0.5
Religion		
Islam	3135	52.3
Christianity	2278	38.0
Others	33	0.6
Missing	546	9.1
Total	**5992**	**100**

Out of the total, 2924 women stated that they were currently breastfeeding (48.8%), 1828 women were not breastfeeding (30.5%) and 1240 women 920.7%) did not state their breastfeeding status. **Table 2** shows a comparison of demographic characteristics between breastfeeding and non-breastfeeding women. Younger and more educated women were more likely to be breastfeeding than older women and less educated ones ($p < 0.05$).

However, only 4636 cards (77%) had correctly filled data on the choice of contraceptives chosen by breastfeeding and non-breastfeeding women. There were more women breast feeding (2854: 61.6%) their children and seeking contraception than women who were not currently breastfeeding (1782: 38.4%). On the whole (irrespective of breastfeeding status), 2126 women (45.9%) choose injectable contraception, 1704 women (36.8%) choose copper-T intrauterine devices, 591 women (12.7%) choose oral contraceptive pills and 215 women (45.9%) choose implants for contraception. While among the 2854 women breast feeding, 1302 (45.6%) choose injectable hormonal contraception, 888 (31.1%) choose intrauterine contraceptive devices, 484 (17%) choose oral contraceptive pills and 180 (6.3%) choose contraceptive implants. There was no record of condom use or use of permanent methods of contraception.

The pattern of preferred methods of contraception was similar among both breast feeding and non-breastfeeding women; uptake of injectable contraception being the highest followed by intrauterine devices, oral contraceptive pills then contraceptive implants (**Figure 1**). However, there was still a significant difference among both groups; breastfeeding women were more likely to take up all the various methods of contraception than non-breastfeeding women (Pearson Chi Square = 212.260, df = 3, p value = 0.000) (**Table 3**).

Table 2. Comparison of demographic characteristics of breastfeeding and non-breastfeeding women.

VARIABLE	BREASTFEEDING Frequency (Row %)	NON-BREASTFEEDING Frequency (Row %)
Age in years (n = 4751)		
<20	80 (85.1)	14 (14.9)
20 - 24	777 (97.9)	17 (2.1)
25 - 29	857 (74.7)	290 (25.3)
30 - 34	813 (60.9)	522 (39.1)
35 - 39	313 (38.9)	492 (61.1)
40 - 44	84 (20.7)	321 (79.3)
45 - 49	0 (0)	130 (100)
≥50	0 (0)	41(100)
$\chi^2 = 1282.062$, df = 7, $p = 0.000$		
Education (n = 4724)		
None	279 (60.0)	186 (40.0)
Some primary	127 (44.7)	157 (55.3)
Completed primary	258 (46.3)	299 (53.7)
Some secondary	392 (79.4)	102 (20.6)
Completed secondary or more	1850 (63.3)	1074 (36.7)
$\chi^2 = 158.816$, df = 4, $p = 0.000$		
Religion (n = 4690)		
Islam	2074 (72.6)	782 (27.4)
Christianity	803 (44.6)	999 (55.4)
Others	32 (100.0)	0 (0.0)
$\chi^2 = 389.000$, df = 2, $p = 0.000$		
Last child birth (n = 4177)		
<6 months	855 (86.5)	133 (13.5)
6 - 15 months	1726 (85.9)	284 (14.1)
>15 months	129 (10.9)	1050 (89.1)
$\chi^2 = 2097.426$, df = 2, $p = 0.000$		

(n = number of valid responses, χ^2 = chi square, df = degree of freedom, p = p value).

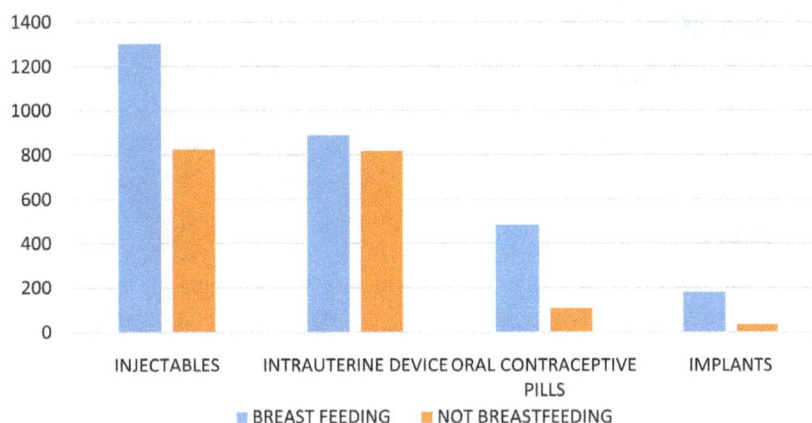

Figure 1. Chart comparing contraceptive methods chosen by breastfeeding and non-breastfeeding women.

Table 3. Cross tabulation of forms on contraception chosen by breast feeding and non-breastfeeding women.

	Injectables	Intrauterine device (copper-T)	Oral contraceptive pills	Implants
Breast feeding	1302 (61.2%)	888 (52.1%)	484 (81.9%)	180 (83.7%)
Not breast feeding	824 (38.8%)	816 (47.9%)	107 (18.1%)	35 (16.3%)
Total	2126 (100%)	1704(100%)	591 (100%)	215 (100%)

(Pearson Chi Square = 212.260, df = 3, p value = 0.000).

4. Discussion

The breastfeeding rate in this population of women attending the family planning clinic was 48% and breastfeeding was commoner among those that were younger and more educated. The 2013 Nigerian Demographic and Health Survey showed that 96% of children aged 6 - 8 months, 91% of children aged 9-11 months and 35% of children aged 20 - 23 months in Nigeria are being breastfed [3].

Injectable contraception was the first method of choice chosen by both breast feeding and non-breastfeeding mothers. This finding is consistent with national surveys which showed that among the modern methods of contraception, injectables (3 percent), male condoms (2 percent), and the pill (2 percent) are the most common methods being used [3]. Anyebe *et al.* [13] also found injectables to be the commonest form of contraception used by 30.2% of 96 respondents. Other authors also found hormonal methods (32%) and condoms (23%) to be the most favourite contraceptive methods during the postpartum period [14] [15]. Injectable contraception such as Depot provera (DMPA) and Noristerat are suitable for women who want a reliable, reversible form of contraception, and has numerous advantages such as; better compliance than like oral contraceptives which requires daily vigilance, unlike barrier contraceptives it is independent of the time of intercourse and It may be more appealing than contraceptive implant or intrauterine devices, as no intervention is required to remove it [16] [17]. It is a suitable choice in the postpartum period and in breastfeeding mothers where oestrogen therapy in the combined oral contraceptive pills may be less desired [16] [17]. Another advantage of the choice of injectable contraception in our environment may be that this form of contraception is not so "obvious" to husbands, especially if the husband may not approve and the woman is still desirous of contraception.

All the other methods chosen are suitable for breast feeding women except for combined hormonal contraception which is classified as a category 4 (unacceptable health risk) for all postpartum women, regardless of breastfeeding status, for the first 21 days [18] due to the risk of thromboembolism.

Condoms have also been found to be popular postpartum contraceptives in a study in Nigeria [3] [19] and has the added advantage of protection against sexually transmitted infections (STI) including HIV/AIDS but was not recorded in this study. This may be because condoms are more commonly distributed free at the STI clinic also within the hospital and in close proximity to the family planning clinic. So while women may be using condoms, the documentation is missed at the family planning clinic. It may be for the same reason that there are no records of permanent methods of contraception (which is more likely to be captured in the theater) documented, though this is a very unpopular choice in Nigeria [3] [13].

5. Conclusion and Recommendations

Breastfeeding rates are high among women seeking contraception. The pattern of contraception is similar among both breastfeeding and non-breastfeeding women, with injectable contraception being the preferred choice. Awareness should be raised on the safety of a wider variety of contraception available for breastfeeding women.

Limitation of Study

This was a retrospective study and some data was lost as they were not properly recorded. Also this made it difficult to delve deeper into reasons affecting choices women made regarding contraceptive methods chosen.

Declaration of Interests

None.

References

[1]   Ronsman, C. and Graham, W.J. (2006) On Behalf of the Lancet Maternal Survival Steering Group. Maternal Mortality: Who, When, Where, and Why? Maternal Survival. *Lancet*, **368**, 1189-1200.

[2]   Mohammed-Durosinlorun, A. and Krishna, R. (2014) A Quantitative Survey on the Knowledge, Attitudes and Practices on Emergency Contraceptive Pills among Adult Female Students of a Tertiary Institution in Kaduna, Nigeria. *Primary Health Care*, **4**, 148.

[3]   National Population Commission (NPC) [Nigeria] and ICF International (2014) Nigeria Demographic and Health Survey 2013. National Population Commission and International ICF, Abuja.

[4]   King, J. (2007) Contraception and Lactation. *Journal of Midwifery and Women's Health*, **52**, 614-620. http://dx.doi.org/10.1016/j.jmwh.2007.08.012

[5]   Dada, O.A., Akesode, F.A., Olanrewaju, D.M., Sule-Odu, O., Fakoya, T.A., Oluwole, F.A., Odunlami, B.V. and WHO (2002) Infant Feeding and Lactational Amennorrhea in Sagamu, Nigeria. *Africa Journal of Reproductive Health*, **6**, 39-50. http://dx.doi.org/10.2307/3583129

[6]   National Health and Medical Research Council (2012) Infant Feeding Guidelines. National Health and Medical Research Council, Canberra.

[7]   Rous, J.J. (2001) Is Breast-Feeding a Substitute for Contraception in Family Planning? *Demography*, **38**, 497-512. http://dx.doi.org/10.1353/dem.2001.0037

[8]   Berens, P., Labbok, M. and The Academy of Breastfeeding Medicine (2015) ABM Clinical Protocol #13: Contraception during Breastfeeding, Revised 2015. Breastfeeding Medicine, **10**, 3-12. http://dx.doi.org/10.1089/bfm.2015.9999

[9]   Truitt, S.T., Fraser, A.B., Grimes, D.A., Gallo, M.F. and Schulz, K.F. (2003) Combined Hormonal versus Nonhormonal versus Progestin-Only Contraception in Lactation. *Cochrane Database of Systematic Reviews*, **2**, Article ID: CD003988.

[10] FFPRHC Guidance (2004) Contraceptive Choices for Breastfeeding Women. *Journal of Family Planning and Reproductive Health Care*, **30**, 181-189. http://dx.doi.org/10.1783/1471189041261429

[11] Kapp, N., Curtis, K. and Naanda, K. (2010) Progestogen-Only Contraceptive Use among Breastfeeding Women: A Systematic Review. *Contraception*, **82**, 17-37 http://dx.doi.org/10.1016/j.contraception.2010.02.002

[12] Queenan, J.T. (2004) Contraception and Breastfeeding. *Clinical Obstetrics and Gynecology*, **47**, 734-739. http://dx.doi.org/10.1097/01.grf.0000139710.63598.b1

[13] Anyebe, E.E., Olufemi, S.K. and Lawal, H.R.N. (2014) Contraceptive Use among Married Women in Zaria, Northwest Nigeria. *Research on Humanities and Social Sciences*, **4**, 69-75.

[14] Cwiak, C., Gellasoh, T. and Zieman, M. (2004) Peripartum Contraceptive Attitudes and Practices. *Contraception*, **70**, 383-386. http://dx.doi.org/10.1016/j.contraception.2004.05.010

[15] Omolulu, A. and Okunowo, A. (2009) Intended Postpartum Contraceptive Use among Pregnant and Puerperal Women at a University Teaching Hospital. *Archives of Gynecology and Obstetrics*, **280**, 987-992. http://dx.doi.org/10.1007/s00404-009-1056-6

[16] Faculty of Sexual and Reproductive Healthcare (2014) Progestogen-Only Injectable Contraception Clinical Guidance.

[17] NICE Clinical Guideline (2014) Long-Acting Reversible Contraception Update.

[18] CDC US (2010) Medical Eligibility Criteria for Contraceptive Use: Adapted from the World Health Organization Medical Eligibility Criteria for Contraceptive Use. 4th Edition, MMWR, No. RR-4, 59.

[19] Adegbola, O. and Okunowo, A. (2009) Intended Postpartum Contraceptive Use among Pregnant and Puerperal Women at a University Teaching Hospital. *Archives of Gynecology and Obstetrics*, **280**, 987-992.
http://dx.doi.org/10.1007/s00404-009-1056-6

22

Investigating Physical Exercise among Jordanians with Diabetes Mellitus

Muhammad W. Darawad[1], Sultan Mosleh[2], Amani A. Khalil[1], Mahmoud Maharmeh[1], Ayman M. Hamdan-Mansour[1], Osama A. Samarkandi[3]

[1]Faculty of Nursing, The University of Jordan, Amman, Jordan
[2]Faculty of Nursing, University of Mutah, Karak, Jordan
[3]Prince Sultan bin Abdulaziz College for Emergency Medical Services, King Saud University, Riyadh, Saudi Arabia
Email: m.darawad@ju.edu.jo, s.mosleh@mutah.edu.jo, a.khalil@ju.edu.jo, m.maharmeh@ju.edu.jo, a.mansour@ju.edu.jo, osamarkandi@ksu.edu.sa

Abstract

This study is aimed to investigate exercise behaviors (frequency and duration) among Jordanian diabetic patients, and their correlation with their physical characteristics and perceived exercise benefits and barriers, exercise self efficacy, and exercise planning. An exploratory descriptive design was utilized using the cross-sectional survey with self-reported questionnaires (Demographics, Charlson Comorbidity Index, Exercise Self-Efficacy Scale, Exercise Benefits and Barriers Scale, and Commitment to a Plan for Exercise Scale). A convenience sample of 115 Jordanians with diabetes mellitus was recruited from diabetes outpatient clinics. Participants reported an average number of 3.2 physical activities per week (average of 2.9 hours), with walking being the most common activity. Participant's body mass index, comorbidity index, and exercise self-efficacy were correlated with both frequency and duration of exercise (r = −0.393, −0.286, 0.219 and −0.272, 0.383, 0.260, respectively). A predictive model of five predictors (age, BMI, CCI, exercise self efficacy, and perceived exercise barriers) that significantly predicted exercise duration (R^2 = 0.34, F = 9.14, P < 0.000) was found. Diabetic patients were found to exercise less than optimum. Illness itself was not a cause of not exercising compared to lack of time and desire. Factors that can enhance or inhibit participants' engagement in exercise should be included in designing tailored exercise educational programs.

Keywords

Physical Exercise, Benefits and Barriers, Self-Efficacy, Diabetes, Jordan

1. Introduction

This Diabetes mellitus (DM) is a stressful chronic disease that is prevalent worldwide with a total number of 371 million adult diabetics in addition to 187 million undiagnosed cases, killing 4.8 million patients, and costing $471.6 billion annually [1]. These numbers are expected to increase by 2030 to affect 439 million, with the speed of 69% affecting new diabetics in the developing countries, which is higher than that expected (20%) in the developed countries [2]. Such difference could be attributed to the limited resources in the developing countries where healthcare utilization is vastly affected by the cost of care, inadequate hospital bed capacity, and low socioeconomic status [3].

According to the International Diabetes Federation [1], 80% of people with diabetes live in low- and middle-income countries. Jordan, as a developing country, has a relatively high diabetes prevalence rate that was reported to be 11.62%, with approximately 2740 deaths annually. This prevalence rate is above the global average (8.3%), above the regional rate of Middle East and North Africa (10.9%), and above those reported in many countries in the region comparable to Jordan such as Iraq (9.71%), Syria (9.63%), and Turkey (7.91%). In addition, a national study found that the age-standardized prevalence of diabetes in Jordan has increased from 13% to 17.1% over 10 years (1994-2004) [4], which indicates that more Jordanians are becoming diabetics at a higher rate.

Jordanian diabetics, like diabetics worldwide, have suffered from many of diabetes-related complications. Such complications include low quality of life [5], high depression rate [6], elevated rates of developing diabetic foot syndrome [7] and diabetic retinopathy [8], and higher rates of sexual dysfunction among men [9] and women [10]. Finally, DM was found to be the leading cause of developing end-stage renal disease necessitating hemodialysis in Jordan [11].

In addition to being a developing country with limited healthcare resources, many factors have potentiated the above mentioned high DM prevalence in Jordan. Such factors include high rate of obesity and physical inactivity [12], elevated lipid profile [13], in addition to the demographic and socio-cultural changes (e.g., aging of the population) that increased the environmental risk factors for diabetes [11].

It is known that DM, as a chronic disease, has no cure. Thus, diabetes management focuses more on controlling blood sugar (medication, diet, and exercise) and strategies to prevent its chronic complications. This absence of cure produces, along with complicated treatment, a state of poor functional and psychosocial status among patients. Accordingly, one strategy that can aid in achieving cost-effective treatment and healthcare utilization by the patient is to teach them self-care behaviors such as physical exercise, which may optimize their treatment and outcomes. Physical exercise is a healthy behavior that has the potential to prevent musculoskeletal disorders and to decrease the risk of developing complications for many chronic illnesses [14] [15].

Even though heavy exercise is contraindicated for diabetic patients as it can precipitate hypoglycemia and death, moderate regular exercises are of great benefit for them both physically and mentally. For instance, a 12-month exercise program was efficient in decreasing diabetic patients' body mass index (BMI), glycosylated hemoglobin (HbA1C) readings, and emotional distress [16]. On the other hand, physical inactivity is a chief problem that can complicate health outcomes of patients with chronic diseases including DM [17] [18].

Although exercise has many advantages for diabetic patients, they were found to exercise significantly less than healthy people. Al-Amer et al. [6] and Khattab, Khader, Al-Khawaldeh, & Ajlouni [19] reported that only 16.4% and 29.9% (respectively) of diabetics in their studies engaged in at least 30 minutes of physical exercise. Knowing such tendency among patients with chronic illnesses (including diabetics) to exercise less than optimum should alarm healthcare providers to integrate exercise among their care plans [20].

Among the factors that may affect patients' adherence to self-care practices, including exercise, are their physical characteristics, mainly BMI, and their health status especially having other comorbidities. For example, a significant negative correlation was reported between patients' BMI and their glycemic control among diabetic patients [19] and with their exercise activity among patients with arthritis [21]. Also, a significant positive correlation between having comorbidities and fluid and diet nonadherence was found among patients with renal failure [22].

Other factors include patients' perception of exercise self-efficacy (confidence in one's ability to perform healthy behaviors in against barriers), exercise benefits and barriers regard their clinical outcomes, and exercise planning [23]. This perception is a significant aspect of the Health Promotion Model that explains health promoting behaviors through causal mechanisms [24]. According to Shin, Hur, Pender, Jang, and Kim [25], perceiving more exercise benefits and less barriers, along with better exercise self-efficacy, can positively promote the commencement and performance of exercise behaviors among patients with chronic illnesses. Also, among Jordanian patients with myocardial infarction, a significant relationship was found between exercise participation and health belief variables [26].

In Jordan, Al-Hassan and Wierenga [27] found that less than 50% of the Jordanian population to perform mild physical exercise. Even Jordanian adolescents were found to be physically inactive [28]. Thus, it is expected that patients with chronic illnesses, including DM, to perceive exercise as a greater challenge compared with the normal population because of their physical limitations. The literature of diabetes in Jordan was interested in diabetes prevalence, complications, and medical treatment. However, the studies that focus on the health promotion behaviors among Jordanian diabetics, such as exercise, are scarce, with no study is found to assess exercise behaviors among Jordanian DM patients.

Therefore, this study came to fill out a gap in this regard so that future studies can build on its outcomes in terms of identifying Jordanian DM patients' exercise behaviors based on the knowledge generated through this study. The aims of this study are to 1) describe exercise behaviors (frequency and duration) among Jordanian diabetic patients; 2) investigate the correlation between exercise behaviors with their physical characteristics (BMI and comorbidities) and perceived exercise benefits and barriers, exercise self-efficacy, and exercise planning; 3) test the differences in exercise behaviors based on their demographics; and 4) explore the predictors of their exercise duration.

2. Methodology

Design: An exploratory descriptive design was utilized using the cross-sectional survey with self-reported questionnaires.

Setting: Data were collected from Jordanian patients diagnosed with DM (both types) at diabetes outpatient clinics of four hospitals representing Jordanian main healthcare sectors including governmental, teaching, and private sectors. The hospitals were randomly selected from the lists of hospitals in each sector.

Sampling: The study used a convenience sample of Jordanian adult diabetic patients. To be included in the study, participant had to be: 1) at least 18 years old, 2) have been diagnosed with DM, 3) able to read and write in Arabic, and 4) accepts participation. On the other hand, exclusion criteria included patients with severe mental, physical, or cognitive deterioration. One hundred fifty diabetic patients met the eligibility criteria and accepted participation, but only 115 returned the filled out questionnaires giving a response rate of 76.7%.

Data collection: The ethical approval was sought before starting the data collection from the Scientific Research Committees at the Faculty of Nursing-the University of Jordan and the participating hospitals. The heads of the participating units were met, and information regarding the study purpose and procedure of data collection were provided to them, and they were asked to facilitate data collection in their units. Then, trained data collectors screened patients for eligibility, and invited those who met the inclusion criteria for voluntarily participation. Those who accepted participation were asked to read the cover letter telling them the purpose of the study along with their rights. Participants were asked either to use the assigned private room for filling out the questionnaires or to take the package home and return it to the head of the unit in a closed envelope. The data collectors were available during filling out the questionnaires to illustrate vague or unclear items. The time needed to finish filling out the questionnaire was approximately 25 - 30 minutes.

Ethical considerations: Participants' right to anonymity and privacy were assured throughout the process of data collection. Participants were given a cover letter to illustrate the study purpose and the rights of participants. However, returning the filled out questionnaire was considered as an implied consent. Each participant was informed that participation was voluntary with no effects for their decision on their medical treatment, and that he/she could withdraw from the study without penalties.

Instruments: The study package had five parts. The first part asked participants to report their demographic characteristics including their age, gender, weight, height, marital status, level of education, smoking status, type of insurance, type of employment, and comorbidities measured by Charlson Comorbidity Index (CCI) [29]. The second part asked participants concerning their exercise behaviors by requesting them to report the number, duration (in hours), and types of exercise activities they perform per week. Also, this part contained three yes/no questions regarding the reasons of not participating in exercise activities.

The third part uses the Exercise Benefits and Barriers Scale (EBBS), which involves 43 items (29 benefits and

14 barriers of exercise) that uses a 4-point Likert scale ranging from 1 "strongly disagree" to 4 "Strongly agree". The benefits (range 29 - 116) and barriers (range 14 - 56) subscales will be separately used. The internal consistency reliability of the EBBS was established with a good Cronbach's alpha 0.95 for the benefits subscale and 0.86 for the barriers subscale [30].

The fourth part evaluated participants' exercise self-efficacy using Exercise Self-Efficacy Scale (ESE). On a 10-unit interval ranging from 0% "cannot do" to 100% "certain can do", the ESE asks participants to rate their confidence of regularly doing 18 exercise routines [23]. The average of the 18 items was considered, with the higher average scores indicating that participants have higher confidence in their abilities to perform exercise. The fifth part asks participants to rate their frequency of doing 20 routines concerning exercise plan using the Commitment to a Plan for Exercise Scale [23]. This scale uses 3-item Likert scale ranging from 1 "Never" to 3 "Often" with a range between 20 - 60, where the greater figures indicate more commitment to a plan for exercise. Shin et al. (2006) utilized the EBBS, ESE, and the Commitment to a Plan for Exercise Scale among patients with osteoporosis and osteoarthritis and reported that Cronbach's alpha was 0.97 for the benefits subscale, 0.89 for the barriers subscale, 0.97 for the ESE, and 0.87 for the exercise commitment scale.

The original questionnaires were translated into the Arabic language using the standard translation and back-translation protocol [31]. Critical problems in backward translation were considered after a pilot testing in the original study, which was carried out to assure clarity and understandability of the instrument prior to introducing it to the participants, along with assessing feasibility of the study.

Data analysis: Data were analyzed using the statistical package for the social sciences (SPSS-version 17.0), using $\acute{a} = 0.05$ (two-tailed). Descriptive statistics were utilized to describe participants' demographic characteristics and variables of the study. In addition, Analysis of Variance (ANOVA) was used to test differences in frequency of exercise and exercise duration based on demographic variables except gender (T-test for independent groups was used). Also, Pearson correlation test was used to test the correlation of exercise behaviors (frequency and duration) with continuous demographics and perceived exercise benefits and barriers, exercise self-efficacy, and exercise planning. Finally, Stepwise linear regression analysis was used to identify predictors of exercise duration.

3. Results

3.1. Demographic Characteristics

A total of 115 patients returned their questionnaires. Participants' age ranged from 19 - 80 years (M = 43.2, SD = 17.1), and comorbidity index ranged from 1 - 3 (M = 1.04, SD = 0.7). Regarding their physical characteristics, the average weight was 75.8 Kg (range 45 - 120) with an average BMI of 26.8 (range 17.9 - 38.1). The majority of the sample was found to be male (63.53%), married (52.2%), educated with less than secondary school (32.1%), full-time employees (32.5%), working sedentary works such as teaching and driving (43.5%) or unemployed (14.8%) including housewives, with a monthly income less than $700 (63.5%), covered with governmental health insurance (43.5%). Regarding their smoking history, only 36.5% of the participants were smokers, with an average of 5.5 years of smoking (range 2 - 5), and 2.1 pack per day (range 1 - 5).

When asked about their physical exercise, participants reported an average number of 3.2 physical activities per week, and an average period of 2.9 hours of physical activity per week. The most common type of physical exercise was walking (45.1%) while the least was performing ball sports (6.2%). Regarding the reasons for not practicing physical exercise, the most common reason was having no desire (32.2%), while having the illness was the least common (12.2%). Regarding the main study variables, participants reported moderate exercise self-efficacy (M = 46.9, SD = 11.7), perception of exercise benefits (M = 2.3, SD = 0.3) and barriers (M = 2.4, SD = 0.3), and exercise planning (M = 1.9, SD = 0.3). Detailed participants' responses regarding physical activity are shown in **Table 1**.

3.2. Correlates of Exercise Behaviors

To achieve the second research aim regarding the relationship between exercise behaviors (frequency and duration) with their physical characteristics (age, BMI, CCI) and perceived exercise variables (exercise benefits and barriers, self-efficacy, and planning), Pearson correlation coefficient test was performed (**Table 2**). Data revealed significant (P < 0.05) correlations between the aforementioned variables, which emphasizes the importance of understanding exercise related factors. For instance, participant's BMI, CCI, and exercise self-efficacy

Table 1. Description of exercise behaviors and perceived exercise variables (N = 115).

Variables	Range	Mean (SD)	% (n)
Type of activity			
Walking			45.1 (51)
Running			16.8 (19)
Physical fitness			12.4 (14)
Ball sports			6.2 (7)
Others			20.5 (22)
Reason for not exercising			
No desire			32.2 (37)
No time			25.2 (29)
Illness (DM)			12.2 (14)
No answer			30.4 (35)
Exercise Self Efficacy	20 - 87	46.9 (11.7)	
Exercise Benefits	1.3 - 2.9	2.3 (0.3)	
Exercise Barriers	2 - 3	2.4 (0.3)	
Exercise Planning	1.2 - 2.5	1.9 (0.3)	
Frequency of exercise per week	0 - 8	3.2 times (2.5)	
Duration of exercise per week	0 - 15	2.9 hours (3.3)	

Table 2. Pearson Correlations of exercise behaviors (frequency and duration) with their physical characteristics and perceived exercise variables.

	1	2	3	4	5	6	7	8	9
1. Age	1.00								
2. BMI	0.053	1.00							
3.CCI	0.191*	0.134	1.00						
4. Exercise Self Efficacy	0.089	−0.026	−0.050	1.00					
5. Exercise Benefits	0.208*	−0.080	0.044	0.212*	1.00				
6. Exercise Barriers	0.201*	0.034	0.020	−0.011	−0.081	1.00			
7. Exercise Planning	−0.042	−0.297**	−0.140	0.141	0.087	0.178	1.00		
8. Frequency of exercise per week	−0.169	−0.393**	−0.286**	0.219*	−0.031	−0.171	0.140	1.00	
9. Duration of exercise per week	0.285**	−0.272**	−0.383**	0.260**	−0.054	−0.292**	0.091	0.677**	1.00

**Correlation is significant at $\alpha = 0.01$ (2-tailed), *Correlation is significant at $\alpha = 0.05$ (2-tailed).

were correlated with both frequency and duration of exercise (r = −0.393, −0.286, 0.219 and −0.272, 0.383, 0.260, respectively). On the other hand, duration of exercise had more correlations (five variables) compared to frequency of exercise (only three variables), with higher correlation for BMI with frequency of exercise (r = −0.393) and for CCI with duration of exercise (r = −0.383) compared to other variables. Interestingly, there was no correlation for exercise self-efficacy with age, BMI, and CCI, however, it had significant relationships with both frequency and duration of exercise (r = 0.219 and 0.260, respectively). To test differences in exercise behaviors (frequency and duration) based on participants' demographics (aim No. 3), Analysis of Variance (ANOVA) and T-test for independent groups (for gender) were used. Results of both tests revealed no differences in both frequency and duration of exercise between various categories of patients' demographics.

3.3. Predictors of Exercise Duration among Diabetics

This section answers the third research question in this study regarding the predictors of exercise duration among diabetics. Stepwise Linear regression analysis was used to estimate the probability of recorded variables including exercise self-efficacy, perceived benefit and barriers, and planning, in addition to significant sample characteristics namely age, BMI, and CCI. Seven variables were entered in the analysis, which consisted of 4 steps model with no missing cases on an entry level of $\acute{a}$ = 0.05 and removal at 0.1. As shown in **Table 3**, results revealed a predictive model of five predictors (age, BMI, CCI, exercise self-efficacy, and perceived exercise barriers) that significantly predicted exercise duration (R^2 = 0.34, F = 9.14, P < 0.000). These factors had a comparable power in their prediction of exercise duration. For instance, CCI, exercise self-efficacy, and perceived exercise barriers had relatively higher predictive effects (β = -0.290, P < 0.000), (β = 0.286, P < 0.01), (β = -0.265, P < 0.01), respectively, compared to age (β = -0.165, P < 0.05) and BMI (β = -0.192, P < 0.05). Consequently, perceived exercise benefits and planning did not have the ability to predict diabetic patient's exercise duration.

4. Discussion

This descriptive study investigated Jordanian diabetics' exercise behaviors and their relationships with different demographic and perceived exercise variables. Of concern is the finding that participants' reported an average of less than three hours of exercise per week, which is way less than the recommended 3.5 hours per week for patients with diabetes and prediabetes [32]. This confirms what have been previously reported about the sedentary life style of Jordanian diabetics [6] [12] [19] and indicates their risk of developing diabetes long term complications. Nonadherence with treatment guidelines is common among patients with chronic illnesses, where patients on hemodialysis were found to be nonadherent to both fluid and diet restriction [33]. This should alarm both healthcare providers and policy maker for the need to integrate physical exercise as part of the routine education in clinics and the media to increase patients' adherence to the prescribed plans.

Regarding the reasons for not exercising, it was noteworthy that illness itself was least common reason, and the lack of desire was the most common. Such a result may indicate that the disease process in DM does not affect the body to exercise as much as it affects patient's cognition leading to lose desire either by being afraid to develop hypoglycemia or to have injuries during exercise. Advanced age and the relatively elevated levels of BMI and CCI constitute other possible factors that can hinder their ability to exercise. While nothing can be done for age, appropriate health stabilization facilitated by primary care providers for both DM and comorbidities can encourage patients to exercise and decrease their BMI, which will be encouraging for further exercise [16]. Other reasons may include the poorly designed communities in Jordan where sidewalks and play grounds are not available in every community. So, efforts to promote patients' physical exercise should consider increasing facilities and areas for exercise including fitness centers and sidewalks. For instance, patient may be advised regarding a customized home-based exercise program that might be beneficial to overcome many of the exercise barriers [34].

Even though participants reported having barriers to exercise, they reported a moderate average of perceived exercise barriers (2.4/4), which was less than that reported among hemodialysis patients (2.66) [35], patients with multiple sclerosis (2.80) [36], and patients with osteoarthritis (2.59) [25]. Such a difference might be attributed to the less acute manifestations of diabetes than other diseases specially if under control.

Regarding the types of exercise activities, as expected, walking was the most common type of exercise. This type of exercise seems to be the safest and the most convenient for patients, where their concerns about comfort

Table 3. Stepwise linear regression analysis of predictors of exercise duration.

Variables	B	SE	β	t	P value
Age	-0.037	0.018	-0.165	-1.995	0.049
CCI	-1.383	0.379	-0.290	-3.646	0.000
BMI	-0.175	0.075	-0.192	-2.353	0.020
Average Self Efficacy	0.082	0.023	0.286	3.559	0.001
Average Plan to Exercise	0.988	0.998	0.084	0.990	0.324
Average Ex Barriers	-2.995	0.922	-0.265	-3.249	0.002
Average Ex Benefits	-1.238	0.939	-0.109	-1.318	0.190

*Predictors of exercise duration final model produced at α = 0.05, F = 52.4, P > 0.001, R^2 = 0.342.

and safety may affect their actual exercise behaviors [37]. On the other hand, walking regularly is still beneficial by helping in reversing metabolic syndrome risk factors better than exercise of moderate intensity [38], and decreased risk of incident diabetes by 28.5% among Indians with impaired glucose tolerance [39]. Therefore, this should be taken in consideration while providing education about the importance of exercise, which means to go with patient's favorites regarding the type of exercise in terms of most interest and fitting into personal schedule [32] [37].

Testing the correlation of variables with patient's exercise behaviors revealed that duration of exercise was correlated (five variables) with more variables than frequency of exercise (three variables), which may indicates the superiority of duration over frequency in assessing the exercise behaviors among patients. Duration of exercise was correlated with patient's age, BMI, CCI, exercise self-efficacy, and perceived exercise barriers, which highlights the importance of considering such factors in understanding patients' exercise behaviors. Also, those with advance age, more BMI and comorbidities, more perceived exercise barriers, and less exercise self-efficacy should be targeted in primary care settings as more vulnerable to become sedentary, which means that they need to be encouraged more about exercise. Similarly, exercise self-efficacy, and perceived exercise barriers were found to be correlated among postmenopausal women [40], and age, BMI, and perceived exercise barriers were correlated among patients with arthritis [21]. Among diabetic patients, variables that were correlated with exercise behavior included exercise self-efficacy [41].

Surprisingly, patients' demographics (except age, BMI, and CCI) did not have any relationship with exercise duration. Many other studies did not find correlation between physical exercise and participants' psychosocial aspects such as insurance in the general population [42], income among patients with arthritis [21], and gender, ethnicity and working status among patients with Parkinson disease [43]. This may indicate that patients with chronic illnesses, including DM, are most commonly overwhelmed by their physical characteristics than their psychosocial aspects. However, this does not mean to neglect patients' differences in designing tailored exercise programs that were found to be beneficial in promoting physical activity [37].

Examining the predictors of exercise duration revealed five significant predictors (CCI, exercise self-efficacy, perceived exercise barriers, age, and BMI, respectively). Similar results were found (age, BMI, and perceived exercise barriers) among patients with arthritis [21]. This indicates that those factors need to be considered in any treatment regimen that includes exercise.

Many implications can be derived from the results of this study regarding encouraging diabetic patients toward promoting their exercise behaviors. For instance, it is highly recommended to have tailored exercise educational programs taking in consideration that patients who are older, overweight, having more comorbidities, perceive exercise as burden and need more encouragement than their counterparts. Also, exercise self-efficacy and perceived exercise barriers were found as significant predictors of patients' exercise behavior, which can be used concurrently while educating patients regarding exercise to increase their self-efficacy and decrease their exercise barriers. However, among the limitations of this study is the small sample size, for which a larger future study is recommended. Also, it is recommended to conduct this study at international level to compare between different cultures so that better understanding of this phenomenon can be achieved. Relying on patient's self-reported exercise behavior constitutes another limitation, for which future studies can use more objective measures (e.g., observation techniques, pedometer) to assess actual patient's exercise behaviors.

5. Conclusion

The current study is among the first to assess Jordanian diabetic patients' exercise behaviors, in which patients are found to exercise less than the recommended time. Illness itself was the least common cause of not exercising compared to lack of time and desire. As expected, age, BMI, CCI, exercise self-efficacy, and perceived exercise barriers were found as significant predictors of exercise duration which should be included in designing tailored exercise educational programs.

Acknowledgements

The authors acknowledge the University of Jordan for funding this study and also, sincere thanks to the participants and to the directors of nursing within the participating hospitals.

References

[1]   International Diabetes Federation (2012) IDF Diabetes Atlas. http://www.idf.org/diabetesatlas

[2]   Shaw, J.E., Sicree, R.A. and Zimmet, P.Z. (2010) Global Estimates of the Prevalence of Diabetes for 2010 and 2030. *Diabetes Research & Clinical Practice*, **87**, 4-14. http://dx.doi.org/10.1016/j.diabres.2009.10.007

[3]   Al-Jauissy, M., Al-Hassan, M. and Akhu-Zaheya, L. (2009) Healthcare Needs of Non-Institutionalized Jordanian Cancer Patients: An Exploratory Descriptive Study. *Cancer Nursing*, **32**, 291-298. http://dx.doi.org/10.1097/NCC.0b013e3181a0221e

[4]   Ajlouni, K., Khader, Y.S., Batieha, A., *et al.* (2008) An Increase in Prevalence of Diabetes Mellitus in Jordan over 10 Years. *Journal of Diabetes & Its Complications*, **22**, 317-324. http://dx.doi.org/10.1016/j.jdiacomp.2007.01.004

[5]   Al-Akour, N., Khader, Y.S. and Shatnawi, N.J. (2010) Quality of Life and Associated Factors among Jordanian Adolescents with Type 1 Diabetes Mellitus. *Journal of Diabetes & Its Complications*, **24**, 43-47. http://dx.doi.org/10.1016/j.jdiacomp.2008.12.011

[6]   Al-Amer, R.M., Sobeh, M.M., Zayed, A.A., *et al.* (2011) Depression among Adults with Diabetes in Jordan: Risk Factors and Relationship to Blood Sugar Control. *Journal of Diabetes & Its Complications*, **25**, 247-252. http://dx.doi.org/10.1016/j.jdiacomp.2011.03.001

[7]   Jbour, A., Jarrah, N., Radaideh, A., *et al.* (2003) Prevalence and Predictors of Diabetic Foot Syndrome in Type 2 Diabetes Mellitus in Jordan. *Saudi Medical Journal*, **24**, 761-764.

[8]   Al-Bdour, M., Al-Till, M. and Abu Samara, K. (2008) Risk Factors for Diabetic Retinopathy among Jordanian Diabetics. *Middle East African Journal of Ophthalmology*, **15**, 77-80. http://dx.doi.org/10.4103/0974-9233.51997

[9]   Khatib, F., Jarrah, N., Shegem, N., *et al.* (2006) Sexual Dysfunction among Jordanian Men with Diabetes. *Saudi Medical Journal*, **27**, 351-356.

[10]   Abu Ali, R.M., Al Hajeri, R.M., Khader, Y.S., *et al.* (2008) Sexual Dysfunction in Jordanian Diabetic Women. *Diabetes Care*, **31**, 1580-1581. http://dx.doi.org/10.2337/dc08-0081

[11]   Abdallah, S., Ahmad, A., Bataieha, A., *et al.* (2007) Diabetes Mellitus: The Leading Cause of Hemodialysis in Jordan. *Eastern Mediterranean Health Journal*, **13**, 803-809.

[12]   Zindah, M., Belbeisi, A., Walke, H., *et al.* (2005) Obesity and Diabetes in Jordan: Findings from the Behavioral Risk Factor Surveillance System, 2004. *Preventing Chronic Disease*, **5**, 1-8.

[13]   Abdel-Aal, N., Ahmad, A., Froelicher, E., *et al.* (2008) Prevalence of Dyslipidemia in Patients with Type 2 Diabetes in Jordan. *Saudi Medical Journal*, **29**, 1423-1428.

[14]   Cheema, B.S.B. (2008) Review Article: Tackling the Survival Issue in End-Stage Renal Disease: Time to Get Physical on Haemodialysis. *Nephrology*, **13**, 560-569. http://dx.doi.org/10.1111/j.1440-1797.2008.01036.x

[15]   Alramly, M., Darawad, M.W. and Khalil, A.A. (2013) Slowing the Progression of Chronic Kidney Disease: Comparison between Predialysis and Dialysis Jordanian Patients. *Renal Failure*, **35**, 1348-1352. http://dx.doi.org/10.3109/0886022X.2013.828260

[16]   Bastiaens, H., Sunaert, P., Wens, J., *et al.* (2009) Supporting Diabetes Self-Management in Primary Care: Pilot-Study of a Group-Based Programme Focusing on Diet and Exercise. *Primary Care Diabetes*, **3**, 103-109. http://dx.doi.org/10.1016/j.pcd.2009.02.001

[17]   Suh, M., Jung, H., Park, J., *et al.* (2002) Effects of Regular Exercise on Anxiety, Depression, and Quality of Life in Maintenance Hemodialysis Patients. *Renal Failure*, **24**, 337-345. http://dx.doi.org/10.1081/JDI-120005367

[18]   Laoutaris, I., Dritsas, A., Brown, M., *et al.* (2007) Immune Response to Inspiratory Muscle Training in Patients with Chronic Heart Failure. *European Journal of Cardiovascular Prevention and Rehabilitation*, **14**, 679-685. http://dx.doi.org/10.1097/HJR.0b013e3281338394

[19]   Khattab, M., Khader, Y.S., Al-Khawaldeh, A., *et al.* (2010) Factors Associated with Poor Glycemic Control among Patients with Type 2 Diabetes. *Journal of Diabetes & Its Complications*, **24**, 84-89. http://dx.doi.org/10.1016/j.jdiacomp.2008.12.008

[20]   Darawad, M. and Khalil, A. (2012) Jordanian Dialysis Patients' Perceived Exercise Benefits and Barriers: A Correlation Study. *Rehabilitation Nursing*, **38**, 315-322. http://dx.doi.org/10.1002/rnj.98

[21]   Brittain, D.R., Gyurcsik, N.C., McElroy, M., *et al.* (2011) General and Arthritis-Specific Barriers to Moderate Physical Activity in Women with Arthritis. *Women's Health Issues*, **21**, 57-63. http://dx.doi.org/10.1016/j.whi.2010.07.010

[22]   Akman, B., Uyar, M., Afsar, B., *et al.* (2007) Adherence, Depression and Quality of Life in Patients on a Renal Transplantation Waiting List. *Transplant International*, **20**, 682-687. http://dx.doi.org/10.1111/j.1432-2277.2007.00495.x

[23]   Bandura, A. (2006) Guide for Constructing Self-Efficacy Scales. In: Pajares, F. and Urdan, T.S., Eds., *Self-Efficacy Beliefs of Adolescents*, Age Information Publishing, Greenwich, 307-337.

[24] Pender, N., Murdaugh, C. and Parson, M. (2002) Health Promotion in Nursing Practice. Prentice-Hall Health, Inc., Upper Saddle River.

[25] Shin, Y.H., Hur, H.K., Pender, N.J., et al. (2006) Exercise Self-Efficacy, Exercise Benefits and Barriers, and Commitment to a Plan for Exercise among Korean Women with Osteoporosis and Osteoarthritis. International Journal of Nursing Studies, 43, 3-10. http://dx.doi.org/10.1016/j.ijnurstu.2004.10.008

[26] Al-Ali, N. and Haddad, L.G. (2004) The Effect of the Health Belief Model in Explaining Exercise Participation among Jordanian Myocardial Infarction Patients. Journal of Transcultural Nursing, 15, 114-121. http://dx.doi.org/10.1177/1043659603262484

[27] Al-Hassan, M. and Wierenga, M. (2000) Exercise Participation Decisions of Jordanian Myocardial Infarction Patients: Application of the Decisional Conflict Theory. International Journal of Nursing Studies, 37, 119-126. http://dx.doi.org/10.1016/S0020-7489(99)00065-6

[28] Obeisat, S. and Gharaibeh, H. (2012) Physical Activity Behaviour of Jordanian Adolescents and Its Associated Factors. European Journal of Scientific Research, 67, 433-443.

[29] Charlson, M., Pompei, P., Ales, K., et al. (1987) A New Method of Classifying Prognostic Comorbidity in Longitudinal Studies: Development and Validation. Journal of Chronic Diseases, 40, 373-383. http://dx.doi.org/10.1016/0021-9681(87)90171-8

[30] Sechrist, K., Walker, S. and Pender, N. (1987) Development and Psychometric Evaluation of the Exercise/Benefit Scale. Research in Nursing and Health, 10, 357-365. http://dx.doi.org/10.1002/nur.4770100603

[31] Guillemin, F., Bombardier, C. and Beaton, D. (1993) Cross-Cultural Adaptation of Health-Related Quality of Life Measures: Literature Review and Proposed Guidelines. Journal of Clinical Epidemiology, 46, 1417-1432. http://dx.doi.org/10.1016/0895-4356(93)90142-N

[32] Hordern, M., Dunstan, D., Prins, J., et al. (2012) Exercise Prescription for Patients with Type 2 Diabetes and Pre-Diabetes: A Position Statement from Exercise and Sport Science Australia. Journal of Science and Medicine in Sport, 15, 25-31. http://dx.doi.org/10.1016/j.jsams.2011.04.005

[33] Khalil, A.A., Darawad, M., Al Gamal, E., et al. (2013) Predictors of Dietary and Fluid Non-Adherence in Jordanian Patients with End-Stage Renal Disease Receiving Haemodialysis: A Cross-Sectional Study. Journal of Clinical Nursing, 22, 127-136. http://dx.doi.org/10.1111/j.1365-2702.2012.04117.x

[34] Ingram, C., Wessel, J. and Courneya, K. (2010) Women's Perceptions of Home-Based Exercise Performed during Adjuvant Chemotherapy for Breast Cancer. European Journal of Oncology Nursing, 14, 238-243. http://dx.doi.org/10.1016/j.ejon.2010.01.027

[35] Darawad, M. and Khalil, A. (2013) Jordanian Dialysis Patients' Perceived Exercise Benefits and Barriers: A Correlation Study. Rehabilitation Nursing, 38, 315-322. http://dx.doi.org/10.1002/rnj.98

[36] Stroud, N., Minahan, C. and Sabapathy, S. (2009) The Perceived Benefits and Barriers to Exercise Participation in Persons with Multiple Sclerosis. Disability & Rehabilitation, 31, 2216-2222. http://dx.doi.org/10.3109/09638280902980928

[37] Wang, H.C., Tsai, J.C., Chao, Y.F., et al. (2013) An Exploration of Beliefs Regarding Exercise among Taiwanese Patients with Chronic Obstructive Pulmonary Disease. Heart and Lung, 42, 133-138. http://dx.doi.org/10.1016/j.hrtlng.2012.12.004

[38] Tjønna, A., Lee, S., Rognmo, Ø., et al. (2008) Aerobic Interval Training versus Continuous Moderate Exercise as a Treatment for the Metabolic Syndrome: A Pilot Study. Circulation, 118, 346-354. http://dx.doi.org/10.1161/CIRCULATIONAHA.108.772822

[39] Ramachandran, A., Snehalatha, C., Mary, S., et al. (2006) The Indian Diabetes Prevention Programme Shows That Lifestyle Modification and Metformin Prevent Type 2 Diabetes in Asian Indian Subjects with Impaired Glucose Tolerance (IDPP-1). Diabetologia, 49, 289-297. http://dx.doi.org/10.1007/s00125-005-0097-z

[40] Barnett, F. and Spinks, W. (2007) Exercise Self-Efficacy and Perceived Barriers of Postmenopausal Women Living in North Queensland. Proceedings of the Australian Conference of Science and Medicine in Sport, Adelaide, 13-16 October 2007.

[41] Didarloo, A., Shojaeizadeh, D., Ardebili, H., et al. (2011) Factors Influencing Physical Activity Behavior among Iranian Women with Type 2 Diabetes Using the Extended Theory of Reasoned Action. Diabetes and Metabolism Journal, 35, 513-522. http://dx.doi.org/10.4093/dmj.2011.35.5.513

[42] Smalley, K., Warren, J. and Klibert, J. (2012) Health Risk Behaviors in Insured and Uninsured Community Health Center Patients in the Rural US South. Rural and Remote Health, 12, 2123.

[43] Ellis, T., Boudreau, J.K., Deangelis, T.R., et al. (2013) Barriers to Exercise in People with Parkinson Disease. Physical Therapy, 93, 628-636. http://dx.doi.org/10.2522/ptj.20120279

23

A Case-Control Study on Leisure Time Physical Activity (LTPA) during the Last Three Months of Pregnancy and Foetal Outcomes in Italy

Guglielmina Fantuzzi, Elena Righi, Gabriella Aggazzotti

Department of Biomedical, Metabolic and Neural Sciences, University of Modena and Reggio Emilia, Modena, Italy

Email: guglielmina.fantuzzi@unimore.it

Abstract

The association between Leisure Time Physical Activity (LTPA) during pregnancy and foetal outcomes has been extensively investigated. However, epidemiological studies specifically referred to LPTA in the last months of pregnancy are scarce. We evaluated the association between LPTA and the risk of both preterm delivery and small for gestational age (SGA) during the last three months of pregnancy in Italy. A nationwide case-control study was performed in nine Italian cities. A total of 299 preterm delivery, 364 SGA and 855 controls were enrolled in the study. A self-administered questionnaire was used to assess socio-demographic variables, medical and reproductive history, life-style habits and LTPA referred to the last three months of pregnancy. Univariate and multivariate regression analyses were performed in order to estimate Odds ratios and 95% CI. LTPA during the last three months of pregnancy decreases the risk of preterm delivery (adjusted OR = 0.56; 95% CI 0.39 - 0.79). Among the different types of physical activity, walking, the most frequently referred activity, appears significantly protective against preterm delivery (adjusted OR = 0.53; 95% CI 0.36 - 0.81). Moreover, a small protective effect of walking was evidenced against SGA (adjusted OR = 0.72; 95% CI 0.51 - 1.00). In conclusion, a mild physical activity such as walking in the last three months of pregnancy seems to reduce the risk of preterm delivery and, at a lesser extent, of SGA, confirming the beneficial effects of physical activity along the whole pregnancy.

Keywords

Leisure Time Physical Activity (LTPA), Preterm Delivery, Small for Gestational Age, Last Three Months of Pregnancy, Case Control Study

1. Introduction

Leisure Time Physical Activity (LTPA) is an important factor to improve and maintain the best conditions of physical well-being. Despite this, pregnant women, especially in the last months of pregnancy, tend to reduce or stop practicing sports and physical exercises, thus contributing to the increase of body weight and other recognized disorders such as gestational diabetes and preeclampsia [1]-[4].

In the last years, an increasing number of epidemiological studies has evaluated the association between LTPA during pregnancy and foetal outcomes, in particular gestational length and infant size for gestational age although with conflicting results. The majority of epidemiological studies found a protective influence of LTPA during pregnancy: a reduced risk of preterm birth among women who were engaged in some kind of exercise in comparison with non-exercisers has been documented [5]-[9]. However, other epidemiological studies didn't find any significant association [10]-[13].

Small for Gestational Age (SGA) birth has been less investigated. Some epidemiological studies, focused on the association between LTPA and birthweight in general, found that LTPA during pregnancy doesn't increase the risk of low birth weight [14] [15]. On the contrary, other studies found an association between the time spent in sport activities and low birthweight [16]. Moreover, epidemiological studies suggest that LTPA may help to normalize birthweight into the healthy range by reducing overweight birth [17].

There is an evidence that women tend to modify their LTPA when they become pregnant: a decline in the intensity of physical activity during pregnancy is observed in women who are involved in vigorous sports activities while, on the contrary, women who are inactive prior to pregnancy sometimes start exercising during pregnancy taking into account the wellness of the baby [18] [19].

LTPA frequency in the last period of pregnancy and during the last three months in particular is not well investigated and epidemiological studies specifically referred to preterm delivery and SGA in late pregnancy are scarce in literature. The aim of the present study was to explore the relationship between LPTA in advanced pregnancy and fetal outcomes such as preterm birth and low birthweight and in particular SGA.

2. Methods

2.1. Study Design and Population

A nationwide case-control study focused on maternal LTPA was carried out as a part of a national study primarily designed to investigate in adverse pregnancy outcomes and life style habits. Data were collected in nine Italian cities as described elsewhere [20]. In five cities the participating obstetric clinics covered nearly 100% of total births that occurred in the municipal areas, while in the four largest cities the coverage ranged from 40% to 60% of total births. Participation rate was 96%.

Preterm birth cases (No. 299) were singleton babiesborn before the end of the 37th week of pregnancy, while SGA cases (No. 364) were births with weight below the 10th percentile for the gestational age, according to Italian standards [21]. Controls (No. 855) were placed on singleton births that occurred in the same hospitals 1 - 2 days after the delivery of the case, with a gestational age > 37th completed week of pregnancy and a birthweight over 2500 g. Only babies born from mothers who were Caucasian, born in Italy and resident in the investigated cities were considered eligible for inclusion in the study. Multiple pregnancies or newborns with congenital malformations were excluded.

2.2. Data Collection and Assessment of LTPA

Mothers of cases and controls were recruited during their hospital stay just after delivery by trained interviewers. After informed consent and before hospital discharge, mothers were asked to complete a structured, self-administrated questionnaire, previously validated regarding some style-life variables [22].

The questionnaire collected information about socio-demographic variables (mother's age, educational level, etc.), reproductive and medical history (parity, miscarriages, stillbirth, hypertension, diabetes, etc.) and life-style habits such as smoking habits, environmental tobacco smoke(ETS) exposure and drinking habits (coffee, beer and alcohol consumption). Maternal and infant medical records were reviewed to obtain clinical data about mother's health and birth outcomes (infant sex, gestational age and infant birthweight).

Information on physical activity, both as working activity and LTPA, was referred to the last three months of pregnancy and based on maternal self-reporting. Working activity was defined as yes (occupational activity with movement) or no (either none or sedentary occupation).

LTPA was referred as follows: "have you played any sport in the last three months (other than that included in the antenatal course)? If yes, which activity have you performed for at least >30 min/day? Gymnastics (times/week), cycling (times/week), swimming in indoor or outdoor pool (times/week), walking >1/2 hour (times/week), other sports, specify (times/week)". The questionnaire also gathered information about domestic physical activity such as house-work and gardening (times/week).

The information about the attendance to antenatal classes was also collected, asking about physical activity performed during the courses, frequency and time length.

2.3. Statistical Analyses

Bivariate and multivariate regression procedures were applied to estimate the associations between LTPA and preterm birth and SGA. Odds ratios (ORs) and 95% Confidence Intervals (95% CI) were calculated.

The following variables were considered as confounders: infant gender, maternal age (years), partner, education, employment during the last three months, parity, previous preterm deliveries, previous SGA, miscarriage, stillbirth, gestational diabetes and hypertension, antenatal class attendance. Among style-life habits, active smoking, alcohol and coffee intake, ETS exposure were taken into account. Confounding variables were assessed both by questionnaire and clinical records, when possible.

The regression models were adjusted for variables significantly associated with case status ($p < 0.05$): statistical analyses were performed with SPSS Statistical Software 18.0 for Windows.

Since no invasive procedures were applied in the study, no Ethics Committee approval was required at the time of enrolment of subjects. However, a positive consensus was subsequently asked and obtained.

3. Results

In **Table 1**, the distribution of socio-demographic variables, medical and reproductive history and life-style habits for preterm births and controls is reported. Among maternal characteristics, only age >40 ys was significantly associated with preterm delivery, while no association was found with marital status, education and working activity during the last three months of pregnancy. Mothers of preterm new borns have had previous preterm deliveries, SGA babies, miscarriages and stillbirth when multipara. Moreover, a history of hypertension and diabetes was shown. Active smoking before and during the last three months but not ETS exposure was more frequent in mothers of preterm babies compared with control subjects. Alcohol and coffee intake were not associated, while antenatal classes attendance was positively associated with a low risk of preterm delivery.

Mothers of SGA babies were more likely to have females and to be primipara (**Table 2**). No association was found with age, marital status, education and employment during the last three months of pregnancy. When multipara, previous preterm deliveries, previous SGA babies and miscarriages were more frequent in mothers of SGA cases, while no difference was observed in stillbirth. Regarding to maternal life-style habits, smoking habits, ETS exposure and coffee intake were more frequent in SGA mothers compared with control subjects, while no association was evidenced in alcohol intake and antenatal classes attendance. Regarding to LTPA within the whole sample (1518 subjects), 26% (400 subjects) declared to practice some kind of physical activity during the last three months of pregnancy.

In **Table 3**, unadjusted and adjusted odds ratios (95% CI) of the association between LTPA in the last three months of pregnancy and preterm delivery are reported. Adjusted odds ratios (95% CI) were calculated after controlling for maternal age, previous preterm deliveries, hypertension, diabetes and active tobacco smoking. Both unadjusted and adjusted analyses showed a protective association of LTPA in general and of walking in particular, on preterm delivery. Other activities such as swimming, sports/exercise, biking, housework and gardening are not associated; however the low number of subjects involved in these activities induces caution. In order to avoid misclassification due to the presence of mothers with previous preterm deliveries, the sensitivity analysis was performed taken into account pregnant women without previous preterm deliveries (No. 251): the same association with LTPA was confirmed.

Regarding to SGA, in **Table 4** unadjusted and adjusted odds ratios (95% CI) of the association between LTPA in the last three months of pregnancy and SGA are reported. After controlling for confounding variables,

Table 1. Distribution of preterm delivery cases and controls according to maternal characteristics, reproductive history and maternal life-style habits in Italy.

	Controls n = 855		Preterm delivery cases n = 299		
	n	%^	n	%^	Unadjusted OR [95% CI]
Maternal characteristics					
Maternal age (years)					
≤20	13	1	7	2	1.52 [0.59 - 3.90]
21 - 30	333	39	118	39	1.00 [Reference]
31 - 40	495	58	162	54	0.92 [0.70 - 1.22]
>40	13	1	12	4	2.60 [1.16 - 5.87]
Partner					
Yes	816	96	279	94	1.00 [Reference]
No	34	4	19	6	1.63 [0.92 - 2.91]
Education					
Primary/middle school	246	29	87	29	1.00 [Reference]
High school	417	49	142	47	0.96 [0.71 - 1.31]
University	191	22	69	23	1.02 [0.71 - 1.50]
Working activity during the last three months					
No	240	29	86	29	1.00 [Reference]
Yes	587	71	204	70	0.97 [0.72 - 1.30]
Reproductive history					
Newborn sex					
Males	413	48	160	54	1.00 [Reference]
Females	442	52	135	46	0.79 [0.60 - 1.03]
Parity					
Primiparae	424	50	153	51	1.00 [Reference]
Multiparae	428	50	145	49	0.94 [0.72 - 1.22]
Previous preterm deliveries[§]					
No	386	91	99	68	1.00 [Reference]
Yes	38	9	46	32	4.72 [2.91 - 7.65]
Previous SGA[§]					
No	343	96	73	74	1.00 [Reference]
Yes	15	4	26	26	8.14 [4.11 - 16.14]
Miscarriages[§]					
No	285	67	76	52	1.00 [Reference]
Yes	140	33	69	48	1.85 [1.26 - 2.71]

Continued

Stillbirth[§]					
No	418	99	137	95	1.00 [Reference]
Yes	5	1	8	5	4.88 [1.57 - 15.17]
Diabetes					
No	838	99	277	94	1.00 [Reference]
Yes	10	1	18	6	5.44 [2.48 - 11.94]
Hypertension					
No	820	96	246	84	1.00 [Reference]
Yes	32	4	45	15	4.69 [2.91 - 7.54]
Maternal life-style habits					
Active smoking before pregnancy					
No	595	70	187	63	1.00 [Reference]
Yes	259	30	110	37	1.35 [1.02 - 1.78]
Active smoking in the last three months of pregnancy					
No	721	85	237	80	1.00 [Reference]
Yes	125	15	60	20	1.46 [1.04 - 2.05]
Environmental tobacco smoke exposure					
No	555	65	186	63	1.00 [Reference]
Yes	295	35	111	37	1.12 [0.85 - 1.48]
Coffee intake					
No	357	42	133	45	1.00 [Reference]
Yes	492	58	160	55	0.87 [0.67 - 1.14]
Alcohol intake					
No	468	56	173	59	1.00 [Reference]
Yes	373	44	119	41	0.86 [0.66 - 1.13]
Antenatal classes attendance					
No	436	51	195	66	1.00 [Reference]
Yes	417	49	102	34	0.55 [0.42 - 0.72]

^Percentage may not add to 100 because of rounding or missing information for some subjects; [§]Only in multiparae.

no significant association was observed between LTPA and SGA: however, a small association between SGA and walking was observed in multivariate analysis.

In **Table 5**, adjusted odds ratios [95% CI] of preterm delivery and SGA related to the frequency of LTPA and walking in particular during the last three months of pregnancy were reported. Preterm deliveries were significantly less frequent in women practicing LTPA, both 1 - 2 times/week and ≥3 times/week. Regarding to walking, a protective relationship against preterm delivery was confirmed, above all in women practicing walking 3 times/week.

After controlling for confounding variables (low birth weight, active smoking, coffee) no significant adjusted ORs were evidenced between LTPA and SGA when the frequency of LTPA and walking (1 - 2 times/week and ≥3 times/week) was taken into account.

Table 2. Distribution of SGA cases and controls according to maternal characteristics, reproductive history and maternal life-style habits in Italy.

	Controls n = 855		SGA cases n = 364		
	n	%^	n	%^	Unadjusted OR [95% CI]
Maternal characteristics					
Maternal age (years)					
≤20	13	1	10	3	1.73 [0.74 - 4.04]
21- 30	333	39	148	41	1.00 [Reference]
31- 40	495	58	198	54	0.90 [0.70 - 1.16]
>40	13	1	7	2	1.21 [0.47 - 3.10]
Partner					
Yes	816	96	342	94	1.00 [Reference]
No	34	4	20	5	1.40 [0.80 - 2.47]
Education					
Primary/middle school	246	29	114	38	1.00 [Reference]
High school	417	49	176	59	0.91 [0.69 - 1.21]
University	191	22	68	23	0.77 [0.54 - 1.10]
Employment during the last three months					
No	240	29	105	30	1.00 [Reference]
Yes	587	71	244	70	0.95 [0.72 - 1.25]
Reproductive history					
Newborn sex					
Males	413	48	157	43	1.00 [Reference]
Females	442	52	207	57	1.29 [1.00 - 1.66]
Parity					
Primiparae	424	50	220	61	1.00 [Reference]
Multiparae	428	50	138	38	0.62[0.48 - 0.80]
Previous preterm deliveries[§]					
No	386	91	108	79	1.00 [Reference]
Yes	38	9	29	21	2.73 [1.61 - 4.63]
Previous SGA[§]					
No	343	96	79	81	1.00 [Reference]
Yes	15	4	19	19	5.50 [2.68 - 11.30]
Miscarriages[§]					
No	285	67	75	55	1.00 [Reference]
Yes	140	33	62	45	1.68 [1.14 - 2.49]
Stillbirth[§]					
No	418	99	134	98	1.00 [Reference]
Yes	5	1	3	2	1.87 [0.44 - 7.93]
Diabetes					
No	838	99	348	99	1.00 [Reference]
Yes	10	1	4	1	0.96 [0.30 - 3.09]
Hypertension					
No	820	96	345	95	1.00 [Reference]
Yes	32	4	19	5	1.41 [0.79 - 2.52]

Continued

Maternal life-style habits					
Active smoking before pregnancy					
No	595	70	228	63	1.00 [Reference]
Yes	259	30	131	36	1.32 [1.02 - 1.71]
Active smoking in the last three months of pregnancy					
No	721	85	256	71	1.00 [Reference]
Yes	125	15	102	28	2.30 [1.71 - 3.10]
Environmental tobacco smoke exposure					
No	555	65	199	58	1.00 [Reference]
Yes	295	35	141	41	1.33 [1.03 - 1.72]
Coffee intake					
No	357	42	116	35	1.00 [Reference]
Yes	492	58	219	65	1.37 [1.05 - 1.78]
Alcohol intake					
No	468	56	203	61	1.00 [Reference]
Yes	373	44	130	39	0.80 [0.62 - 1.08]
Antenatal classes attendance					
No	436	51	181	51	1.00 [Reference]
Yes	417	49	175	49	1.01 [0.79 - 1.29]

^Percentage may not add to 100 because of rounding or missing information for some subjects. §Only in multiparae.

Table 3. Unadjusted and adjusted odds ratios (OR) [95% confidence intervals] of preterm delivery related to LTPA during the last three months of pregnancy.

	Controls n = 853		Cases n = 299		Unadjusted ORs [95% CI]	Adjusted ORs* [95% CI]
	n	%^	n	%^		
LTPA						
No	604	71	244	82	1.00 [Reference]	1.00 [Reference]
Yes	249	29	54	18	0.54 [0.39 - 0.75]	0.56 [0.39 - 0.79]
Swimming						
No	763	89	279	94	1.00 [Reference]	1.00 [Reference]
Yes	90	11	19	6	0.58 [0.35 - 0.96]	0.71 [0.42 - 1.21]
Walking						
No	678	79	261	88	1.00 [Reference]	1.00 [Reference]
Yes	175	21	37	12	0.55 [0.37 - 0.80]	0.53 [0.36 - 0.81]
Sports/exercise						
No	833	98	296	99	1.00 [Reference]	1.00 [Reference]
Yes	20	2	2	1	0.28 [0.06 - 1.21]	0.28 [0.06 - 1.16]
Biking						
No	839	98	293	98	1.00 [Reference]	1.00 [Reference]
Yes	14	2	5	2	1.02 [0.36 - 2.86]	1.32 [0.46 - 3.82]
House-work and gardening						
No	791	93	276	93	1.00 [Reference]	1.00 [Reference]
Yes	57	7	20	7	1.00 [0.59 - 1.70]	0.96 [0.54 - 1.70]

*adjusted for maternal age, previous preterm deliveries, hypertension, diabetes and active tobacco smoke during pregnancy.

Table 4. Unadjusted and adjusted odds ratios (OR) [95% confidence intervals] of SGA related to LTPA during the last three months of pregnancy.

	Controls n = 853		Cases n = 364		Unadjusted ORs [95% CI]	Adjusted ORs* [95% CI]
	n	%^	n	%^		
LTPA						
No	604	71	261	73	1.00 [Reference]	1.00 [Reference]
Yes	249	29	97	27	0.90 [0.68 - 1.19]	0.87 [0.65 - 1.16]
Swimming						
No	763	89	314	88	1.00 [Reference]	1.00 [Reference]
Yes	90	11	44	12	1.19 [0.81 - 1.74]	1.17 [0.78 - 1.75]
Walking						
No	678	80	299	83	1.00 [Reference]	1.00 [Reference]
Yes	175	20	59	17	0.76 [0.55 - 1.06]	0.72 [0.51 - 1.00]
Sports/exercise						
No	833	98	349	97	1.00 [Reference]	1.00 [Reference]
Yes	20	2	9	3	1.07 [0.48 - 2.38]	1.05 [0.47 - 2.38]
Biking						
No	839	98	354	99	1.00 [Reference]	1.00 [Reference]
Yes	14	2	4	1	0.68 [0.22 - 2.07]	0.78 [0.25 - 2.44]
House-work and gardening						
No	791	93	331	93	1.00 [Reference]	1.00 [Reference]
Yes	57	7	25	7	1.05 [0.64 - 1.71]	1.11 [0.67 - 1.84]

*adjusted for maternal age, previous preterm deliveries, hypertension, diabetes and active tobacco smoke during pregnancy.

Table 5. Adjusted odds ratios [95% CI] of preterm delivery and SGA related to the frequency of LTPA and walking in particular during the last three months of pregnancy.

	Controls		Preterm delivery			SGA		
LTPA (times/week)	n	%	n	%	Adjusted ORs° [95% CI]	n	%	Adjusted ORs* [95% CI]
No	604	71	244	82	1.00 [Reference]	261	73	1.00 [Reference]
1, 2 times/week	83	10	16	5	0.50 [0.27 - 0.90]	32	9	0.96 [0.61 - 1.51]
≥3 times/week	166	19	38	13	0.59 [0.39 - 0.88]	65	18	0.82 [0.59 - 1.16]
Walking (times/week]								
No	678	72	261	88	1.00 [Reference]	299	83	1.00 [Reference]
1, 2 times/week	43	5	14	5	0.85 [0.44 - 1.67]	12	3	0.65 [0.33 - 1.26]
≥3 times/week	132	15	23	8	0.44 [0.27 - 0.71]	47	13	0.74 [0.51 - 1.07]

°adjusted for age, active smoking, other preterm delivery, hypertension, diabetes; *adjusted for other low birth weight, active smoking, coffee.

4. Discussion

The present study shows that women who have performed physical activity as LTPA mainly walking in the late period of pregnancy are at substantially lower risk of preterm delivery compared to women who are less active.

The results of our study are in agreement with some large prospective cohorts when comparing the same period of pregnancy. Findings from a study performed in Brazil on preterm delivery showed that LTPA during the third trimester was associated with a lower chance of preterm birth [6]. Moreover, mild physical activity during the second trimester of pregnancy such as walking shows an independent protective effect on low birth weight, preterm birth, and intrauterine growth restriction [9].

In Europe, the Norwegian Mother and Child Cohort Study showed that women exercising three to five times per week at 30th week of gestation had significantly reduced risk of preterm birth (adjusted OR = 0.74, 95% CI = 0.65 - 0.83) compared to non-exercisers [8]. Very similar results have been observed also in the Danish National Birth Cohort where a reduced risk of preterm birth among women who engaged in some kind of exercise during pregnancy, even at the lowest level, in comparison with non-exercisers was evidenced (hazard ratio: 0.82, 95% C.I.: 0.76 - 0.88) [5].

In our study, the slight but not significant protective effect against the risk of SGA is in agreement with the results from the Danish National Birth Cohort where in the exercising women a slightly decreased risk of having a child small for gestational age (hazard ratio = 0.87, 95% CI 0.83 - 0.92) was observed [23]. Other studies suggest that recreational physical activity is associated with a protective effect against SGA when practiced at a medium range of frequency (for instance 3 - 4 times a week) while either a high or low frequency of physical activity may be at risk of SGA [16]. A recent cohort study among predominantly Puerto Rican women evidenced that a high total physical activity in mid-pregnancy was associated with a decreased risk of SGA (RR = 0.42; 95% CI 0.21 - 0.82) as compared to those with low total activity: however, high levels of sports/exercise were associated with an increased SGA risk (RR = 2.14, 95% CI 1.04 - 4.39) [23]. No association between sports and LTPA and low-birthweight was recently found in a large population based study in Sweden where 4458 healthy women who delivered after 37th completed gestational weeks were involved [14].

Our study has some strengths. First of all, it has been carried out nationwide involving Italian subjects from North to South and Sicily, resident in Italy. Moreover, the enrolment of cases and controls has reached a high coverage (100% of births in 5 cities and from 40 to 60% in the remaining 4) and the participation rate was high as well (96%), with no difference between cases and controls. In this way, selection bias was controlled.

Within our sample, LTPA was practiced in 29% of control subjects: this value is in agreement with the data reported in the Danish cohort by Juhl et al. [5] while higher than those reported by Haastad et al. in Norway, where less than 11% were defined as regular exercisers in the third trimester [24]. A very low prevalence value (4%) of LTPA during the 3 trimester was reported in a Brazil cohort study [6]. However, women characteristics such as race, income and style-life habits could explain the observed differences. Information bias in the classification of cases could be excluded as preterm delivery and SGA cases were confirmed by medical records. Moreover this kind of data may suffer from reporting bias because of social desirability and/or poor recall: however, the interlapsed time is short and misclassification may be not significant.

In the present study a variety of potential confounding factors was taken into account; however, residual confounding may still be present. First of all the assessment of LTPA is based on self-reported questionnaire. It is well known that it may be an important source of potential bias: however, our results are similar to those provided by other investigators. They suggest that the relation between physical activity and pregnancy outcomes is robust, and can be detected even when physical activity is measured using relatively imprecise techniques. Of particular concern, we cannot exclude that the observed association between LTPA and pregnancy outcomes is confounded by maternal weight gain during pregnancy, variable which we were not able to control for in the analysis.

A limitation of any study on physical activity during pregnancy is that women whose previous pregnancies resulted in preterm birth or other negative outcomes are more likely to avoid physical efforts. In our study when the sensitivity analysis was performed taken into account women without previous preterm deliveries only, the results of the study were confirmed: however residual confounding could exist and not controlled for.

Moreover, women who are active during the third trimester may represent a very specific group of women who are willing to exercise and likely to adopt several other healthy habits. Unfortunately, these aspects cannot be controlled for in this study. Regarding to biological plausibility, LTPA during pregnancy could decrease the risk of preterm delivery by improving placentation and vascularization while reducing oxidative stress [25] [26].

5. Conclusion

In conclusion, because no harm or risk increase was detected among women who exercised, and physical activity throughout life is considered a healthy behaviour, LTPA during the whole pregnancy, the last period included, should be encouraged during prenatal care visits. This is in agreement with the American College of Obstetricians and Gynaecologists guidelines (2002) that recommend that women with no contraindications should be advised to practice physical activity during the whole pregnancy [27].

Acknowledgements

This study was partially supported by the Italian Ministry of University, Technology and Research (grant No. 9806171176/98).

Conflict of Interest

The authors declare that they have no conflict of interest.

References

[1]   Borodulin, K., Evenson, K.R., Wen, F., Herring, A. and Benson, A. (2008) Physical Activity Patterns during Pregnancy. *Medicine & Science in Sports & Exercis*, **40**, 1901-1908. http://dx.doi.org/10.1249/MSS.0b013e31817f1957

[2]   Hegaard, H.K., Pedersen, B.K., Nielsen, B.B. and Damm, P. (2007) Leisure Time Physical Activity during Pregnancy and Impact on Gestational Diabetes Mellitus, Pre-Eclampsia, Preterm Delivery and Birth Weight: A Review. *Acta Obstetricia et Gynecologica Scandinavica*, **86**, 1290-1296. http://dx.doi.org/10.1080/00016340701647341

[3]   Downs, D.S., Chasan-Taber, L., Evenson, K.R., Leiferman, J. and Yeo, S. (2012) Physical Activity and Pregnancy: Past and Present Evidence and Future Recommendations. *Research Quarterly for Exercise & Sport*, **83**, 485-502. http://dx.doi.org/10.1080/02701367.2012.10599138

[4]   Mudd, L.M., Owe, K.M., Mottola, M.F. and Pivarnik, J.M. (2013) Health Benefits of Physical Activity during Pregnancy: An International Perspective. *Medicine & Science in Sports & Exercise*, **45**, 268-277. http://dx.doi.org/10.1249/MSS.0b013e31826cebcb

[5]   Juhl, M., Andersen, P.K., Olsen, J., Madsen, M., Jorgensen, T., Nohr, E.A. and Nybo Andersen, A. (2008) Physical Exercise during Pregnancy and the Risk of Preterm Birth: A Study within the Danish National Birth Cohort. *American Journal of Epidemiology*, **167**, 859-866. http://dx.doi.org/10.1093/aje/kwm364

[6]   Domingues, M.R. and Barros, A.J. (2007) Leisure-Time Physical Activity during Pregnancy in the 2004 Pelotas Birth Cohort Study. *Revista de Saude Publica*, **41**, 173-180. http://dx.doi.org/10.1590/S0034-89102007000200002

[7]   Hegaard, H.K., Hedegaard, M., Damm, P., Ottesen, B., Petersson, K. and Henriksen, T.B. (2008) Leisure Time Physical Activity Is Associated with a Reduced Risk of Preterm Delivery. *American Journal of Obstetrics and Gynecology*, **198**, 180-185. http://dx.doi.org/10.1016/j.ajog.2007.08.038

[8]   Owe, K.M, Nystad, W., Skjaerven, R., Stigum, H. and Bø, K. (2012) Exercise during Pregnancy and the Gestational Age Distribution: A Cohort Study. *Medicine & Science in Sports & Exercise*, **44**, 1067-1074. http://dx.doi.org/10.1249/MSS.0b013e3182442fc9

[9]   Takito, M.Y. and Benício, M.H. (2010) Physical Activity during Pregnancy and Fetal Outcomes: A Case-Control Study. *Revista de Saúde Públic*, **44**, 90-101. http://dx.doi.org/10.1590/s0034-89102010000100010

[10]   Leiferman, J.A. and Evenson, K.R. (2003) The Effect of Regular Leisure Physical Activity on Birth Outcomes. *Maternal and Child Health Journal*, **7**, 59-64. http://dx.doi.org/10.1023/A:1022545718786

[11]   Barakat, R., Stirling, J.R. and Lucia, A. (2008) Does Exercise Training during Pregnancy Affect Gestational Age? A Randomised Controlled Trial. *British Journal Sports Medicine*, **42**, 674-678. http://dx.doi.org/10.1136/bjsm.2008.047837

[12]   Barakat, R., Pelaez, M., Montejo, R., Refoyo, I. and Coteron, J. (2014) Exercise throughout Pregnancy Does Not Cause Preterm Delivery. A Randomized, Controlled Trial. *Journal of Physical Activity & Health*, **11**, 1012-1017. http://dx.doi.org/10.1123/jpah.2012-0344

[13]   Currie, L.M., Woolcott, C.G., Fell, D.B., Armson, B.A. and Dodds, L. (2014) The Association between Physical Activity and Maternal and Neonatal Outcomes: A Prospective Cohort. *Maternal and Child Health Journal*, **18**, 1823-1833. http://dx.doi.org/10.1007/s10995-013-1426-3

[14]   Hegaard, H.K., Petersson, K., Hedegaard, M., Ottesen, B., Dykes, A.K., Henriksen, T.B. and Damm, P. (2010) Sports and Leisure-Time Physical Activity in Pregnancy and Birth Weight: A Population-Based Study. *Scandinavian Journal of Medicine & Science in Sports*, **20**, e96-e102. http://dx.doi.org/10.1111/j.1600-0838.2009.00918.x

[15]   Juhl, M., Olsen, J., Andersen, P.K., Nøhr, E.A. and Andersen, A.M. (2010) Physical Exercise during Pregnancy and Fetal Growth Measures: A Study within the Danish National Birth Cohort. *American Journal of Obstetrics & Gyne-

cology, **202**, 63.e1-63.e8. http://dx.doi.org/10.1016/j.ajog.2009.07.033

[16] Campbell, M.K. and Mottola, M.F. (2001) Recreational Exercise and Occupational Activity during Pregnancy and Birth Weight: A Case-Control Study. *American Journal of Obstetrics and Gynecology*, **184**, 403-408. http://dx.doi.org/10.1067/mob.2001.109392

[17] Alderman, B.W., Zhao, H., Holt, V.L., Watts, D.H. and Beresford, S.A. (1998) Maternal Physical Activity in Pregnancy and Infant Size for Gestational Age. *Annals of Epidemiology*, **8**, 513-519. http://dx.doi.org/10.1016/S1047-2797(98)00020-9

[18] Petersen, A.M., Leet, T.L. and Brownson, R.C. (2005) Correlates of Physical Activity among Pregnant Women in the United States. *Medicine & Science in Sports & Exercise*, **37**, 1748-1753. http://dx.doi.org/10.1249/01.mss.0000181302.97948.90

[19] Haakstad, L.A., Voldner, N., Henriksen, T. and Bo, K. (2007) Physical Activity Level and Weight Gain in a Cohort of Pregnant Norwegian Women. *Acta Obstetricia et Gynecologica Scandinavica*, **86**, 559-564. http://dx.doi.org/10.1080/00016340601185301

[20] Aggazzotti, G., Righi, E., Fantuzzi, G., Biasotti, B., Ravera, G., Kanitz, S., Barbone, F., Sansebastiano, G., Battaglia, M., Leoni, V., Fabiani, L., Triassi, M. and Sciacca, S. (2004) Chlorination By-Products (CBPs) in Drinking Water and Adverse Pregnancy Outcomes in Italy. *Journal of Water and Health*, **2**, 233-247.

[21] Parazzini, F., Cortinovis, I., Bortolus, R., Fedele, L. and Decarli, A. (1995) Weight at Birth by Gestational Age in Italy. *Human Reproduction*, **10**, 1862-1963.

[22] Barbone, F., Valent, F., Brussi, V., Tomasella, L., Triassi, M., Di Lieto, A., Scognamiglio, G., Righi, E., Fantuzzi, G., Casolari, L. and Aggazzotti, G. (2002) Assessing the Exposure of Pregnant Women to Drinking Water Disinfection By-Products. *Epidemiology*, **13**, 540-544. http://dx.doi.org/10.1097/00001648-200209000-00009

[23] Gollenberg, A.L., Pekow, P., Bertone-Johnson, E.R., Freedson, P.S., Markenson, G. and Chasan-Taber, L. (2011) Physical Activity and Risk of Small-for-Gestational-Age Birth among Predominantly Puerto Rican Women. *Maternal and Child Health Journal*, **15**, 49-59. http://dx.doi.org/10.1007/s10995-009-0563-1

[24] Haakstad, L.A., Voldner, N., Henriksen, T. and Bø, K. (2009) Why Do Pregnant Women Stop Exercising in the Third Trimester? *Acta Obstetricia et Gynecologica Scandinavica*, **88**, 1267-1275. http://dx.doi.org/10.3109/00016340903284901

[25] Clapp, F., Kim, H., Burciu, B. and Lopez, B. (2000) Beginning Regular Exercise in Early Pregnancy: Effect on Feto-Placental Growth. *American Journal of Obstetrics and Gynecology*, **183**, 1484-1488. http://dx.doi.org/10.1067/mob.2000.107096

[26] Clapp, J.F., Stephanchak, W., Tomaselli, J., Kortan, M. and Faneslow, S. (2000) Portal Vein Blood Flow—Effects of Pregnancy, Gravity, and Exercise. *American Journal of Obstetrics and Gynecology*, **183**, 167-172.

[27] American College of Obstetricians and Gynecologists (ACOG Committee) (2002) Opinion No. 267: Exercise during Pregnancy and the Postpartum Period. *Obstetrics & Gynecology*, **99**, 171-173. http://dx.doi.org/10.1016/S0029-7844(01)01749-5

24

The Brunel Mood Scale Rating in Mental Health for Physically Active and Apparently Healthy Populations

Ricardo Brandt[1,2], Dafne Herrero[3], Thaís Massetti[4], Tânia Brusque Crocetta[2,5], Regiani Guarnieri[5], Carlos Bandeira de Mello Monteiro[4,5], Maick da Silveira Viana[2], Guilherme Guimarães Bevilacqua[2], Luiz Carlos de Abreu[5], Alexandro Andrade[2]

[1]State University of West Parana, Marechal Cândido Rondon, Brazil
[2]Laboratory of Sport and Exercise Psychology, Santa Catarina State University, Florianópolis, Brazil
[3]Faculty Public Health, São Paulo, Brazil
[4]Post-Graduate Program in Rehabilitation Sciences, Faculty of Medicine, University of São Paulo, São Paulo, Brazil
[5]Department of Morphology and Physiology, Faculty of Medicine of ABC, Santo André, Brazil
Email: ricabrandt@gmail.com

Abstract

There is a positive relationship between mood states and mental health. The aim of the present study was to investigate the construct validity and internal consistency of the Brunel Mood Scale (BRUMS) for use with different populations, which are physically active and apparently healthy. Measures were obtained from 1295 male (N = 709, 34 ± 20 years, mean ± SD) and female (N = 576, 43 ± 24 years, mean ± SD) volunteers. Factor analysis was used, verifying that six factors (components) accounted for 62.65% of the total variance of the scale. The Varimax method with Kaiser Normalization for the rotation of the factors for the main components, and it was observed that the 24 scale items loaded on six mood factors (anger, depression, tension, vigor, fatigue, and confusion). Internal consistency was good for all the factors identified. We suggest that the results provide some support for validity of the BRUMS for use with different populations, which are physically active and apparently healthy.

Keywords

Mental Health, Mood States, Psychometrics, Brunel Mood Scale, BRUMS

1. Introduction

Over the past few decades, there has been a growing body of literature on mental health [1]. However, there is still a need to develop related research into the association between physical activity and mental health [2], as problems in this context are a worldwide concern in public health [3], affecting all age groups and accounting for significant expenditure by governments [4].

There is a positive relationship between mood states and mental health [5] [6]. It is considered that the high level of vigor associated with lower levels of tension, depression, anger, fatigue and confusion is related to a better mental health condition [7] [8].

Among the instruments that evaluate moods, the POMS (Profile of Mood States) stands out as one of the most widely used in different populations [9] [10]. The Brunel Mood Scale (BRUMS), derived from the POMS, the validation of which in Brazil was performed by Rohlfs *et al.* [11], was presented as a tool for detection of the over-training syndrome. In addition, such scales have been used in different populations and contexts in Brazil [12]-[14] and other countries [15]-[17].

The 24-item BRUMS measures six identifiable mood states (Tension, Depression, Anger, Vigor, Fatigue, and Confusion) through a self-report inventory. The respondents rating a list of adjectives, on a 5-point Likert scale from 0 (not at all) to 4 (extremely), on the basis of how they had been feeling in the previous week, or in the moment of evaluation [12] [18]. The six affective mood states subscales are not diagnostic indicators, but refer to sub-clinical psychological states (mood states) [19].

This study aims to investigate the construct validity and internal consistency of the BRUMS for different populations, which are physically active and apparently healthy.

2. Method

This is a descriptive cross-sectional study with non-probability sampling (Sample size calculation was not conducted before sampling). The participants in the study were 1,295 individuals from Santa Catarina state, south of Brazil, of both sexes, physically active and apparently healthy: 709 (54.7%) men with a mean age of 34 years (±20) and 586 (45.3%) women, with a mean age of 43 years (±24). Data were collected during 2013 year, from February to November.

The BRUMS [11] has 24 items arranged into six subscales: anger, confusion, depression, fatigue, tension and vigor (**Table 1**), each with four items. The research participant selects, from a numerical rating scale of zero to four (0 = not at all, 1 = a bit, 2 = moderate, 3 = enough; 4 = extremely), the option they believe best represents the situation at that time, using questions such as "How do you feel now?", "How have been feeling in the past week, including today?", or "How have you been feeling?".

The items on each subscale are:

- Anger: annoyed, bitter, angry, bad-tempered;
- Confusion: confused, muddled, mixed-up, uncertain;
- Depression: depressed, downhearted, unhappy, miserable;
- Fatigue: worn out, exhausted, sleepy, tired;
- Tension: panicky, anxious, worried, nervous;
- Vigor: lively, energetic, active, alert.

Table 1. Dimensions of BRUMS.

DIMENSION	DEFINITION
Tension	State of musculoskeletal tension and worry.
Depression	Emotional state of despondency, sadness, unhappiness.
Anger	State of hostility, for others.
Vigor	State of energy, physical force.
Fatigue	State of tiredness, low energy.
Confusion	State of feeling stunned, instability in emotions.

Reference: Brandt *et al.* [20].

The sum of the responses of each subscale results in a score that ranges from zero to 16. The questionnaire does not generate an overall score, and each scale should be examined individually, although the constructs are related.

Survey participants were characterized with respect to other variables, based on the study of Brandt et al. [12], regarding self perception of sleep quality and self-related health. Self perceived health status and quality of sleep, composed Likert scale with responses from 0 ("very bad") to 4 ("excellent") [20]. These questions were used to compare means of moods, depending on the variables mentioned in the literature, allowing the visualization of the use of the scale in the research.

All survey participants signed an informed consent and it was approved by the Research Ethics Committee (44/2011), according to Resolution 196/96 of the National Health Council. A previously trained researcher administered the sample individually. The research procedures were explained and the participants asked to point out if the matter was not clear. For elderly participants, a printed sheet was presented with the response options. The response time was no longer than six minutes.

Data were tabulated and analyzed using SPSS software version 21.0. The internal consistency of the subscales was assessed using Cronbach's alpha. The authors of the original instrument [21], found the alpha to be greater than 0.76, so it is considered an instrument with good internal consistency.

Construct validity was assessed through exploratory factor analysis, which identified the common components in a large number of variables. The factor analysis was performed according to the steps proposed by Dancey and Reidy [22].

We used the principal components method for extracting the factors and considered only those that presented an eigenvalue of one. For selected factors, a correlation matrix was generated, where relationships between items and factors were observed through factor loadings. For the purposes of the matrix, the orthogonal rotation Varimax method was applied, which maximizes high correlations and minimizes casualties, facilitating analysis.

To analyze the results of the mood states, descriptive and inferential statistics (mean and standard deviation) were used (Kruskal-Wallis and Mann-Whitney).

3. Results

In order to confirm the theoretical factors, factor analysis was used, verifying that the six factors (components) accounted for 62.65% of the total variance of the scale (**Table 2**). The KMO (Kaiser-Mayer-Olkin) test ($X^2 = 0.909$, $p < 0.001$) indicated the proportion of the data variance and their values can be considered suitable, as well as the Bartlett sphericity test ($X^2 = 11259.9$, $p < 0.05$), concerning the correlation between the data.

Table 3 shows the correlations (factor loadings) for each item with each factor, respectively. We used the method of the main components with the Varimax method rotation of the factors, with Kaiser normalization. The saturation with values was greater than 0.30 and the items appear ordered by factor.

It is observed that the 24 scale items loaded on six mood factors (anger, depression, tension, vigor, fatigue and confusion), corresponding to the analyses found by Rohlfs et al. [11] in the BRUMS validation to search for Brazilian athletes and non-athletes.

Table 2. Eigenvalues and explained variance components of the BRUMS.

COMPONENT	Eigenvalues initials		
	Total	% Variance	% cumulative
1 (Anger)	7.27	30.33	30.33
2 (Depression)	2.62	10.92	41.25
3 (Tension)	1.68	7.03	48.28
4 (Vigor)	1.41	5.91	54.20
5 (Fatigue)	1.13	4.72	58.92
6 (Confusion)	1.01	3.73	62.65

Extraction method: Principal component analysis.

Table 3. Exploratory factor load for each item in the six factors extracted from the BRUMS.

Component	1	2	3	4	5	6	Cronback Alfa
ITENS	Anger	Depression	Tension	Vigor	Fatigue	Confusion	
Annoyed	0.722						0.830
Bitter	0.785						0.826
Angry	0.813						0.831
Bad tempered	0.671						0.830
Depressed		0.648					0.831
Downhearted		0.621					0.831
Unhappy		0.647					0.832
Miserable		0.440					0.832
Panicky			0.388				0.829
Anxious			0.806				0.831
Worried			0.724				0.834
Nervous			0.741				0.831
Lively				0.725			0.851
Energetic				0.773			0.851
Active				0.789			0.851
Alert				0.639			0.852
Worn out					0.776		0.830
Exhausted					0.803		0.829
Sleepy					0.491		0.835
Tired					0.785		0.831
Confused						0.693	0.828
Muddled						0.486	0.828
Mixed-up						0.614	0.832
Uncertain						0.601	0.828

Extraction method: Principal component analysis. Rotation Method: Varimax, with Kaiser normalization.

Anger and Vigor had factor loadings above 0.63 in all items, without existing cross-loading. In Depression, the items, "depressed", "downhearted", and "unhappy" showed high factor loadings, greater than 0.62. The item "miserable" showed a lower factor loading (0.440). There was cross-loading with the item "confused". For Tension, the items "anxious", "worried", and "nervous" obtained factor loadings higher than 0.72, with no cross-loading. Fatigue items obtained factor loadings above 0.70 except for "sleepy", which showed a lower factor loading (0.491). Confusion presented three items with factor loadings above 0.60. The item "muddled" had a lower factor loading and introduced cross-loading with the Depression factor.

The internal consistency of the 24 items was high ($\alpha = 0.85$). Internal consistency was good for all the factors identified: Anger $\alpha = 0.65$; Confusion $\alpha = 0.63$; Depression $\alpha = 0.66$; Fatigue $\alpha = 0.60$; Tension $\alpha = 0.65$, and Vigor $\alpha = 0.81$.

The participants, both men and women, showed high levels of Vigor and low levels of Tension, Depression, Anger, Fatigue and Confusion (**Figure 1**), and there are significant differences in the variables Anger, Vigor and Fatigue between men and women.

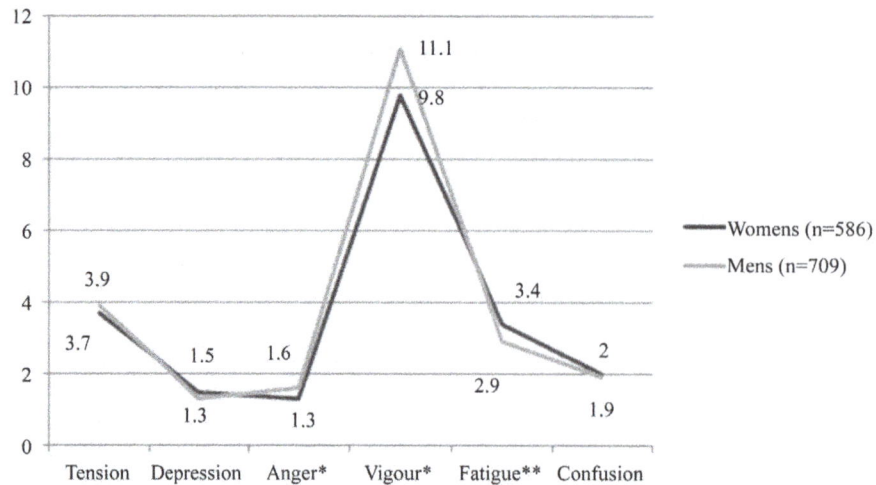

Figure 1. Mood states of men and women engaged in physical activity, apparently healthy.
*Significant difference at p < 0.05. **Significant difference at p < 0.001.

Separating the participants into age groups (**Table 4**), there is a significant difference between the moods of the youngest participants (under 18), adults (between 18 and 60 years) and the elderly (over 60 years).

By analyzing the mood depending on self-perceived health status, participants who showed better perception had lower levels of Depression, Fatigue and Confusion and Vigor, when compared to those with poorer self-rated health. With the relationship between sleep and moods, all factors are significantly different between those with a better perception of quality of sleep.

4. Discussion

The aim of this study was to investigate the construct validity and internal consistency of the BRUMS, so as to recognize it as an instrument for measuring mental health in different populations, which are physically active and apparently healthy.

The BRUMS has been used in different populations of athletes and non-athletes, young people and adults [12] [23], with heart disease [24], and with fibromyalgia [13] [14], among others. Its validation for physically active and apparently healthy populations showed consistent results, with good reliability and construct validity, as evidenced by the alpha coefficient and factor loadings, found to be higher than other instrument validation studies [25].

Generally, the factors were properly loaded in their respective domains. The low cross-existence between the loading factors is a positive element in the present study, given that other validations showed a higher amount of cross-loading which does not compromise their results [26]. It has been found that there are six factors with eigenvalues above one, similar to those found in Rohlfs et al. [11]. A high internal consistency was observed, with values of 0.85, whereas all areas had values appropriate for its validation.

In the analysis of the results for the BRUMS application, it is evident that there is a difference in the moods of men and women, already presented in other studies, as well as for the different age groups [7] [12] [14] [27]. Moreover, in the latter, there is a significant difference in all mood factors. When analyzing the results of the mood states, it is suggested that researchers investigate these characteristic differences in their populations, thereby reducing the possibility of error in the data analysis.

In analyzing the results of the self-assessment of health and sleep, it is clear who has a tendency to better health and sleep, has a mood with greater vigor and less tension, depression, anger, fatigue and confusion. This would be consistent with the proposed profile by Morgan [8] entitled the 'iceberg' profile (**Figure 1**), this being an ideal mental health model. Corroborating this study demonstrates the importance of sleep to mental health, in the sense of insufficient or poor sleep can cause mental disorders, impairing cognitive function and performance [28] [29].

From these analyses it is evident that the use of BRUMS beyond the detection of the over-training syndrome [11], where it has been used in research to delineate the mood profile of different populations, is that it may also

Table 4. Factors of mood about age, self perceived health status and self perception of sleep quality in physically active subjects, apparently healthy.

Associated factors	Tension $\bar{x}$	±	Depression $\bar{x}$	±	Anger $\bar{x}$	±	Vigor $\bar{x}$	±	Fatigue $\bar{x}$	±	Confusion $\bar{x}$	±
Age group	**		**		**		**		**		**	
Less than 18 years (n = 271)	4.8	2.9	1.1	1.2	1.4	2.2	10.7	2.8	3.1	2.7	2.4	2.6
Between 18 and 60 (n = 624)	4.4	3.2	1.6	2.6	1.9	2.9	10.9	3.1	3.6	3.4	2.1	2.6
More than 60 years (n = 385)	2.1	2.4	1.2	2.1	0.7	1.7	9.7	2.8	2.5	2.9	1.1	1.9
Health assessment			**				**		*		*	
Excellent (n = 292)	3.7	3.2	0.8	1.7	1.2	2.3	11.6	2.9	2.7	3.1	1.4	2.1
Good (n = 589)	4.1	2.9	1.3	2.2	1.6	2.5	10.6	2.7	3.2	3.1	2.2	2.4
Regular (n = 134)	3.7	3.1	1.9	2.9	1.7	2.8	9.8	3.1	3.5	3.1	2.1	2.6
Poor (n = 11)	5.7	4.5	3.9	3.5	2.3	3.1	8.7	3.8	4.8	3.8	2.6	3.9
Very bad (n = 5)	2.2	1.6	1.2	2.1	0.6	1.3	10.4	2.9	1.4	1.9	1.0	1.7
Sleep quality perception	*		**		**		**		**		**	
Excellent (n = 105)	4.1	3.0	0.8	1.6	1.4	2.0	12.0	3.1	2.6	2.5	1.5	2.0
Good (n = 419)	4.3	2.9	1.2	2.1	1.5	2.4	11.1	2.7	3.1	2.9	1.9	2.2
Regular (n = 231)	4.8	3.0	1.4	2.4	1.9	2.7	10.5	3.1	3.9	3.6	2.4	2.7
Poor (n = 44)	5.5	3.9	2.7	3.8	3.7	4.2	10.4	2.9	5.3	3.6	3.4	3.4
Very bad (n = 5)	6.2	5.7	7.2	3.9	5.8	4.8	8.0	2.2	6.4	3.7	6.8	4.9

*Significant difference at $p < 0.05$. **Significant difference at $p < 0.001$.

be used as a mental health indicator.

5. Conclusion

From the above, considering that researchers are in different contexts and with different populations, their use of the BRUMS can investigate mental health in different populations, which are physically active and apparently healthy.

Authors' Contributions

All authors participated in the acquisition of data and revision of the manuscript. All authors determined the design, interpreted the data and drafted the manuscript. All authors read and gave final approval for the version submitted for publication.

Declaration of Interest

The authors report no conflict of interest. All authors were responsible for the content and writing of this paper.

References

[1] Takacs, J. (2014) Regular Physical Activity and Mental Health. The Role of Exercise in the Prevention of, and Intervention in Depressive Disorders. *Psychiatr Hung*, **29**, 386-397.

[2] Asare, M. and Danquah, S.A. (2015) The Relationship between Physical Activity, Sedentary Behaviour and Mental Health in Ghanaian Adolescents. *Child and Adolescent Psychiatry and Mental Health*, **9**, 11. http://dx.doi.org/10.1186/s13034-015-0043-x

[3]   Whiteford, H.A., Degenhardt, L., Rehm, J., Baxter, A.J., Ferrari, A.J., Erskine, H.E., Charlson, F.J., Norman, R.E., Flaxman, A.D., Johns, N., Burstein, R., Murray, C.J. and Vos, T. (2013) Global Burden of Disease Attributable to Mental and Substance Use Disorders: Findings from the Global Burden of Disease Study 2010. *Lancet*, **382**, 1575-1586. http://dx.doi.org/10.1016/S0140-6736(13)61611-6

[4]   Sarmento, M. (2015) A "Mental Health Profile" of Higher Education Students. *Procedia-Social and Behavioral Sciences*, **191**, 12-20. http://dx.doi.org/10.1016/S0140-6736(13)61611-6

[5]   Sarkin, A.J., Groessl, E.J., Carlson, J.A., Tally, S.R., Kaplan, R.M., Sieber, W.J. and Ganiats, T.G. (2013) Development and Validation of a Mental Health Subscale from the Quality of Well-Being Self-Administered. *Quality of Life Research*, **22**, 1685-1696. http://dx.doi.org/10.1007/s11136-012-0296-2

[6]   Yoshihara, K., Hiramoto, T., Sudo, N. and Kubo, C. (2011) Profile of Mood States and Stress-Related Biochemical Indices in Long-Term Yoga Practitioners. *BioPsychoSocial Medicine*, **5**, 6. http://dx.doi.org/10.1186/1751-0759-5-6

[7]   Monteagudo, M., Rodriguez-Blanco, T., Pueyo, M.J., Zabaleta-del-Olmo, E., Mercader, M., Garcia, J., Pujol, E. and Bolibar, B. (2013) Gender Differences in Negative Mood States in Secondary School Students: Health Survey in Catalonia (Spain). *Gac Sanit*, **27**, 32-39. http://dx.doi.org/10.1016/j.gaceta.2012.01.009

[8]   Morgan, W.P. (1980) Test of Champions the Iceberg Profile. *Psychology Today*, **14**, 92.

[9]   Sakano, K., Ryo, K., Tamaki, Y., Nakayama, R., Hasaka, A., Takahashi, A., Ebihara, S., Tozuka, K. and Saito, I. (2014) Possible Benefits of Singing to the Mental and Physical Condition of the Elderly. *BioPsychoSocial Medicine*, **8**, 11. http://dx.doi.org/10.1186/1751-0759-8-11

[10]   Takarada, T., Asada, T., Sumi, Y. and Higuchi, Y. (2014) Effect of a Rotation Training System on the Mental Health Status of Postgraduate Dental Trainees at Kyushu University Hospital, Fukuoka, Japan. *Journal of Dental Education*, **78**, 243-249.

[11]   de Miranda Rohlfs, I.C.P., Rotta, T.M., Luft, C.D.B., Andrade, A., Krebs, R.J. and de Carvalho, T. (2008) Brunel Mood Scale (BRUMS): An Instrument for Early Detection of Overtraining Syndrome (A Escala de Humor de Brunel (Brums): Instrumento para detecção precoce da síndrome do excesso de treinamento). *Revista Brasileira de Medicina do Esporte*, **14**, 176-181.

[12]   Brandt, R., de Liz, C.M., Crocetta, T.B., Arab, C., Bevilacqua, G., Dominski, F.H., Vilarino, G.T. and Andrade, A. (2014) Mental Health and Associated Factors in Athletes during the Open Games of Santa Catarina. *Revista Brasileira de Medicina do Esporte*, **20**, 276-280. http://dx.doi.org/10.1590/1517-86922014200401607

[13]   Steffens, R. de A.K., de Liz, C.M., Viana, M. de S., Brandt, R., de Oliveira, L.G.A. and Andrade, A. (2011) Walking Improves Sleep Quality and Mood Status of Women with Fibromyalgia Syndrome (Praticar caminhada melhora a qualidade do sono e os estados de humor em mulheres com síndrome da fibromialgia). *Revista Dor*, **12**, 327-331. http://dx.doi.org/10.1590/S1806-00132011000400008

[14]   Brandt, R., Fonseca, A.B.P., de Oliveira, L.G.A., Steffens, R. de A.K., Viana, M. de S. and Andrade, A. (2011) Profile's Mood in Women with Fibromyalgia (Perfil de humor de mulheres com fibromialgia). *Jornal Brasileiro de Psiquiatria*, **60**, 216-220. http://dx.doi.org/10.1590/S0047-20852011000300011

[15]   Zhang, C.Q., Si, G., Chung, P.K., Du, M. and Terry, P.C. (2014) Psychometric Properties of the Brunel Mood Scale in Chinese Adolescents and Adults. *Journal of Sports Sciences*, **32**, 1465-1476.

[16]   van Wijk, C.H. (2011) Mental Health Measures in Predicting Outcomes for the Selection and Training of Navy Divers. *Diving and Hyperbaric Medicine Journal*, **41**, 22-26.

[17]   Kennedy, H., Unnithan, R. and Wamboldt, M.Z. (2015) Assessing Brief Changes in Adolescents' Mood: Development, Validation, and Utility of the Fast Assessment of Children's Emotions (FACE). *Journal of Pediatric Health Care*, **29**, 335-342. http://dx.doi.org/10.1016/j.pedhc.2015.01.004

[18]   van Wijk, C.H., Martin, J.H. and Hans-Arendse, C. (2013) Clinical Utility of the Brunel Mood Scale in Screening for Post-Traumatic Stress Risk in a Military Population. *Military Medicine*, **178**, 372-376. http://dx.doi.org/10.7205/MILMED-D-12-00422

[19]   Van Wijk, C.H. (2011) The Brunel Mood Scale: A South African Norm Study. *South African Journal of Psychiatry*, **17**.

[20]   Brandt, R., Viana, M. de S., Segato, L. and Andrade, A. (2010) Mood States Sail Athletes during the Pre-Pan-American. *Motriz-Revista De Educacao Fisica*, **16**, 834-840.

[21]   Rohlfs, I., Rotta, T., Andrade, A., Terry, P., Krebs, R. and Carvalho, T. (2005) The Brunel of Mood Scale (BRUMS): Instrument for Detection of Modified Mood States in Adolescents and Adults Athletes and Non Athletes. *FIEP Bulletin*, **75**, 281-284.

[22]   Dancey, C.P. and Reidy, J. (2006) Statistics without Maths for Psychology: Using SPSS for Windows (Estatística sem matemática para psicologia: Usando SPSS para Windows). 3rd Edition, Artmed Bookman, Porto Alegre.

[23]   Vieira, J.L.L., de Rocha, P.G.M. and Porcu, M. (2008) Physical Exercise's Influence in Mood and Clinical Depression

in Women (Influência do exercício físico no humor e na depressão clínica em mulheres). *Motriz: Revista de Educação Física*, **14**, 179-186.

[24] Sties, S.W., Gonzales, A.I., Netto, A.S., Wittkopf, P.G., Lima, D.P. and de Carvalho, T. (2014) Validation of the Brunel Mood Scale for Cardiac Rehabilitation Program. *Revista Brasileira De Medicina Do Esporte*, **20**, 281-284. http://dx.doi.org/10.1590/1517-86922014200401999

[25] Lan, M.F., Lane, A.M., Roy, J. and Hanin, N.A. (2012) Validity of the Brunel Mood Scale for Use with Malaysian Athletes. *Journal of Sports Science and Medicine*, **11**, 131-135.

[26] Terry, P.C., Lane, A.M., Lane, H.J. and Keohane, L. (1999) Development and Validation of a Mood Measure for Adolescents. *Journal of Sports Sciences*, **17**, 861-872. http://dx.doi.org/10.1080/026404199365425

[27] Kataoka, M., Ozawa, K., Tanioka, T., Okuda, K., Chiba, S., Tomotake, M. and King, B. (2015) Gender Differences of the Influential Factors on the Mental Health Condition of Teachers in the A University. *Journal of Medical Investigation*, **62**, 56-61. http://dx.doi.org/10.2152/jmi.62.56

[28] Song, H.T., Sun, X.Y., Yang, T.S., Zhang, L.Y., Yang, J.L. and Bai, J. (2015) Effects of Sleep Deprivation on Serum Cortisol Level and Mental Health in Servicemen. *International Journal of Psychophysiology*, **96**, 169-175. http://dx.doi.org/10.1016/j.ijpsycho.2015.04.008

[29] Hashizume, Y. (2014) The Importance of Sleep in the Mental Health. *Nihon Rinsho*, **72**, 341-346.

Permissions

All chapters in this book were first published in Health, by Scientific Research Publishing; hereby published with permission under the Creative Commons Attribution License or equivalent. Every chapter published in this book has been scrutinized by our experts. Their significance has been extensively debated. The topics covered herein carry significant findings which will fuel the growth of the discipline. They may even be implemented as practical applications or may be referred to as a beginning point for another development.

The contributors of this book come from diverse backgrounds, making this book a truly international effort. This book will bring forth new frontiers with its revolutionizing research information and detailed analysis of the nascent developments around the world.

We would like to thank all the contributing authors for lending their expertise to make the book truly unique. They have played a crucial role in the development of this book. Without their invaluable contributions this book wouldn't have been possible. They have made vital efforts to compile up to date information on the varied aspects of this subject to make this book a valuable addition to the collection of many professionals and students.

This book was conceptualized with the vision of imparting up-to-date information and advanced data in this field. To ensure the same, a matchless editorial board was set up. Every individual on the board went through rigorous rounds of assessment to prove their worth. After which they invested a large part of their time researching and compiling the most relevant data for our readers.

The editorial board has been involved in producing this book since its inception. They have spent rigorous hours researching and exploring the diverse topics which have resulted in the successful publishing of this book. They have passed on their knowledge of decades through this book. To expedite this challenging task, the publisher supported the team at every step. A small team of assistant editors was also appointed to further simplify the editing procedure and attain best results for the readers.

Apart from the editorial board, the designing team has also invested a significant amount of their time in understanding the subject and creating the most relevant covers. They scrutinized every image to scout for the most suitable representation of the subject and create an appropriate cover for the book.

The publishing team has been an ardent support to the editorial, designing and production team. Their endless efforts to recruit the best for this project, has resulted in the accomplishment of this book. They are a veteran in the field of academics and their pool of knowledge is as vast as their experience in printing. Their expertise and guidance has proved useful at every step. Their uncompromising quality standards have made this book an exceptional effort. Their encouragement from time to time has been an inspiration for everyone.

The publisher and the editorial board hope that this book will prove to be a valuable piece of knowledge for researchers, students, practitioners and scholars across the globe.

List of Contributors

Kaliyaperumal Karunamoorthi
Division of Medical Entomology and Vector Control, Department of Environmental Health Science & Technology, College of Public Health and Medical Sciences, Jimma University, Jimma, Ethiopia
Unit of Tropical Diseases, Faculty of Public Health and Tropical Medicine, Jazan University, Jazan, KSA

Buzuna Beyene and Argaw Ambelu
Division of Medical Entomology and Vector Control, Department of Environmental Health Science & Technology, College of Public Health and Medical Sciences, Jimma University, Jimma, Ethiopia

Vagner Rosa Bizarro, Tatiane Andreazza Lucchese, Amanda Maia Breis, Karine Rucker, Minelli Salles Alves Fernandes, Mikele Torino Paletti, Ana Luísa Conceição de Jesus and Denise Rosso Tenório Wanderley Rocha
Division of Endocrinology, IPEMED Medical School, Rio de Janeiro, Brazil

Raphael Calafange Marques Pereira
Division of Rehabilitation Sciences, UNISUAM, Rio de Janeiro, Brazil

Alberto Krayyem Arbex
Division of Endocrinology, IPEMED Medical School, Rio de Janeiro, Brazil
Harvard School of Public Health, Harvard University, Boston, USA

Palaniappan Marimuthu
Department of Biostatistics, National Institute of Mental Health Neuro Sciences, Bangalore, India

Grish N. Rao
Department of Epidemiology, National Institute of Mental Health Neuro Sciences, Bangalore, India

Manoj Kumar Sharma
Department of Clinical Psychology, National Institute of Mental Health Neuro Sciences, Bangalore, India

Ramasamy Dhanasekara Pandian
Department of Psychiatry Social Work, National Institute of Mental Health Neuro Sciences, Bangalore, India

Hossein Jenaabadi
Faculty of Educational Sciences and Psychology, University of Sistan and Baluchestan, Zahedan, Iran

Bahareh Azizi Nejad
Department of Educational Science, Payame Noor University, Tehran, Iran

Fatemeh Saeidi Mahmoud Abadi
Islamic Azad University, Tehran, Iran

Rezvan Haghi
Allameh Tabatabai University, Tehran, Iran

Maryam Hojatinasab
MA of Educational Research, University of Sistan and Baluchestan, Zahedan, Iran

Salime Donida Chedid Lisboa, Cláudia Gomes Bracht, Alexandra Ferreira Vieira, Luiz Fernando Martins Kruel andThais Reichert
Universidade Federal do Rio Grande do Sul, Porto Alegre, Brazil

Rodrigo Sudatti Delevatti
Universidade Federal do Rio Grande do Sul, Porto Alegre, Brazil
Faculdade Sogipa de Educação Física, Porto Alegre, Brazil

Ana Carolina Kanitz
Universidade Federal do Rio Grande do Sul, Porto Alegre, Brazil
Universidade Federal de Uberlândia, Uberlândia, Brazil

Adamos Vrachimis
School of Human & Life Sciences, Roehampton University, London, UK
Department of Life & Health Sciences, University of Nicosia, Nicosia, Cyprus

Marios Hadjicharalambous
Department of Life & Health Sciences, University of Nicosia, Nicosia, Cyprus

Chris Tyler
School of Human & Life Sciences, Roehampton University, London, UK

Saki Tadenuma
Department of Environmental Health and Public Health, Faculty of Medicine, Shimane University, Shimane, Japan
Department of Anesthesiology, Faculty of Medicine, Shimane University, Shimane, Japan

Hideyuki Kanda
Department of Environmental Health and Public Health, Faculty of Medicine, Shimane University, Shimane, Japan

Shizukiyo Ishikawa and Eiji Kajii
Division of Community and Family Medicine, Center for Community Medicine, Jichi Medical University, Tochigi, Japan

Kazunori Kayaba,
Graduate School of Saitama Prefectural University, Saitama, Japan

Tadao Gotoh
Wara National Health Insurance Clinic, Gifu, Japan

Yosikazu Nakamura
Department of Public Health, Jichi Medical University, Tochigi, Japan

Ada C. Nwaneri, Ijeoma Okoronkwo and Patricia Uzor Okpala
Department of Nursing, University of Nigeria, Enugu Campus, Nsukka, Nigeria

Eunice Ogonna Osuala
Department of Nursing Science, Nnamdi Azikiwe University, Nnewi Campus, Awka, Nigeria

Anthonia Chidinma Emesowum
Department of Nursing, Imo State University, Orlu Campus, Owerri, Nigeria

Fatma Kizilay and Aysegul Beykumul
PMR Department, Turgut Ozal Medical Center, Inonu University, Malatya, Turkey

Cengiz Arslan
Faculty of Sports Science, Firat University, Elazıg, Turkey

Fatma İ. Kerkez
School of Physical Education and Sports, Mugla Sıtkı Kocman University, Mugla, Turkey

Egemen Kizilay
PMR Clinic, Malatya State Hospital, Malatya, Turkey

Rachel J. Shulder, Eric E. Hall and Paul C. Miller
Department of Exercise Science, Elon University, Elon, USA

Takuji Yamaguchi and Ailing Hu
Center of Advanced Kampo Medicine and Clinical Research, Juntendo Graduate School of Medicine, Bunkyo-ku, Japan

Masakazu Azuma and Senichi Suzuki
Lion Implant Center, Ebina-shi, Japan
Department of Hospital Administration, Juntendo University Graduate School of Medicine, Bunkyo-ku, Japan

Masaki Sawa and Tomoko Yoshizawa
Department of Hospital Administration, Juntendo University Graduate School of Medicine, Bunkyo-ku, Japan

Hiroyuki Kobayashi
Department of Hospital Administration, Juntendo University Graduate School of Medicine, Bunkyo-ku, Japan
Center of Advanced Kampo Medicine and Clinical Research, Juntendo Graduate School of Medicine, Bunkyo-ku, Japan

Ruth-Maria Korth
Practice and Research in General Medicine FiDA, Munich, Germany

Graciela Freyermuth-Enciso
Centro de Investigaciones y Estudios Superiores en Antropología Social (CIESAS) sede SURESTE, San Cristóbal de las Casas, México

Mónica Carrasco-Gómez
Cátedras CONACYT/Centro de Investigaciones y Estudios Superiores en Antropología Social sede SURESTE, San Cristóbal de las Casas, México

Martín Romero-Martínez
National Public Health Institute's Research Center in Evaluations and Surveys, Cuernavaca, México

Samantha Ismaile, Seham Al-Enezi, Wajdan Otaif, Albandari Al-Mahadi, Nada Bingorban, Nourah Barayaan
The College of Nursing, Princess Nourah Bint Abdulrahman University, Riyadh, Saudi Arabia

Marianne K. Thygesen and Ole Mogensen
Institute of Clinical Research, Faculty of Health Sciences, University of Southern Denmark, Odense, Denmark
Department of Obstetrics and Gynaecology, Odense University Hospital, Odense, Denmark

René De Pont Christensen
Research Unit of General Practice, University of Southern Denmark, Odense, Denmark

Lone Hedemand
Institute of Clinical Research, Faculty of Health Sciences, University of Southern Denmark, Odense, Denmark

Susanna Geidne, Ingela Fredriksson, Koustuv Dalal and Charli Eriksson
School of Health and Medical Sciences, Örebro University, Örebro, Sweden

Kazumitsu Nawata
Graduate School of Engineering, University of Tokyo, Tokyo, Japan

Koichi Kawabuchi
Graduate School of Medical and Dental Sciences, Tokyo Medical and Dental University, Tokyo, Japan

Adhikari Ramil
Massey University, Wellington, New Zealand

Junko Mitoma, Masami Kitaoka, Hiroki Asakura, Enoch Olando Anyenda, Daisuke Hori, Nguyen Thi Thu Tao, Toshio Hamagishi, Koichiro Hayashi, Fumihiko Suzuki, Yukari Shimizu, Hiromasa Tsujiguchi, Yasuhiro Kambayashi, Yuri Hibino, Takiko Sagara, Aki Shibata and Hiroyuki Nakamura
Department of Environmental and Preventive Medicine, Graduate School of Medical Science, Kanazawa University, Ishikawa, Japan

Tadashi Konoshita
Third Department of Internal Medicine, Fukui University School of Medicine, Fukui, Japan

Bryan Paul
Faculty of Science, University of Alberta, Edmonton, Canada

Wai Liang Tham
Faculty of Medicine, University of British Columbia, Vancouver, Canada

A. Mohammed-Durosinlorun, A. Abubakar, J. Adze, S. Bature, C. Mohammed and M. Taingson
Department of Obstetrics and Gynaecology, Faculty of Medicine, Kaduna State University, Kaduna, Nigeria

A. Ojabo
Department of Obstetrics and Gynaecology, College of Health Sciences, Benue State University, Makurdi, Nigeria

Muhammad W. Darawad, Amani A. Khalil, Mahmoud Maharmeh and Ayman M. Hamdan-Mansour
Faculty of Nursing, The University of Jordan, Amman, Jordan

Sultan Mosleh
Faculty of Nursing, University of Mutah, Karak, Jordan

Osama A. Samarkandi
Prince Sultan bin Abdulaziz College for Emergency Medical Services, King Saud University, Riyadh, Saudi Arabia

Guglielmina Fantuzzi, Elena Righi and Gabriella Aggazzotti
Department of Biomedical, Metabolic and Neural Sciences, University of Modena and Reggio Emilia, Modena, Italy

Ricardo Brandt
State University of West Parana, Marechal Cândido Rondon, Brazil
Laboratory of Sport and Exercise Psychology, Santa Catarina State University, Florianópolis, Brazil

Dafne Herrero
Faculty Public Health, São Paulo, Brazil

Thaís Massetti
Post-Graduate Program in Rehabilitation Sciences, Faculty of Medicine, University of São Paulo, São Paulo, Brazil

Tânia Brusque Crocetta
Laboratory of Sport and Exercise Psychology, Santa Catarina State University, Florianópolis, Brazil
Department of Morphology and Physiology, Faculty of Medicine of ABC, Santo André, Brazil

Regiani Guarnieri and Luiz Carlos de Abreu
Department of Morphology and Physiology, Faculty of Medicine of ABC, Santo André, Brazil

Carlos Bandeira de Mello Monteiro
Post-Graduate Program in Rehabilitation Sciences, Faculty of Medicine, University of São Paulo, São Paulo, Brazil
Department of Morphology and Physiology, Faculty of Medicine of ABC, Santo André, Brazil

Maick da Silveira Viana, Guilherme Guimarães Bevilacqua and Alexandro Andrade
Laboratory of Sport and Exercise Psychology, Santa Catarina State University, Florianópolis, Brazil